Surgery of
FACIAL BONE FRACTURES

Surgery of
FACIAL BONE FRACTURES

Edited by

CRAIG A. FOSTER, M.D., D.D.S.

Associate Professor of Otolaryngology and
Head and Neck Surgery, New York
Medical College, Valhalla; Associate
Attending Surgeon (Plastic Surgery),
Manhattan Eye, Ear, and Throat Hospital;
Director, Facial Plastic Surgery, New York
Eye and Ear Infirmary, New York, New York

JOHN E. SHERMAN, M.D.

Assistant Clinical Professor of Surgery (Plastic
Surgery), Mount Sinai School of Medicine of
the City University of New York; Associate
Attending Surgeon, Beth Israel Medical
Center; Adjunct Attending Surgeon,
Memorial Sloan-Kettering Cancer Center,
New York, New York

Illustrated by

Elizabeth Roselius, M.S., A.M.I.

Churchill Livingstone

New York, Edinburgh, London, Melbourne

1987

Library of Congress Cataloging-in-Publication Data

Surgery of facial bone fractures.

Includes bibliographies and index.
1. Face — Surgery. 2. Facial bones — Fractures. 3. Skull — Fractures.
I. Foster, Craig A.   II. Sherman, John E. [DNLM: 1. Facial Bones — injuries.
2. Facial Injuries — surgery. 3. Skull Fractures — surgery. WE 706 S961]
RD523.S84   1987   617'.52'059   86-24481
ISBN 0-443-08436-X

Distributed in the United Kingdom by Churchill Livingstone, Robert Stevenson
House, 1-3 Baxter's Place, Leith Walk, Edinburgh EH1 3AF, and by associated
companies, branches, and representatives throughout the world.

Accurate indications, adverse reactions, and dosage schedules for drugs are provided
in this book, but it is possible that they may change. The reader is urged to review
the package information data of the manufacturers of the medications mentioned.

Sponsoring Editor: *Linda Panzarella*
Copy Editor: *Nancy Terry*
Production Designer: *Rosalie Marcus*
Production Supervisor: *Sharon Tuder*

Printed in the United States of America

First published in 1987

This book is dedicated to our wives, Susan
and Randi, and to our families for their
much needed and appreciated support.
We also recognize our teachers and
students and continually learn from both.

Contributors

Daniel C. Baker, M.D.

Associate Professor of Surgery (Plastic Surgery), Institute of Reconstructive Plastic Surgery, New York University School of Medicine; Associate Attending Surgeon, Manhattan Eye, Ear, and Throat Hospital; Associate Attending Surgeon, Bellevue Hospital, New York, New York

Lanny Garth Close, M.D.

Associate Professor and Vice Chairman, Department of Otorhinolaryngology, The University of Texas Health Science Center at Dallas, Dallas, Texas

Louis R. M. Del Guercio, M.D.

Professor and Chairman, Department of Surgery, New York Medical College; Chief of Surgery, Westchester County Medical Center, Valhalla, New York

F. Ronald Feinstein, D.M.D., M.D.

Clinical Assistant Professor of Surgery (Plastic Surgery), University of Southern California School of Medicine; Chief, Department of Plastic Surgery, Kaiser Permanente Medical Center, Los Angeles, California

Craig A. Foster, M.D., D.D.S.

Associate Professor of Otolaryngology and Head and Neck Surgery, New York Medical College, Valhalla; Associate Attending Surgeon (Plastic Surgery), Manhattan Eye, Ear, and Throat Hospital; Director, Facial Plastic Surgery, New York Eye and Ear Infirmary, New York, New York

Joseph S. Gruss, M.B., F.R.C.E.(C)

Assistant Professor, Department of Surgery, University of Toronto Faculty of Medicine; Head, Division of Plastic Surgery, Sunnybrook Hospital, Toronto, Ontario, Canada

Peter A. Hilger, M.D.

Assistant Professor of Otolaryngology, University of Minnesota Medical School, Minneapolis; Attending Staff, Department of Otolaryngology, Saint Paul-Ramsey Hospital and Medical Center, St. Paul, Minnesota

Stephen C. Hill, D.D.S.

Associate Professor, Division of Oral and Maxillofacial Surgery, The University of Texas Health Science Center at Dallas, Dallas, Texas

Glenn W. Jelks, M.D.

Assistant Professor of Surgery (Plastic Surgery), Institute of Reconstructive Plastic Surgery, New York University School of Medicine; Attending Staff, Bellevue Hospital, Manhattan Eye, Ear, and Throat Hospital, Veterans Administration Hospital, and New York Eye and Ear Infirmary, New York, New York

Haim Y. Kaplan, M.D.

Lecturer, Department of Plastic and Maxillofacial Surgery, Hadassah Hebrew University School of Medicine, Jerusalem, Israel; Clinical Instructor in Surgery (Plastic Surgery), Institute of Reconstructive Plastic Surgery, New York University School of Medicine, New York, New York

Thomas J. Krizek, M.D.

Professor of Surgery and Chairman, Section of Plastic and Reconstructive Surgery, University of Chicago Pritzker School of Medicine, Chicago, Illinois

Paul Hak Joo Kwon, D.D.S., Ph.D.

Associate Professor of Oral and Maxillofacial Surgery, University of Minnesota School of Dentistry; Attending Staff, University of Minnesota Hospital, Hennepin County Medical Center, and Fairview Hospital, Minneapolis, Minnesota

Gregory La Trenta, M.D.

Clinical Instructor in Surgery (Plastic Surgery), Institute of Reconstructive Plastic Surgery, New York University School of Medicine, New York, New York

Richard Dean Lisman, M.D.

Assistant Clinical Professor of Ophthalmology, Mount Sinai School of Medicine of the City University of New York; Clinic Co-Chief, Department of Ophthalmic Plastic Surgery, and Associate Attending Surgeon, Manhattan Eye, Ear, and Throat Hospital; Associate Attending Surgeon, Mount Sinai Hospital; Assistant Adjunct Surgeon, New York Eye and Ear Infirmary, New York, New York

Robert H. Mathog, M.D.

Professor and Chairman, Department of Otolaryngology, Wayne State University School of Medicine; Chief, Department of Otolaryngology, Harper-Grace Hospitals; Chief, Department of Otolaryngology, Detroit Receiving Hospital, Detroit, Michigan

William L. Meyerhoff, M.D., Ph.D.

Professor and Chairman, Department of Otorhinolaryngology, The University of Texas Health Science Center at Dallas, Dallas, Texas

Othella T. Owens, M.D.

Assistant Professor of Otolaryngology, Wayne State University School of Medicine, Detroit; Chief, Section of Otolaryngology, Department of Surgery, Veterans Administration Hospital, Allen Park, Michigan

Richard A. Pollock, M.D.

Clinical Instructor of Surgery (Plastic Surgery), Emory University School of Medicine; Director, Center for Facial Reconstruction, Regional Trauma Unit, Georgia Baptist Medical Center; Director, International Center for Reconstructive Surgery, Atlanta, Georgia

John A. Savino, M.D.

Associate Professor of Surgery, New York Medical College; Chief of Trauma/Critical Care, Westchester County Medical Center, Valhalla, New York

John E. Sherman, M.D.

Assistant Clinical Professor of Surgery (Plastic Surgery), Mount Sinai School of Medicine of the City University of New York; Associate Attending Surgeon, Beth Israel Medical Center; Adjunct Attending Surgeon, Memorial Sloan-Kettering Cancer Center, New York, New York

Douglas P. Sinn, D.D.S.

Professor and Chairman, Division of Oral and Maxillofacial Surgery, The University of Texas Health Science Center at Dallas, Dallas, Texas

Henry M. Spinelli, M.D.

Chief Resident in Ophthalmology, Manhattan Eye, Ear, and Throat Hospital; Resident in Surgery, Presbyterian Hospital, New York, New York

Walter G. Sullivan, M.D.

Assistant Professor of Surgery, Wayne State University School of Medicine; Chief, Division of Plastic and Reconstructive Surgery, and Director, Craniofacial Anomalies and Cleft Palate Clinic, Children's Hospital of Michigan, Detroit, Michigan

Daniel E. Waite, D.D.S., M.S., A.A., F.A.C.D.

Professor and Chairman, Department of Oral and Maxillofacial Surgery, and Assistant Dean for Hospital Affairs, Baylor College of Dentistry, Dallas, Texas

Stephen W. Watson, D.D.S., M.D.

Clinical Faculty, Division of Oral and Maxillofacial Surgery, The University of Texas Health Science Center at Dallas, Dallas, Texas

Foreword

Given the current plethora of plastic surgery publications, it is unusual to be able to identify an area that has not been adequately updated. The discerning among us have realized that the one glaring deficiency in what is available for the plastic surgeon's library is a North American book describing the modern management of facial trauma. It has been somewhat disappointing that until now only the new edition of Rowe and Williams from the United Kingdom has filled that gap. This deficiency has now been answered, and those dealing with facial trauma have an authoritative source to consult rather than the sadly outdated Kazanjian and Converse. Foster and Sherman have come to our academic and legal rescue with the assistance of their able publisher, Churchill Livingstone.

To be asked to write the foreword to a book that is actually required by the profession, rather than the publisher, is indeed an honor and a pleasant change. These feelings are enhanced by the fact that the book itself is well planned and the chapters, although written by different individuals, follow a set and logical pattern of anatomy, assessment, treatment, early complications, late complications, and treatment of the latter. The writing is clear and the information given is up-to-date and concise. At long last a twentieth-century approach to trauma is presented. Discussion includes the coronal flap for direct exposure of fractures, accurate fixation with wires and plates, immediate bone grafting, use of cranial bone grafts, and an emphasis on CT scanning as the most useful vehicle for treatment-related diagnosis.

A unique feature of the book is the admixture of specialists. Plastic surgery, oral surgery, otorhinolaryngology, and ophthalmology are represented, each adding its own particular flavor and each contributing pearls that have been gathered from extensive experience in the area. Perhaps in this representation of disciplines is the important message that we should cooperate more frequently in the management of these very complex problems. The plastic surgeon frequently will call the ophthalmologist when he fears an injury to the eye or to the ocular adnexa is beyond his expertise, but he will neglect to seek the cooperation of the oral surgeon in difficult fractures involving inter-dental relationships. This illustrates a certain lack of consistency. The same criticism, however, can be leveled at oral surgery and otorhinolaryngology. Perhaps the question should be asked more often — do our patients deserve better? This book points the way. I applaud and endorse the concept.

For all plastic surgeons involved in head and neck trauma, whether nascent or experienced, there is now a guide on the modern treatment of facial fractures. It heralds a new era; it encourages and virtually demands a movement away from traditional methods. It is long overdue and much welcomed.

It is my pleasure to be able to contribute in a very small way. I congratulate the authors and their illustrious team, and I commend the publisher for agreeing to produce this work.

Ian T. Jackson
Mayo Clinic
Rochester, Minnesota

Preface

Almost no endeavor of surgical practice imparts or carries with it more emotional distress than facial trauma. Disruption of many critical functions ensues, as this area is responsible for vision, hearing, respiration, mastication, and deglutition and is the cornerstone of the cosmetic expressive system.

This volume is for the resident-in-training and the practitioner involved in the care of the facially injured. It is intended as a concise and quick source of reference for standard and advanced methods used in the repair of these injuries.

Maxillofacial traumatology is a continually evolving science. No fewer than nine medical and dental disciplines intersect at the head and neck. Despite this clinical overlap, best results are usually obtained by cooperative efforts between allied specialties. It is in that spirit of cooperation that we dedicate this book. The authorship of this volume is multidisciplined and broadly based geographically. The three major specialties dealing with maxillofacial trauma (plastic surgery, otolaryngologic surgery, and oral-maxillofacial surgery) are represented. The text concentrates on maxillofacial trauma, with emphasis on facial injury, because these injuries require the most sophistication and expertise.

Craig A. Foster
John E. Sherman

Acknowledgements

This text represents two years of effort by many individuals, and the editors gratefully acknowledge their contribution. We congratulate our contributing authors, all of whom found time in their busy schedules to produce complete and concise chapters on the varied facets of maxillofacial trauma.

The continuity and quality of this book is also due in large part to the skills of our medical illustrator Elizabeth Roselius, who worked with patience and perseverance with the authors and editors.

Many productive hours were spent with Linda Panzarella, our sponsoring editor, whose unending patience and hard work were invaluable. We also wish to thank Lynn Herndon, whose initial enthusiasm for our concept was infectious and most appreciated, and Nancy Terry, our copy editor, for her sustained effort.

We would be remiss if we did not express our great appreciation to our office staff, Cynthia Jardiolin and Alice Cruz, for their daily support in working, compiling, and coordinating the manuscripts.

We are saddened by the recent death of Dr. Reed O. Dingman. We wish to acknowledge his life-long contribution to the specialty of plastic surgery and, in particular, to the treatment of facial injuries. This book was inspired and supported by Dr. Dingman. Drs. Dingman and Natvig's *Surgery of Facial Fractures* has been well-worn on our bookshelves and will continue to serve as a classic in the field.

The editors would also like to thank Dr. Ian. T. Jackson for writing the foreword. Dr. Jackson's contributions to the field of maxillofacial surgery are widely recognized, and we are honored by his contribution.

Contents

Initial Evaluation of the Trauma Patient

1

John A. Savino
Louis R. M. Del Guercio

The primary objectives of trauma management must be rapid and accurate assessment of the injured patient's condition and provision of resuscitation and stabilization on a priority basis in order to increase survival. Death from trauma is known to have a trimodal distribution.[1] The first peak in the incidence of death is within minutes of initial injury, and primary causes of these mortalities are related to lacerations of the brain, brain stem, high spinal cord, heart, and aorta or other large vessel. The second death peak occurs within minutes to a few hours after injury. This period is usually referred to as the "golden hour" when rapid assessment and resuscitation, if adequately provided, reduce mortality. These deaths are usually secondary to subdural and epidural hematoma, hemopneumothorax, ruptured spleen, lacerations of the liver, fractured femur, and multiple injuries associated with significant blood loss. The third death peak occurs days or weeks after initial injury and is usually due to sepsis and organ failure.

The goal of this chapter is to provide a standardized method of evaluation and treatment of trauma victims in the immediate post-injury period so that more patients survive the second period of threat. Sequential steps in rapidly assessing and treating patients during the golden hour should follow an order related to priority of injuries. The most obvious injuries must not be treated (particularly in the maxillofacial region and extremities) until all body systems have been evaluated. During the primary survey, life-threatening conditions are identified, and simultaneous management is begun. Airway maintenance with cervical spine control and pulmonary status take precedence. Subsequently, an estimation should be made of blood loss and cardiac status. A brief neurologic exam should then be performed to establish the patient's level of consciousness, pupillary size, and reaction. Finally, the patient should be completely undressed to facilitate thorough examination and assessment.

During early care of critically injured patients, shock management is initiated, oxygenation is provided when necessary, and hemorrhage control is reevaluated. Continuous monitoring of life-threatening conditions that have been identified is an absolute necessity.

The secondary survey, which includes head-to-toe evaluation of the trauma patient, begins only after life-threatening conditions have been stabilized. This in-depth evaluation of the body by sections includes assessment of the head, neck, chest, abdomen, and extremities and an in-depth neurologic examination.

Clinical manifestations, mechanisms of injury, and physical examination form the basis for investigating and identifying internal injuries. It is also essential to obtain a history of the event from the patient, family, bystanders, and ambulance personnel.

PRIMARY ASSESSMENT AND RESUSCITATION

Airway and Cervical Spine

During the initial rapid survey, the examiner must determine whether the patient has a patent, unobstructed airway by looking, listening, and palpating. The examiner should be able to document the status of the upper airway. The presence, rapidity, and strength of respiratory effort should be observed. Evidence of gasping, stridor, or wheezing should be sought. The chest wall should be evaluated for symmetrical movement, splinting or paradoxical movement, use of accessory muscles, and relative duration of inspiration and expiration. The examiner should be attentive to the patient's ability (or inability) to breathe and maximize ventilation in the supine position. If this evaluation indicates that the patient is apneic or the airway totally obstructed, immediate attention must be directed to this area. Upper airway obstruction may be due to the tongue (most commonly), foreign bodies (including blood, vomitus, and dentures), edema of the glottic area, or injury to the larynx.[2]

In the unconscious patient, tone is lost in those muscles that normally maintain the tongue away from the posterior pharyngeal wall. Laxity of these muscles, with the unconscious patient in the supine position, allows the tongue to prolapse back and obstruct the upper airway. Airway obstruction by the tongue can be alleviated by maneuvering the mandible anteriorly, thereby moving the tongue

anteriorly. This maneuver can be accomplished either by the chin-lift or jaw-thrust technique. With the patient in the supine position, the fingers of one hand are placed under the symphysis (chin) of the mandible, which is lifted forward. The thumb of the same hand lightly depresses the lower lip to open the mouth. The thumb may also be placed behind the lower incisors as (the chin is gently lifted.) This maneuver is the method of choice for trauma victims, as it does not risk compromising a possible cervical spine fracture.

An alternative method is the jaw-thrust maneuver, which is performed by grasping the angles of the mandible and displacing the mandible forward. Mechanical methods for opening and maintaining the airway include use of an oropharyngeal airway, nasopharyngeal airway, and endotracheal tube. If difficulty occurs in establishing ventilation with a mask, intubation should be performed without delay. An endotracheal tube can be inserted either orally or nasally.[3] After intubation, position of the tube should be verified by listening to the right and left lung fields to ensure that both are equally ventilated. The more direct path of the right main stem bronchus from the trachea can often cause the endotracheal tube to slip into the right bronchus, with exclusion of the left lung, resulting in ventilation perfusion abnormalities. Auscultating the epigastrium ensures that the tube has not been placed in the esophagus and the stomach is not being distended with air. After proper position of the tube has been confirmed, the cuff should be inflated with 5 to 10 cc of air. Hyperextension of the neck is avoided to prevent cord injury in patients with suspected or present cervical spine fracture. An axiom in trauma management is to assume a cervical spine fracture is present in any patient with an injury above the clavicles. The head must be maintained in neutral position. Performance of nontraumatic intubation is essential, as traumatic insertion causes increased intracranial pressure.

Inability to intubate the trachea, edema of the glottis secondary to injury, fracture of the larynx, and severe oropharyngeal hemorrhage obstructing airway visibility are the primary indications for cricothyroidotomy or tracheotomy.[4] Needle cricothyroidotomy is an acceptable alternative to surgery and may be preferred over tracheotomy in emergency situations involving children under the age of 12.[5]

Use of the jet insufflation technique will provide 45 minutes of oxygenation, allowing tracheotomy to be performed under safer conditions. This technique is performed by placing a large bore plastic cannula, #14 gauge, in the trachea below the level of obstruction. The cannula is subsequently connected to a high flow oxygen source with a Y connector attached between the oxygen source and the plastic cannula. Intermittent ventilation, using the rhythm of 1 second on and 4 seconds off, can be achieved by placing the thumb over the open end of the Y connector. During the 4 seconds that oxygen is not delivered under pressure, some exhalation will occur, and the patient may be adequately oxygenated for approximately 30 to 45 minutes. Inadequate exhalation of carbon dioxide limits this technique.

Surgical cricothyroidotomy may be readily performed through the cricothyroid membrane (Fig. 1-1). Access to the cricothyroid membrane is more rapid due to its proximity to the skin surface and requires minimal retraction for exposure. Subglottic stenosis or vocal cord dysfunction following this procedure has been demonstrated in recent series to be an infrequent complication.[4] A transverse incision 2 to 3 cm in length is made directly over the cricothyroid membrane. The membrane is incised transversely over the anterior third of the tracheal circumference. A curved clamp is inserted and spread to define the opening. A #5 to #7 curved (60°) tracheotomy tube is inserted and the cuff inflated. With suspected cervical spine fracture, one must decide which is the greater liability—the obstructed airway or possible cervical spine injury. The airway always has priority. If the patient is not facing a life-threatening situation, cervical spine injury can be ruled out by a portable cross table lateral cervical-spine view or Swimmers view that visualizes all seven cervical vertebrae. The complications of oral and nasal endotracheal intubation are listed in Table 1-1.[1] Incidence of these complications increases with the inexperience of the practitioner who is inserting the tube. Cricothyroidotomy is also associated with a number of complications including asphyxia, aspiration, cellulitis, creation of false passage into tissues, subglottic ste-

nosis/edema, laryngeal stenosis, hemorrhage or hematoma formation, laceration of the esophagus, laceration of the trachea, mediastinal emphysema, and vocal cord paralysis with secondary hoarseness.[1,6]

Pulmonary Status

Once an airway has been established, assessment of ventilatory status should follow. The examiner should perform a careful inspection involving palpation and auscultation of the thorax. If the patient is not breathing, artificial ventilation should be instituted either by a bag-mask unit or by connecting the endotracheal tube to a time-cycled, positive pressure breathing device.

Injuries to the chest wall and parenchyma may be subdivided into two categories: immediately life threatening and potentially life threatening. With the exception of airway obstruction, which has already been discussed, the remaining injuries that require immediate treatment include: open pneumothorax, flail chest, tension pneumothorax, massive hemothorax, and pericardial tamponade. The six potentially life-threatening injuries that do not require immediate treatment include: rupture of the tracheobronchial tree, pulmonary contusion, diaphragmatic rupture, esophageal perforation, myocardial contusion, and great vessel injuries.[2,7]

Either penetrating or blunt trauma can produce an open pneumothorax. Inability to generate negative intrathoracic pressure collapses the lung and leads immediately to ventilatory insufficiency. Concomitant pulmonary parenchymal injury can exist. Treatment consists of immediate application of petrolatum gauze or another clean air-tight dressing over the opening in the chest wall. A thoracotomy tube should be inserted through a separate incision as soon as it is feasible. The most important aspect of immediate treatment is closure of the chest wall opening. Reexpansion of the affected lung is of secondary importance. After the chest wall opening has been closed, close monitoring is imperative to avoid tension pneumothorax.

Flail chest results in paradoxical movement of a portion of the chest wall when there are multiple

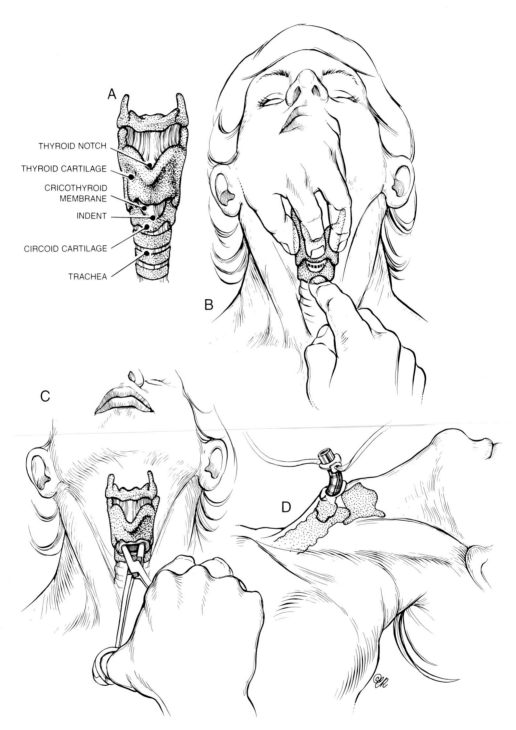

THYROID NOTCH

THYROID CARTILAGE

CRICOTHYROID
MEMBRANE

INDENT

CIRCOID CARTILAGE

TRACHEA

Fig. 1-1. Steps in performing surgical cricothyroidotomy. **(A)** Cartilaginous and membranous anatomy of the anterior neck. **(B)** A tranverse incision 2 to 3 cm in length is made over the cricothyroid membrane, and **(C)** a curved clamp is inserted and spread to define the opening. **(D)** A curved tracheostomy tube is inserted and the cuff inflated.

Table 1-1. Complications of Oral and Nasal Endotracheal Intubation

1. Esophageal intubation leading to hypoxia and death.
2. Right mainstem bronchus intubation, resulting in left lung collapse and pneumothorax.
3. Inability to intubate, leading to hypoxia and death.
4. Induction of vomiting leading to aspiration.
5. Dislocation of the mandible.
6. Fracture of the epiglottis.
7. Airway hemorrhage secondary to trauma.
8. Avulsion-tear of the vocal cords (usually secondary to the stylet).
9. Chipping or loosening of the teeth (secondary to levering of the laryngoscope against the teeth.)
10. Rupture and leak of the endotracheal tube cuff, resulting in loss of seal during ventilation and necessitating reintubation.
11. Absence of the tube adapter leading to mouth-to-tube ventilation.
12. Dislocation of the cervical spine during hyperextension or hyperflexion.
13. Neck strain during hyperextension.
14. Atlanto-occipital dislocation.
15. Potential fracture of an anterior cervical fusion.
16. Conversion of a cervical spine without neurological deficit to a C-spine with neurological deficit.

(Committee on Trauma, American College of Surgeons: Advanced Trauma Life Support Course. American College of Surgeons, Chicago, 1984.)

rib fractures and usually when individual ribs are fractured at multiple sites. Respiratory difficulty occurs because the chest wall is unstable, moving inward with inspiration and outward with expiration. Development of negative intrathoracic pressure is prevented, and normal gas flow via the trachea does not occur. This problem is compounded by severe pain and splinting associated with rib fractures. Under emergency circumstances, simply preventing movement of the chest wall relieves severe respiratory distress and is most easily accomplished by turning the patient onto the affected side. If distress continues, immediate intubation and positive pressure ventilation are necessary to achieve internal stabilization of the fractures and to ventilate the lungs.

Massive hemothorax usually results from injuries to the aortic arch, pulmonary hilum, or systemic vessels such as the internal mammary or intercostal arteries. Most patients with continuous pleural bleeding following thoracic injuries are not bleeding from the lungs, because the pulmonary vasculature is a low-pressure system. Early placement of thoracotomy tubes in a patient showing evidence of intrathoracic blood loss is essential. Monitoring blood loss determines blood volume replacement and provides continuous assessment of the patient's hemodynamic status. Blood loss greater than 1,000 to 1,500 ml or more than 300 ml/hr for 2 to 3 hours usually indicates need for thoracotomy.

Lacerations of the pulmonary parenchyma occasionally function as flap valves and create a tension pneumothorax because air enters the pleural space and is unable to escape. Pleural pressure rises, the lung collapses, the mediastinum shifts toward the opposite hemithorax, and the vena cava is narrowed at the diaphragm and thoracic inlet, thus interfering with venous return. In addition, the normal lung is severely compressed. The combination of these factors may lead rapidly to death. Treatment is immediate tube thoracostomy.

Cardiac tamponade is a collection of blood in the pericardial sac, usually resulting from direct injury to the myocardium. Patients with pericardial tamponade typically present with hypotension due to decreased cardiac output. Blunt chest trauma may also produce tamponade, caused by laceration of the proximal portion of the aorta and subsequent bleeding into the pericardium. The criteria for a clinical diagnosis of cardiac tamponade are a wound in a suspiciously close area, elevated central venous pressure reflected by distended neck veins, decreased systolic arterial pressure, and muffled heart sounds. Other conditions that present similarly in the injured patient are tension pneumothorax and myocardial failure secondary to myocardial contusion or coronary air embolism. Pericardiocentesis should be performed to temporarily relieve tamponade.

Circulation

Assessment of the degree of shock is of critical importance in the initial management of acutely traumatized patients. This determination should be based on the time elapsed since injury. If injury occurred within 15 minutes of arrival in the emergency room and the patient is in profound shock, one must consider this presentation consistent with massive hemorrhage. Conversely, if the patient is in mild shock and the accident occurred several hours previously, less aggressive volume resuscitation is required to replace blood loss.

Indicators that are commonly utilized to assess degree of shock in the emergency setting include blood pressure, pulse rate, skin perfusion (color, temperature, moisture), urine output, mental status, and central venous pressure.[2] Although blood pressure is a time-honored parameter in defining volume loss, it is less accurate than pulse rate, skin perfusion, and urine output. Response of the blood pressure to intravascular depletion is nonlinear. Compensatory mechanisms of increased cardiac rate and contractility, and venous arteriolar vasoconstriction can offset the initial 15 to 20 percent of intravascular volume loss in the healthy young adult. When volume loss increases above 20 percent, decline in blood pressure is more precipitous. In the elderly patient less able to compensate by the aforementioned mechanisms, decline in blood pressure starts at 10 to 15 percent volume loss and will proceed to the point of arrest by 40 percent loss. In poorly monitored patients blood pressure will suddenly drop reflecting decompensation rather than acute bleeding. Clearly, blood pressure does not have an absolute level of normality, with 120 mmHg systolic representing profound shock in the hypertensive trauma victim, whereas levels of 85 to 90 mmHg systolic represent acceptable levels in young, healthy athletic patients.[7]

Pulse rate is the second most commonly used indicator of shock; however, its value is limited by its lack of specificity. Emotionalism, pain, and excitement surrounding the usual trauma situation may result in tachycardia without hypovolemia. Tachycardia above levels of 120/min should be considered an indicator of hypovolemia until proven otherwise. In young patients with severe volume depletion, the heart rate may accelerate to 160 to 180/min. The older patient is unable to accelerate to this degree and rarely will sustain rates greater than 140/min.

Skin perfusion is a more accurate indicator in evaluating trauma patients. The first level physiologic compensation for volume loss is vasoconstriction of vessels to the skin and muscle, manifested by paleness and coolness of the skin, which rapidly develops. The release of epinephrine, which accompanies hypovolemia, is reflected by cool skin and moisture on the trunk and extremities. The body's second level compensation for hypovolemia is visceral vasoconstriction, which results in decreased flow to the gastrointestinal tract, liver, and kidneys. Any patient with significant trauma should have an indwelling urinary bladder catheter inserted to monitor urine output; this should be recorded every 15 minutes. Urine output will immediately reflect decreases in renal blood flow. A urine output of 0.5 ml/kg/hr is considered minimally adequate, and resuscitative fluids should be rapidly administered until this level is reached. If urine output exceeds 1 ml/kg/hr, the fluid administration rate can be diminished. During resuscitation and surgery, urine output is the best indicator of the adequacy of volume resuscitation.

The next indicator of hypovolemia, alteration in mental status, is rarely observed until pre-terminal levels of hypovolemia are reached. Compensatory mechanisms maintain flow to the myocardium and brain with great tenacity; therefore, one does not observe cerebral hypoperfusion until blood pressure reaches the 30 to 60 mmHg systolic range or less. The patient becomes irrational, anxious, and uncooperative. Such states are also commonly produced by alcohol, hypoxia, hypoglycemia, and drugs administered in the emergency setting. There is no absolute method to resolve this problem except to retain a high index of suspicion and to be aware that the agitated patient must be evaluated carefully to exclude hypovolemia as a cause for his or her behavior.

The last parameter, central venous pressure, is an inaccurate indicator of hypovolemia, as the normal levels of 3 to 8 mmHg are relatively difficult to distinguish from hypovolemic levels of 0 to 5 mmHg, particularly when one is initially estimating the pressure only by inspection of external jugular neck veins.

Resuscitation

Oxygen therapy should be provided and immediately followed by vigorous intravenous therapy with a balanced salt solution. Placement of peripheral IV lines and/or cutdowns may be quicker, safer, and less complicated than central lines.

Shock associated with trauma is most often hypovolemic in nature.[8] After initiation of fluid therapy, type-specific blood may be used as necessary while properly crossmatched blood is being prepared. If type-specific blood is not available, consideration should be given to the use of low-titer type-O blood. For life-threatening blood loss, the use of unmatched, type-specific whole blood can be life saving and is preferred over type-O blood. Hypovolemic shock is not treated by vasopressors, steroids, or sodium bicarbonate.[9]

Adequate resuscitation is best assessed by quantitative improvement of physiologic parameters (i.e., ventilatory rate, pulse, blood pressure, arterial blood gases, and urinary output) rather than the qualitative assessment performed in the primary survey. When a state of shock is identified, the pneumatic antishock garment may be applied, inflated, and used in conjunction with IV fluid resuscitation. Other indications for its use include systolic blood pressure less than 90 mmHg, intraabdominal hemorrhage with hypotension, stabilization of suspected pelvic and lower extremity fractures, and neurogenic shock with hypotension.[10] When inflated, the device increases systolic blood pressure, probably by acting as a local vasoconstrictor and increasing peripheral resistance.

If the patient is already wearing an antishock suit, vital signs should be checked and IV fluids administered before it is removed. The device should be deflated gradually, beginning with the abdominal sections and followed by each leg. If blood pressure falls, deflation should be halted.

THE SECONDARY ASSESSMENT

The secondary survey is an assessment to determine additional injuries. The patient should be examined systematically for both external and internal injuries. Obvious injuries may be examined initially, but in the subsequent sequence the patient is evaluated from head to feet.

Head

The secondary survey begins with evaluation of the head and identification of all related and significant injuries. The eyes should be reevaluated for pupillary size and penetrating injuries, then the fundi for hemorrhages, lens for dislocation, anterior chambers for hyphema, and conjunctiva for hemorrhages. A quick visual confrontation examination of both eyes is done by having the patient read either a Snelling chart or words on the side of an IV container. This frequently identifies optic injuries not otherwise apparent.

Blunt or penetrating trauma to the head can cause injury to the scalp, skull, and brain tissue. The head should be examined for lacerations, contusions, and entry and exit wounds.

Maxillofacial Trauma

Maxillofacial trauma not associated with airway obstruction should only be treated after the patient is completely stabilized and is not suffering major life-threatening injuries. Patients with midfacial fractures may have a fracture of the cribriform plate. For these patients, gastric intubation should be performed via the oral route or through a soft nasopharyngeal airway, rather than transnasally, to avoid intracranial penetration through the fractured cribriform plate.

Ecchymosis around the mastoid area (Battle's sign) may suggest a temporal bone fracture. Raccoon's eyes, or sharply demarcated ecchymosis around the eyelids, may indicate an anterior basal skull fracture. Signs of cerebrospinal fluid leakage from either nose or ears may suggest a communication between the subarachnoid space and the external environment.

Cervical Spine/Neck

Patients with maxillofacial trauma produced by blunt injury should be presumed to have a cervical spine fracture. Examination of the neck includes visual examination and palpation. Absence of neurological deficit does not rule out injury to the cervical spine; such an injury should be presumed until ruled out by radiograph. In penetrating trauma, wounds that extend through the platysma should not be manually explored in the emergency department. This type of injury requires surgical evaluation and consultation. Nonoperative measures include observation, arteriography, laryngoscopy, bronchoscopy, esophagoscopy, and esophagography.

Chest

Visual evaluation of the chest, both anteriorly and posteriorly, will identify sucking chest injuries and perhaps a large flail chest. A complete evaluation of the chest wall requires palpation of the entire thorax, in which each rib and clavicle is felt individually. Blunt sternal pressure will be painful if any attached ribs are fractured.

Evaluation of internal structures is best done with the stethoscope. Breath sounds are auscultated at the apex for pneumothorax and at the base for hemothorax and pulmonary contusion. Distant heart sounds and distended neck veins may indicate cardiac tamponade. Distant heart sounds may be difficult to appreciate in a noisy emergency department, and distended neck veins may be absent because of associated hypovolemia. A narrow pulse pressure may be the only reliable indication of cardiac tamponade.

Abdomen

Any abdominal injury is potentially dangerous and must be diagnosed and treated aggressively. The specific diagnosis is not as important as the fact that an abdominal injury exists and surgical intervention may be needed. Initial examination of the abdomen may not be representative of the patient's condition one to several hours later. Close observation and frequent reevaluation of the abdomen by inspection, palpation, and auscultation is impor-

tant in the management of blunt abdominal trauma. Indications for peritoneal lavage are discussed below.

Patients with neurological injury, impaired sensorium secondary to alcohol or drugs, or equivocal abdominal findings should be considered candidates for peritoneal lavage. Fractures of the pelvis or the lower thorax may also hinder adequate diagnostic examination of the abdomen.

Rectum

A rectal examination is an essential part of the secondary survey. The physician should look for the presence of blood within the bowel lumen, a high-riding prostate, pelvic fractures, integrity of the rectal wall, and quality of sphincter tone.

Fractures

Extremities should be visually evaluated for contusions and deformity. Palpation of the bones with rotational or three-point pressure to assess tenderness, crepitation, or abnormal movement along the shaft helps identify fractures, where alignment has been maintained. Downward pressure with the heels of the hands on both anterior-superior iliac spines and on the symphysis pubis can identify pelvic fractures. In addition, all peripheral pulses should be assessed and their presence or absence documented.

Neurological Examination

An in-depth neurological examination includes not only motor and sensory evaluation of the extremities but also reevaluation of the patient's level of consciousness and pupils. The pupils should be examined for size, shape, equality, and reactivity to light. One nonreactive and dilated pupil may indi-

Table 1-2. Glasgow Coma Scale

Eye Opening		Verbal Response		Motor Response	
Spontaneous	4	Oriented	5	Obeys command	6
To voice	3	Confused	4	Localizes pain	5
To pain	2	Inappropriate words	3	Withdraw (pain)	4
None	1	Incomprehensible words	2	Flexion (pain)	3
		None	1	Extension (pain)	2
				None	1

(Modified from Teasdale G, Jennett B: Assessment of coma and impaired consciousness. A practical scale. Lancet 2:81, 1974.)

cate pressure on the third cranial nerve (oculomotor), possibly secondary to a supratentorial herniation of the brain's temporal lobe over the tentorium cerebelli. A numerical evaluation such as the Glasgow Coma Scale facilitates detection of early changes (Table 1-2).[11]

The patient's motor and sensory functions of spinal and cranial nerves should be routinely tested. Decerebrate and decorticate posturing are ominous signs of significant cranial injury. Deep tendon reflexes should be checked for symmetry. Any evidence of paralysis or paresis suggests major injury to the spinal column or peripheral nervous system.[12] Adequate immobilization using short or long spine boards and a semirigid cervical collar must be established initially. Patient transport to a facility capable of spinal cord injury management requires the same type of adequate immobilization.

Acute epidural and subdural hematomas, depressed skull fractures, and other intracranial emergencies are best treated by the neurosurgeon. Changes in intracranial status may be associated with alterations in the level of consciousness. Serious sequelae of head injuries include cerebral edema, increased intracranial pressure, hypoxemia, and an increase in PCO_2. If a patient with a head injury deteriorates neurologically, the management and treatment priorities may change. Oxygenation and perfusion of the brain and adequacy of ventilation should be reassessed. If these latter parameters are unchanged, intracranial surgical intervention may be indicated. Computed tomography (CT) is the diagnostic procedure of choice in the assessment of the head-injured patient to determine if more sophisticated monitoring, such as intracranial monitoring of pressure or surgery to decompress and stop bleeding, is necessary.

HISTORY AND MECHANISMS OF INJURY

A history of the event or knowledge of the patient's association with an injury-producing mechanism may be helpful in the diagnosis of certain injuries. Generally, the greater the speed of the vehicle (automobile or object striking the patient) the greater the injury. A bent or collapsed steering wheel should lead one to consider abdominal and chest injuries, fractured ribs or sternum, laryngotracheal injuries, fractures of the spine at any level, and possible tears of the thoracic aorta (deceleration injury).

Improperly worn lap seat belts will often produce abdominal injuries that may be suspected by an abrasive mark on the abdominal wall. Shoulder strap seat belts may cause clavicular fractures or shoulder dislocations. A history of a broken windshield and damaged dashboards is associated with head and cervical spine trauma, maxillofacial injuries, laryngotracheal injuries, knee injuries, and posterior fracture dislocation of the head of the femur from the acetabulum. Broken inside door latches or window handles often produce penetrating wounds or possible sucking chest wounds. Lateral impacts can produce rib fractures, acetabular fractures, and intrathoracic deceleration injuries.

With penetrating trauma, the caliber of gun or size of knife is important information. Gunshot wounds will be commonly associated with internal bleeding and visceral organ perforations as well as fractures. Burns of the nose, mouth, and pharynx should alert one to the dangers of smoke inhalation and carbon monoxide poisoning.

If the patient is conscious, the examiner should determine the location of major symptoms and focus the examination on those areas. Internal thoracic and abdominal injuries do not produce reliable physical findings, unlike injuries to the extremities, spine, and chest wall. A clear statement by the patient that there is absence of pain or tenderness in the neck or back and in the arms and legs, either at rest or with movement, can immediately eliminate the need for extensive and time-consuming x-ray studies. The examiner should also obtain a medical history regarding allergies, medications currently taken by the patient, past medical illnesses and surgical procedures, the time of the last meal, and the events that preceded the injury.

Table 1-3. Tetanus Prophylaxis of the Wounded Patient

History of Tetanus Immunization (doses)	Clean, Minor Wounds		Tetanus-Prone Wounds	
	TD[a]	TIG	TD[a]	TIG[b]
Uncertain	Yes	No	Yes	Yes
0–1	Yes	No	Yes	Yes
2	Yes	No	Yes	No[c]
3 or more	No[d]	No	No[e]	No

[a] For children less than 7 years old DTP (DT, if pertussis vaccine is contraindicated) is preferred to tetanus toxoid alone. For persons 7 years old and older, TD is preferred to tetanus toxoid alone.

[b] When TIG and TD are given concurrently, separate syringes and separate sites should be used.

[c] Yes, if wound is more than 24 hours old.

[d] Yes, if more than 10 years since last dose.

[e] Yes, if more than 5 years since the last dose. (More frequent boosters are not needed and can accentuate side effects.)

(Committee on Trauma, American College of Surgeons: Advanced Trauma Life Support Course. American College of Surgeons, Chicago, 1984.)

TETANUS IMMUNIZATION AND DIAGNOSTIC PROCEDURES

Attention must be directed to adequate tetanus prophylaxis in the multiply injured patient, particularly if open extremity trauma is present. Standard immunization in adults requires at least three injections of toxoid. A routine booster of absorbed toxoids (TD) is indicated every 10 years thereafter. Passive immunization with human tetanus globulin (TIG, 250 units) must be individually considered for each patient. Recommendations for tetanus prophylaxis are based on the condition of the wound and the patient's immunization history. Wounds with any one of the following features are considered tetanus prone: gunshot or stab wounds, wounds 6 hours old, stellate avulsion, crush injury, burn injury, frostbite, evidence of devitalized tissue, signs of infection, or heavy contamination (dirt, feces, soil, saliva). Tetanus prophylaxis for the wounded patient is listed in Table 1-3.[1]

The placement of urinary and gastric catheters should now be considered, if not already placed, provided urethral transection or cribriform plate fractures do not contraindicate their insertion. If the cribriform plate is fractured, a nasogastric tube may be inadvertently inserted into the intracranial cavity. For victims of blunt trauma resulting in suspected urethral transection, insertion of a urinary catheter should not be attempted before a rectal examination has been performed. Urinary catheter insertion, without a preceding urethrogram is usually contraindicated if there is (1) blood at the meatus, (2) blood in the scrotum, or (3) if the prostate cannot be palpated or is high-riding.

The principal diagnostic studies in the emergency department are radiographic. Laboratory testing contributes minimally, with the exception of arterial blood gases to assess respiratory dysfunction, hematocrit to assess blood loss, and serum amylase to assess pancreatic injury. Unless a prior history exists to suggest a problem, studies of electrolytes, liver function, and clotting are rarely abnormal and, in most situations, are not indicated. Careful electrocardiogram monitoring of all trauma patients is required. Incidences of arrhythmias, such as atrial fibrillation, premature ventricular contractions, and ST segment changes, may be observed.

The most commonly performed radiographic study is the chest roentgenogram. The chest roentgenogram provides the greatest immediate information regarding intrathoracic injury and allows pneumothorax, hemothorax, rib fractures, mediastinal injury, and occasionally, diaphragmatic injury to be quickly defined.

In contrast to the chest roentgenogram, a plain

film of the abdomen usually contributes minimally to the therapeutic management of trauma patients. Intravenous pyelography, excretory urography, cystography, and urethrography are the mainstays for preliminary evaluation of injuries to the genitourinary tract.

Computed tomography of the abdomen assists in evaluation of hemodynamically stable patients subjected to blunt trauma to the lower chest or abdomen, especially patients with equivocal indications for celiotomy or patients difficult to evaluate because of obtundation or spinal cord damage. CT detects intra- and retroperitoneal bleeding and identifies the damaged organ. CT is accurate in assessing the organs most likely to be damaged with blunt trauma (i.e., liver, spleen, kidneys, and pancreas). It is also accurate in detecting retroduodenal air or edema associated with duodenal disruptions and free intraperitoneal air associated with rupture of the small or large intestine.

Indications for peritoneal lavage in the stable patient are similar to those for CT of the abdomen (equivocal findings on abdominal examination or neurologic abnormalities that preclude abdominal examination).[13] To perform a lavage, the bladder must be decompressed by passing a Foley catheter. The skin below the umbilicus is infiltrated with a local anesthetic, and an incision is made to the fascia. A catheter is then inserted through the fascia into the peritoneal cavity. The peritoneal cavity is infused with 1,000 ml of Ringer's lactate and drained. The lavage is considered technically adequate if more than 500 ml are recovered. A red blood cell count greater than 50,000/mm or a white blood cell count greater than 500/mm suggests injury to abdominal viscera.[13]

SOPHISTICATED MONITORING TECHNIQUES

During the acute phase of injury, the attention of the trauma team is directed toward resuscitation. Precision in maintaining cardiopulmonary function is an essential feature of therapy at this time and in subsequent phases of management in the operating room. Detailed assessment of hemodynamic, respiratory and circulatory function of the traumatized patient can be performed at the bedside and in the operating room with the automated physiologic profile.[14,15] Patients requiring physiologic assessment undergo right heart cardiac catheterization at the bedside by the use of a disposable balloon flotation catheter inserted by a percutaneous technique via either the internal jugular or subclavian vein. Serial pressure measurements within the right atrium, right ventricle, pulmonary artery, and pulmonary artery wedge position are recorded. Following pressure recordings and thermal dilution studies, blood samples are obtained for arterial and pulmonary artery blood gas analysis, carboxyhemoglobin saturation, hemoglobin, hematocrit, and lactate determinations. In addition the patient's age, height, weight, and rectal temperature are noted.

All data are entered into a programmable calculator. Primary and derived data include cardiac index, pulse rate, stroke index, left ventricular stroke work, peripheral vascular resistance, right ventricular stroke work, and pulmonary vascular resistance. Arteriovenous oxygen difference, oxygen consumption, and venoarterial admixture are calculated; these aid in the description of respiratory function. Serum lactate and arterial base excess allow assessment of the integration of hemodynamic and respiratory functions within the integrity of metabolic requirements. Routine measurements of carboxyhemoglobin concentration have been found to be useful in the management of trauma and burn patients. Intracardiac and intravascular pressure measurements as well as a ventricular function diagram are also recorded.

Cardiac output, the actual amount of blood ejected by the heart, is related to contractility of the myocardium, preload, afterload, and pulse rate. Myocardial contractility refers to the state of health of heart muscle and the rate at which muscle fibers shorten circumferentially around the bolus of blood within the ventricles. The preload is the degree of muscle fiber stretch imposed by filling of the ventricles during diastole. This varies directly with cardiac output. The afterload is the impedance to cardiac ejection during systole imposed by vascular resistance, blood pressure, and blood viscosity. The stroke output of the heart varies inversely with afterload. Cardiac output varies directly with pulse rate up to a rate of 160, at which point there is insufficient time for complete ventricular filling. The Sarnoff ventricular function curve plots stroke work (blood pressure) against ventricular end diastolic pressure or end diastolic volume. It provides a good evaluation of myocardial contractility because it includes consideration of afterload and preload. The automated physiologic profile clearly assesses all of these factors, and is rapidly displayed on a preprinted format by means of an analog plotter. Through use of the programmable calculator system, data reduction and analysis of derived data are routinely performed and readily available. Bar graphs displaying recorded and derived data are provided with indications of normal ranges for recorded values. Intracardiac pressures are recorded adjacent to the cardiac silhouette to provide a clear pictorial representation of intracardiac dynamics.

REFERENCES

1. Committee on Trauma, American College of Surgeons: Advanced Trauma Life Support Course. American College of Surgeons, Chicago, 1984
2. Trunkey DD, Lewis FR: Current Therapy of Trauma. C.V. Mosby, St Louis, 1984
3. Danzl DF, Thomas DM: Nasotracheal Intubation in the Emergency Department, Crit Care Med 8:667, 1980
4. Brantigan CO, Grow JB: Cricothyroidotomy: Elective use in respiratory problems requiring tracheotomy. J Thorac Cardiovasc Surg 71:72, 1976
5. Levinson MM, Scuderi PE, Gibson RL, Comer PB: Emergency percutaneous and transtracheal ventilation. JACEP/Ann Emerg Med 8(10):396, 1979
6. Greene R, Stark P: Trauma of the larynx and trachea. Radiol Clin North AM 16:309, 1978
7. Jones KW: Thoracic Trauma. Surg Clin North Am 60:957, 1980
8. Shires GT, Canizaro PC, Carrico CJ: Shock. p. 116. In Schwartz SI (ed): Principles of Surgery, 4th Ed. McGraw-Hill, New York, 1984
9. Virgilio RW, Rice CL, Smith DE, et al: Crystalloid vs colloid resuscitation: Is one better? A randomized clinical study. Surgery 85:129, 1979
10. Committee on Trauma, American College of Surgeons: Early Care of the Injured Patient. Philadelphia. W.B. Saunders, pp. 48–55, 1982
11. Teasdale G, Jennett B: Assessment of coma and impaired consciousness. A practical scale. Lancet 2:81, 1974
12. Weiss MH: Head trauma and spinal cord injuries: Diagnostic and therapeutic criteria. Crit Care Med 2:311, 1974
13. Fischer RP, Beverlin BC, Engrav LH, et al: Diagnostic peritoneal lavage—Fourteen years and 2,586 patients later. Am J Surg 136:701, 1976
14. Cohn JD, Engler PE, Del Guercio LRM: The automated physiologic profile. Crit Care Med 3:51, 1975
15. Del Guercio LRM: Physiologic Monitoring of the Surgical Patient. p. 524. In Schwartz SI (ed): Principles of Surgery. 3rd Ed. McGraw-Hill, New York, 1979

Frontal Sinus Fractures

2

Othella T. Owens
Robert H. Mathog

Frontal sinus fractures are among the least common injuries affecting the facial skeleton, representing 5 to 15 percent[1,2] of all facial fractures. These injuries are usually related to accidents and assaults. Windshields on automobiles, motorcycles, and snowmobiles are inches from the area of impact on the frontal bone. Seat belts alone will not help, and shoulder restraints are necessary to prevent the head from hitting the upper part of the steering wheel or dashboard. Because so much traumatic force can be transmitted to the frontoethmoid complex, injuries to this area, as well as associated injuries, are severe.

ANATOMY

The frontal bone is composed of paired vertical portions and a single horizontal portion. In the adult the vertical parts are called anterior and posterior tables, which with the floor inferiorly enclose the frontal sinuses. These sinuses are separated by a midline septum, are pyramidal in shape, and vary considerably in size and symmetry.

In addition to forming the anterior aspect of the cranial vault, the frontal bone forms the superior part of the facial skeleton. Frontal bone contours produce forehead landmarks, including the frontal eminence superiorly and superciliary arches. The glabella is that flat area of bone separating the arches, which lies above the orbits. The horizontal portion of the frontal bone consists of the thin orbital plates separated medially by the ethmoid notch in which lie the ethmoid bones.

Frontal sinuses develop from the frontal recess, an evagination of the anterior-superior portion of the middle meatus. By age 6 years the frontal sinuses are demonstrable on plain radiographs and continue to develop through puberty. By age 12 the sinuses are of sufficient size to become significant in terms of trauma. Approximately 10 percent of the population has unilateral development of the frontal sinuses, and in 4 percent of the population there is agenesis.

The anterior wall of the frontal sinus is composed of cancellous bone and is generally stronger than the posterior wall, which is made of compact bone and is thinner and closely adherent to dura. Generally, larger sinuses have weaker walls. The degree of damage from trauma, then, depends on size and extent of pneumatization.

Each frontal sinus drains into the nose. In most instances, the frontal sinus drains directly into the frontal recess of the nasal cavity. In other individuals, a well-formed duct starts at the posterior-medial portion of the sinus floor at the junction of the ethmoid and nasal components and passes into the middle meatus, a distance of few millimeters to a centimeter. This position of the duct makes it prone to injury from posterior-inferior fractures. The longer ducts, surrounded by thin-walled ethmoid cells, are especially susceptible to traumatic rupture. In 15 percent of subjects, the duct drains into the infundibulum ethmoidale.[3]

The ethmoid notch, separating the two orbital plates or horizontal parts of the frontal sinus floor, is filled by the cribriform plate of the ethmoid. This structure transmits small olfactory nerve endings and is tightly adherent to dura.[4] Injury here is often associated with permanent loss of smell and cerebrospinal fluid (CSF) leak.

CLASSIFICATION

Rowe and Killey outlined a classification of frontal sinus fractures based on injury to the anterior and posterior sinus walls and nasofrontal duct.[5]

Anterior sinus wall fractures can be simple linear, simple depressed, compound linear, compound linear depressed, or compound comminuted.
Posterior sinus wall fractures with or without anterior wall fractures can be simple linear, compound linear, compound and/or comminuted depressed.
Finally, sinus floor (nasofrontal duct) injuries can be associated with any of the previously mentioned fractures, or with naso-orbital fracture.

Fractures of the floor will often involve the nasofrontal duct and cause obstruction of the duct from edema, displaced bone fragments, or blood clot.

These fractures can also extend to the cribriform plate, and if a sufficient dural tear occurs, they can cause CSF leak.

ASSESSMENT

Preliminary evaluation of patients with frontal sinus fractures should proceed so that an efficient and thorough history of events coincident with the trauma is obtained. A physical examination should be performed with particular attention to airway and circulatory functions. The central nervous system (CNS) should be evaluated to ascertain the extent of head injury. The frontal bone is then assessed for comminution, cosmetic deformity, and CSF leaks.

Plain skull films taken during early assessment will identify clouding, air-fluid levels, fractures, pneumocephalus, sinus size, and symmetry (Fig. 2-1). Often posterior table fractures and floor fractures involving the nasofrontal duct cannot be appreciated on plain films, and polytomography is required (Fig. 2-2). Computed tomography (CT) (Fig. 2-3) is valuable for defining complex bone and soft tissue injuries involving the paranasal sinuses, nasofrontal duct, cribriform plate, orbit, optic nerve, and brain.[6,7] The site of CSF leaks can be detected by plain x-ray film successfully in 20 percent of cases, according to Lenzt et al.[8] By adding tomography they are able to identify the fistula site in 50 percent of cases. Recent experience with CT scans shows even better resolution and often permits identification of small fracture sites and areas of minimal soft tissue injury.

Computed tomography scans are rapidly replacing polytomography and plain films as the diagnostic procedure of choice in head and neck trauma. Due to the forces involved with frontal bone fractures, concomitant brain injuries are frequent, necessitating brain CT scanning for evaluation. Additional scanning can easily be performed to delineate frontal sinus pathology.

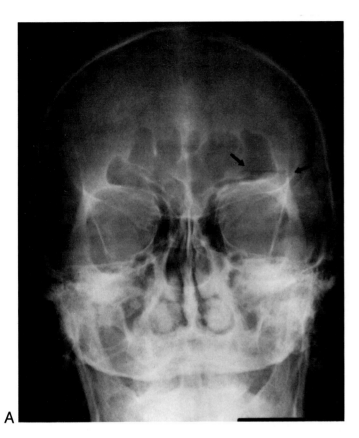

A

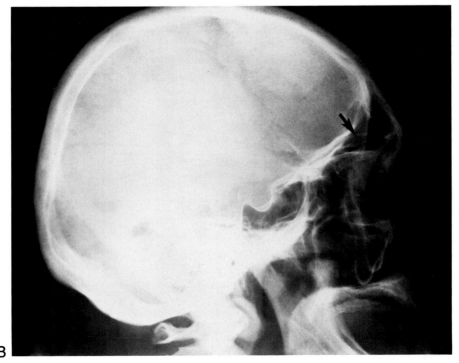

B

Fig. 2-1. Radiographs of the skull in the (**A**) posterior-anterior and (**B**) lateral projections showing a linear horizontal fracture of the posterior wall of the frontal sinus (arrows).

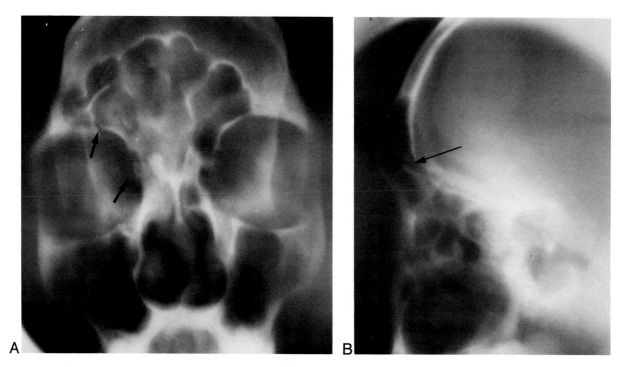

Fig. 2-2. Tomograms in the **(A)** frontal and **(B)** lateral projections showing fractures extending along the floor of the frontal sinus, with a blowout defect of the posterior wall (arrows).

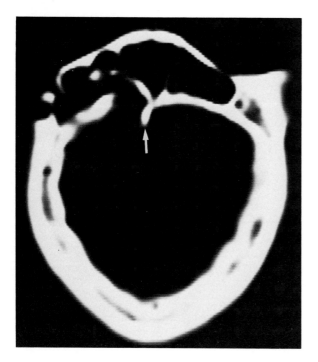

Fig. 2-3. Computed tomography (CT) scan taken in a horizontal plane of the same patient as in Figure 2-2. A "trap door" defect of the posterior wall is apparent (arrow).

TREATMENT

General

Definitive management can be planned once initial evaluation of the sinus fracture has been completed. All patients with frontal sinus fractures should be treated prophylactically with intravenous antibiotics. For comminuted or extensive fractures one should choose aqueous penicillin with an antistaphylococcal penicillin, since penicillins cross the blood-brain barrier and provide excellent prophylaxis for intracranial contamination. If lacerations are present, a limited exploration of the sinus wall can be performed to assess the extent of injury.

After the initial exam and appropriate radiographs, one should decide on conservative management with antibiotics, radiographic follow-up with limited exploration through lacerations, or, if needed, more detailed radiographic and extensive surgical evaluation.

Definitive surgery can be delayed 2 to 5 days to allow stabilization of vital signs (see Chapter 1). With additional time, a decrease in soft tissue swelling will permit better assessment of cosmetic defects and opportunity for additional radiographic studies.

Anterior Table

Injury to the anterior table is more common and less complex than injury to other frontal bone sites. With intact skin and a nondisplaced fracture by radiographic examination, the patient can be followed expectantly. If the anterior wall is depressed, trephine through the sinus floor is performed and fragments may be elevated to anatomical position (Fig. 2-4).

If a laceration exists and the anterior wall alone is involved, the fracture may be explored through the laceration. Extension of the laceration may be nec-

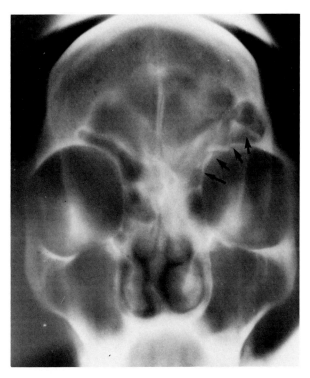

Fig. 2-4. Tomogram showing fractures of the anterior table of the frontal bone that required exploration and elevation of fragments into appropriate positions (arrows).

essary for better exposure. Nondisplaced fractures are left intact and the skin repaired by plastic surgery technique. If fragments are displaced, a hook may be used to elevate them. Often after reduction, the fragments are stable and fixation is not necessary.

For depressed anterior table fractures in which injury is believed to extend to the nasofrontal duct or in which unstable fragments are present, the frontal sinus can be explored by the standard frontoethmoidectomy approach (Lynch incision). The floor of the sinus is perforated with a small burr, and a Kerrison rongeur is used to enlarge the opening. This exposure provides direct visualization of the nasofrontal duct and anterior wall. If necessary, the incision may be extended and the skin over the sinus elevated, taking care to leave the periosteum attached to all fragments. If suturing the periosteum over the fragments does not provide adequate stabilization, Gelfoam may be placed in the

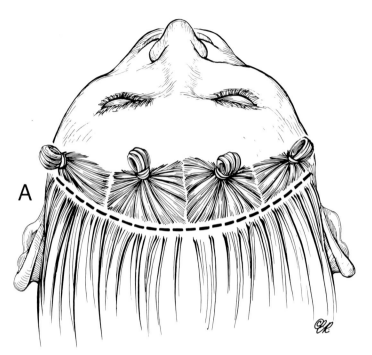

A

Fig. 2-5. Surgical approach to fractures of the posterior table. (**A**) The line of incision is posterior to the hairline and anterior to the ear. (**B**) The coronal flap is elevated and the x-ray template marked. (*Figure continues.*)

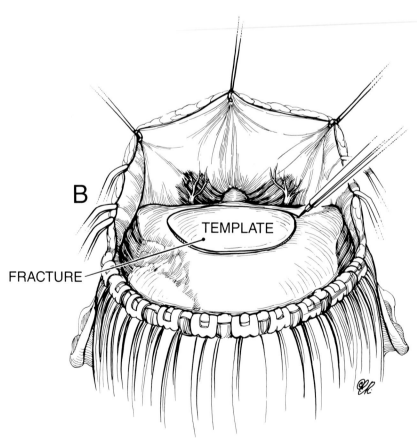

B

TEMPLATE

FRACTURE

Fig. 2-5 *(Continued).* **(C)** The bone flap is elevated and the intersinus septum and mucosa are removed with a cutting burr. **(D)** Fat is implanted and the bone flap returned.

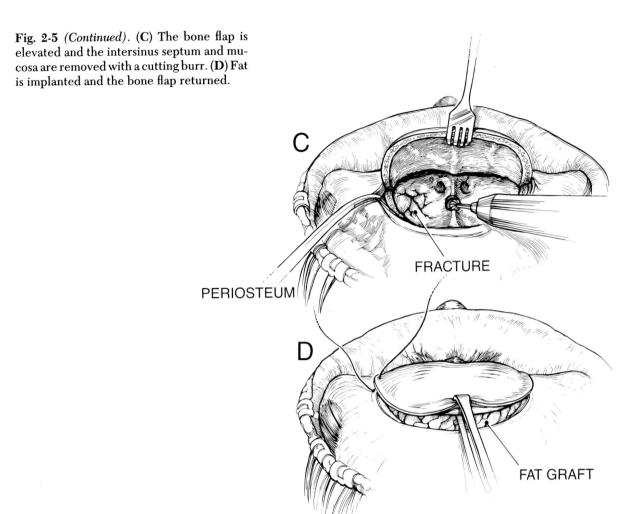

sinus to support bone fragments. Davini et al.[9] have used autogeneous bone dust and butyl-2-cyanoacrylate (Histoacryl-Blau) with apparent success for some frontal sinus injuries.

Posterior Table and Floor

Fractures of the posterior table and floor and more extensive fractures of the anterior table require greater exposure in order to be approached. Although traditionally exposed through a coronal incision, these fractures can be approached through a butterfly incision, provided the sinus is shallow and the anterior table is not severely comminuted. When a posterior fracture is recognized, neurosurgical exploration is needed, and the coronal approach is preferred.

A frontal sinusotomy by frontal osteoplastic flap can be performed through either the butterfly or coronal approach. Either technique allows assessment and repair of CSF leaks and direct visualization of the posterior table and nasofrontal duct.

The coronal incision should be made at least 1.5 cm behind the hairline. (Fig. 2-5A). A solution of epinephrine 1 : 200,000 can be injected into the line of incision to aid hemostatic control.

The flap is elevated in a subgaleal plane, preserving the integrity of the periosteum. Raney clips may be used on the scalp margins for hemostasis. The flap is elevated forward to the nasion and supraorbital rims, carefully preserving the nerve and blood supply to these areas (Fig. 2-5B).

To determine the site of the osteotomy, a template is constructed from an outline of the frontal sinus on a Caldwell radiograph taken 6 feet from the subject. The template, which has been autoclaved or cold sterilized at the start of the procedure, is placed over the frontal bone. The periosteal incision should be outlined with methylene blue several millimeters outside the intended osteotomy incisions to prevent indentation after healing (Fig. 2-5B). The periosteum is incised and elevated a few millimeters over the edge of the intended bone flap. A Stryker saw is used to perform most of the osteotomy. A 2 mm osteotome is then used to perforate the bone over the orbital rims and nasion, so that the bone flap can be easily reflected forward and remain attached to the overlying periosteum (Fig. 2-5C).

The posterior table is completely examined, and if there are nondisplaced fragments and the nasofrontal ducts are intact, one can replace the flap or proceed with an obliteration procedure. If the nasofrontal duct is damaged, the intersinus septum can be removed to allow the unaffected duct to function for both sides (Fig. 2-5C).

Pollack and Payne[10] do not advocate obliteration even in the presence of repairable dural injury. Schultz[1] found that CSF leaks stopped spontaneously with reduction of posterior table fractures. Obvious leaks however should be repaired with closure of the dura with 4-0 silk or a patch of temporalis fascia or lyophilized dura.

When the posterior table is depressed or comminuted, Hybels[11] advocates fat obliteration in which a dense fibrous barrier between the respiratory tract and intracranial contents is sought.

Once it has been decided to obliterate the sinus, all mucosa must be meticulously removed. Starting at an edge, an elevator is used to dissect mucosa intact, since piecemeal removal should be avoided. Displaced fragments can then be elevated into position and stabilized with 28-gauge interosseus wire. Under magnification a cutting burr is used to remove any remaining elements of mucosa and prepare a vascular bony surface. Mucosa at the nasofrontal ducts is pushed inferiorly, and the intersinus septum is completely removed.

Abdominal fat is harvested through a left McBurney incision with minimal handling of fat. Temporalis fascia, fascia lata, or pericranium obtained at the same time is used to cover the nasofrontal ducts. Fat is placed in the sinus and the bone flap replaced. Periosteum is approximated with 3-0 chromic or vicryl suture (Fig. 2-5D). Placement of a drain and light dressing is optional.

Alternatively, in the Riedel procedure the walls of the frontal sinus are removed and the frontal soft tissues collapsed onto the posterior table or dura. A secondary reconstructive procedure must be considered to correct the resulting cosmetic defect.

Donald and Bernstein[12] advocate obliteration by frontal sinus cranialization (Fig. 2-6). This method of obliteration is reserved for instances of severe frontal sinus injury. Meticulous removal of debris, posterior table, mucosa, nonviable brain, and covering of the nasofrontal ducts are mandatory.

When fractures of the sinus floor are extensive and obliteration is not feasible, because of difficulty in removing mucosa, an anterior frontoethmoidectomy with reconstruction of the duct can be considered. (Fig. 2-7) This method calls for exenteration of the ethmoid complex and enlargement

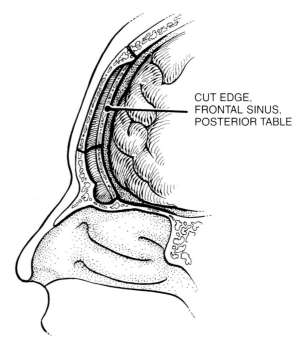

CUT EDGE,
FRONTAL SINUS,
POSTERIOR TABLE

Fig. 2-6. Cranialization of frontal sinus after removal of the posterior sinus wall.

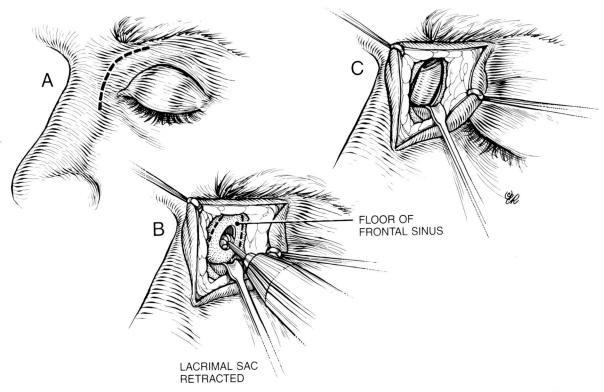

FLOOR OF
FRONTAL SINUS

LACRIMAL SAC
RETRACTED

Fig. 2-7. Anterior frontoethmoidectomy. **(A)** A frontoethmoidal incision (Lynch type) is made. **(B)** The anterior ethmoid bone and floor of the sinus are removed with a cutting burr. **(C)** A large Silastic tube is used to reconstruct the nasofrontal duct.

of the nasofrontal duct. The duct can be layered with a mucosal flap from the nose and is stented with a #28 chest tube or #8 endotracheal tube left in place for 6 weeks. The intersinus septum should be removed so that the contralateral nasofrontal duct may function for the entire sinus.

EARLY COMPLICATIONS

Sinusitis

Sinusitis can be an immediate complication of frontal sinus fractures. This should be treated with appropriate antibiotics and oral and topical decon-

gestants. If infection persists, frontal sinus trephine for external drainage through the floor should be performed. The patient should be carefully observed and followed with serial radiographs until there is complete resolution of pathology. Persistent or recurrent infections indicate the need for exploratory sinusotomy.

Cerebrospinal Fluid Rhinorrhea

Cerebrospinal fluid rhinorrhea (CSF) may also occur immediately after injury. If leakage persists after reduction of frontal sinus fractures or after repair of the dura with suturing and/or fascia, the patient should undergo studies to localize and assess the need for repair. The patient should be treated with antibiotics to prevent development of meningitis. A delay of 2 to 3 weeks after injury is an acceptable period to allow for spontaneous cessation of the leak. Various imaging studies are useful in localizing CSF leaks, but if there are no obvious defects of the frontal bone or no accumulation of fluid in the sinus to suggest the site of leak, dye studies should be performed. Intrathecal fluoroscein dye preoperatively or intraoperatively has been advocated.[13–15] Neurotoxicity precludes the use of indigo carmine and methylene blue. Intrathecal metrizamide with coronal display tomography can be used.[6] Radioactive isotopes can be used, but diffusion into the mucous secretions confounds their analysis. Radioactively tagged albumin is no longer considered safe for intrathecal administration.

Intracerebral Pneumocephalus

Intracerebral pneumocephalus most commonly occurs after fractures of the frontal sinus, anterior ethmoid, or cribriform plate area.[16] The potential for infection and intracranial complications should be appreciated.

proached through the frontal osteoplastic flap approach with obliteration as described above. A Riedel procedure may well be advocated for treatment of mucopyoceles, if the patient has had a previous obliteration procedure.

Delayed CSF leaks, with or without associated intracranial sepsis, strongly point toward continued communication between the sinus and intracranial cavity. The site of leakage must be determined, as many patients will require dural repair and obliteration.

Contour Defects

Late contour defects may result from poorly reduced fractures or bone resorption of the osteoplastic flap. Reconstruction should be delayed 6 to 12 months. Schultz[17] and Merville[18] advocate onlay bone grafts of iliac crest or split rib for some depressed deformities of the supraorbital and glabella regions. Methyl methacrylate has proven suitable for complex contour irregularities, as has solid dimethylpolysiloxane (Silastic) for gross frontal bone defects.

LATE COMPLICATIONS

Any patient who has had more than minor trauma to the frontal sinus is subject to delayed complications. Late occurring infections, if persistent or recurrent, strongly suggest the need for exploratory sinusotomy and obliteration.

Mucoceles or Mucopyoceles

Mucoceles or mucopyoceles result from obstruction of the nasofrontal duct and may occur many years after initial injury. Rarely, they are seen as a late complication of obliteration procedures in which a nidus of secreting mucosa was not removed. Management of mucoceles is best ap-

REFERENCES

1. Schultz RC: Supraorbital and glabellar fractures. Plast Reconstr Surg 45:227, 1980
2. May MH, Ogura JH, Schramm V: Nasofrontal duct in frontal sinus fractures. Arch Otolaryngol 92:534, 1970
3. Montgomery WW: Surgery of the frontal sinus in Surgery of the Upper Respiratory System, 2nd Ed., Vol. 1. Lea & Febiger, Philadelphia, 1979
4. Goss CM: Osteology in Gray's Anatomy, 29th Ed. Lea and Febiger, Philadelphia, 1973
5. Rowe NL, Killey HC: Fractures of the facial skeleton, 2nd Ed. Williams & Wilkins, Baltimore, 1970
6. Noyek AM, Kassel EE: Computerized tomography in frontal sinus fractures. Arch Otolaryngol 108:378, 1982

7. Kassel EE, Noyek AM, Cooper PW: CT in facial trauma. J Otolaryngol 12:2, 1982
8. Lentz E, Forbes G, Brown M, Law C: Radiology of cerebrospinal fluid rhinorrhea. Am J Radiol 135:23, 1980
9. Davini V, Rivano C, Borzone M, Tercero E: Bone duct and adhesive material for closing bony breaches of the skull — A new method. J Neurosurg Sci 25:117, 1981
10. Pollack K, Payne EE: Fractures of the frontal sinus. Otolaryngol Clin North Am 9:517, 1976
11. Hybels RC: Posterior table fractures of the frontal sinus. II. Clinical Aspects. Laryngoscope 87:1740, 1977
12. Donald PJ, Bernstein L: Compound frontal sinus injuries with intracranial penetration. Laryngoscope 88:225, 1978
13. Calcaterra TC: Extracranial surgical repair of cerebrospinal rhinorrhea. Ann Otol Rhinol Laryngol 89:8, 1980
14. Kirchner F, Proud G: Method of identification and localization of cerebrospinal fluid rhinorrhea and otorrhea. Laryngoscope 70:94, 1960
15. Duckert L, Mathog R: Diagnosis in persistent cerebrospinal fluid fistulas. Laryngoscope 87:18, 1977
16. Ramsden RT, Block J: Traumatic pneumocephalus. J Laryngol Otol 90:345, 1976
17. Schultz RC: Frontal sinus and supraorbital fractures from vehicle accidents. Clin Plast Surg 2:93, 1975
18. Merville LC, Derome P, de Saint-Jorre G: Fronto-orbito-nasal dislocations: secondary treatment. J Maxillofac Surg 11:71, 1983

Nasal Fractures

3

Lanny Garth Close
William L. Meyerhoff

The nose is the most prominent and fragile structure of the facial skeleton. It is not surprising, therefore, that the bones of the nose are fractured more frequently than any other bony structure of the face. In one series, nasal fractures comprised 39 percent of all facial fractures.[1] Untreated or poorly treated nasal fractures can result in deformity of the bony and cartilaginous framework of the nose, resulting in a defect in cosmesis and distortion of normal respiratory physiology. Obstruction of the nasal airway, chronic crust formation in the nose, snoring, sinusitis, increased incidence of throat infections, and even serous otitis media may be sequelae of this altered physiology. It is well known that nasal fractures in children can also result in delayed or abnormal growth of the nose and midfacial skeleton as well as malalignment of the teeth.

Although nasal fractures occur at all ages, they are especially common in children. It is estimated that approximately 25 percent of all nasal fractures occur in patients less than 12 years of age.[2] Fractures can occur during the fetal period secondary to intrauterine pressure stress, especially during the first stage of labor in the primipara. At delivery, particularly when forceps are used, the nasal skeleton is again at risk. The incidence of nasal fracture in the newborn has been reported to range from 1 to 7 percent.[3] Incidental trauma during infancy as well as known injury during later childhood and teenage years can also result in nasal fractures. Unfortunately, unless the injury in children is severe enough to cause a moderate amount of swelling or an obvious cosmetic deformity, airway obstruction, or epistaxis, the physician may not be consulted. In adults, on the other hand, the majority of nasal fractures occur as a result of automobile accidents or physical assaults. In addition, sports injuries and accidents both at home and at work commonly result in nasal fractures. In one comprehensive study, 36 percent of adults suffering nasal fractures were under the influence of ethanol.[1]

ANATOMY

The skin of the nose has an excellent blood supply. Injuries to the nose, therefore, usually result in marked bleeding and formation of hematoma and ecchymosis. Since the skin of the upper nose is thin and freely moveable over the underlying bone and cartilage, and since the adjoining skin of the eyelids and cheeks is also loose, bleeding may extend laterally causing the well-known "black eye."

By contrast, the skin of the lower nose is thick and rich in sebaceous glands. This skin is intimately attached to the underlying cartilage that determines the configuration of the nostril margin. Thus, lacerations in this area may lead to retraction and notching of the nostril borders, unless properly treated.

The supporting framework of the proximal nose is rigid and bony, while that of the caudal nose is cartilaginous and more pliable (Fig. 3-1). The opening in the bony portion of the nose is termed the pyriform aperture. The bones of the nasal dorsum include the paired nasal bones, the nasal process of the frontal bone, and the frontal process of the maxilla. The frontal process of the maxilla projects upward and medially from the body of the maxilla to approximate the nasal bones, and it is frequently involved in fractures of the nose secondary to lateral blows. The nasal bones themselves join in the midline and are supported posteriorly by the nasal process of the frontal bone and laterally by the frontal process of the maxilla. The nasal bones are quadrangular, being thick and narrow above, and thin and wide below (Fig. 3-2). It is probably because of this disparity in thickness that fractures of the nasal bones rarely involve the proximal portion. In fact, fractures in this area are generally a result of violent impact forces resulting in fractures of the entire nasoethmoidal complex. In such cases, the bones are often comminuted and impacted posteriorly.

The upper lateral cartilages are paired and firmly attached to both the inner aspect and inferior border of the nasal bones. These cartilages form the framework for the middle third of the external nose and are intimately attached to the septum in the midline. The lower lateral (alar) cartilages are paired and composed of a lateral and medial crus. They form the framework of the caudal third of the external nose. The medial crura support and make up the framework of the columella. Together the medial and lateral crura of the lower lateral cartilages contour and shape the external nares and nostrils. These cartilages are resilient and normally un-

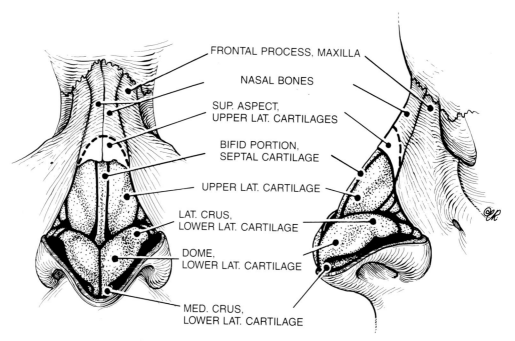

FRONTAL PROCESS, MAXILLA
NASAL BONES
SUP. ASPECT, UPPER LAT. CARTILAGES
BIFID PORTION, SEPTAL CARTILAGE
UPPER LAT. CARTILAGE
LAT. CRUS, LOWER LAT. CARTILAGE
DOME, LOWER LAT. CARTILAGE
MED. CRUS, LOWER LAT. CARTILAGE

Fig. 3-1. Schematic representation of nasal framework.

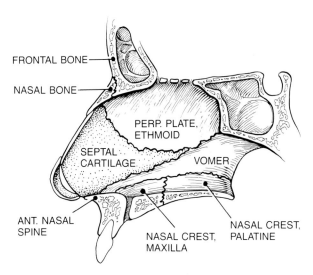

FRONTAL BONE

NASAL BONE

PERP. PLATE, ETHMOID

SEPTAL CARTILAGE

VOMER

ANT. NASAL SPINE

NASAL CREST, MAXILLA

NASAL CREST, PALATINE

Fig. 3-2. Bony and cartilaginous nasal septum. Note that in sagittal section the nasal bone has a thick upper portion and thinner lower portion.

damaged by blunt injury. Nevertheless, they are often displaced in nasal fractures owing to their attachment to the septal cartilage and bony dorsum. Usually, when the bony and septal fractures are reduced, the cartilages follow suit, and no further attention to these structures is required.

Perhaps the most important supporting framework of the nose is the septum (Fig. 3-2). Posteriorly, it is bony and solid; anteriorly and caudally, it is cartilaginous and semimobile. There are four bony components to the septum. The perpendicular plate of the ethmoid forms the superior-posterior septum and is extremely thin and often dehiscent in several areas. It is thicker anteriorly at its junction with the cartilaginous septum. The vomer is a quadraterally shaped bone and forms the inferior-posterior septum. It articulates superiorly with the ethmoid bone and the septal cartilage. Two bones, the nasal crest of the palatine bone and the nasal crest of the maxilla, make up the most inferior portion (floor) of the septum.

The septal cartilage is the anterior supporting structure of the septum. Posteriorly, it articulates with the perpendicular plate of the ethmoid and the vomer (Fig. 3-2). Anteriorly, the free border of the septal cartilage joins the membranous septum. Inferiorly, the cartilage sits in a groove in the crest

of the maxilla. The junction between the cartilage and maxillary crest is easily disrupted by trauma, and a dislocation of the septum in this area results in a large spur along the floor of the nose.

CLASSIFICATION

The type of nasal injury incurred is largely a result of the direction and intensity of the force sustained by the nose. In general, the nose is more resistent to direct frontal blows than it is to lateral forces.

In adults, the great majority of nasal fractures occurs secondary to a lateral blow. When an isolated blow of moderate force is sustained, a fracture of one nasal bone may occur (Fig. 3-3). This fracture often involves the frontal process of the maxilla on the side that sustained the blow. A lateral blow of greater force commonly results in a fracture of both nasal bones along with both frontal processes of the maxilla. The fragments are displaced to one side, and the septum is also shifted

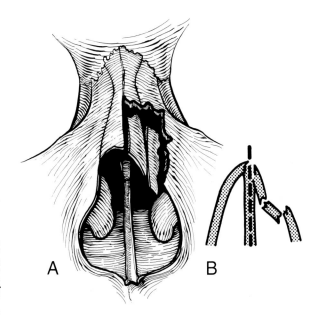

A   B

Fig. 3-3. (A & B) Depressed fracture of one nasal bone.

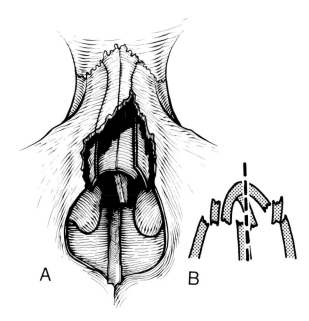

Fig. 3-4. (A & B) Depressed fracture of both nasal bones and nasal septum.

and/or fractured laterally (Fig. 3-4). When either one or both of the nasal bones are fractured, the fracture will occur at the junction of the thick and thin portions of the nasal bones approximately 80 percent of the time.[4]

The septal cartilage can be likened to the sup-porting pole of a tent. Because of its position, the septum is almost always moved out of its proper position when a fracture to the nasal bones occurs. In simple dislocations of the septum, the septal cartilage is displaced from the maxillary crest, resulting in an obstructive spur in at least one side of the nasal cavity (Fig. 3-5A). Such a dislocation is often accompanied by a widening of the nasal tip. Fractures of the septal cartilage occur when the septum buckles and its bending capacity is exceeded. Vertical fractures of the septum occur at variable levels, usually at the junction of the thinner caudal and thicker cephalad portions (Fig. 3-5B). Such vertical fractures may result in an angulation of the anterior septum and dislocation of the caudal septum into one of the nostrils. Horizontal fractures of the septal cartilage can also occur and usually appear to be parallel to the vomerine groove (Fig. 3-5C). A combination of vertical and horizontal fractures can accompany more severe trauma. Whenever the septal cartilage is fractured, tele-scoping with duplication and thickening of the septum can occur. The nose is subsequently shortened and the columella is often retracted.

Nasal fractures less commonly result from direct or anterior-posterior blows to the nose. Such blows cause the septal cartilage to be forced back against the perpendicular plate of the ethmoid, which is usually fractured. The cartilage is then telescoped

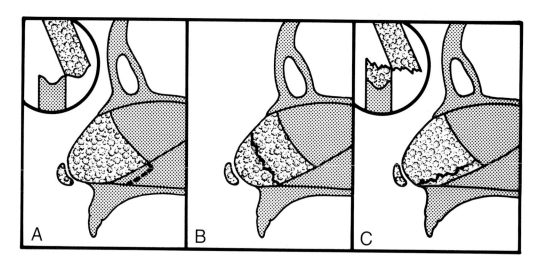

Fig. 3-5. Dislocation and fractures of the septal cartilage. **(A)** Dislocation. **(B)** Vertical fracture. **(C)** Horizontal fracture.

backward and overlaps this bone. This injury results in shortening of the nose.

Blows of moderate intensity may fracture the thin inferior portion of the nasal bones, leaving the thicker superior portion uninvolved. In adults the nasal bones tend to remain attached in the midline even when fractured. More severe direct trauma to the nose may result in a nasofrontal disarticulation in which the entire external nose is comminuted or disengaged in the posterior and cephalad direction. The most intense anterior blows result in the most severe fractures in which the nasal bones are usually comminuted and accompanied by fractures of the lacrimal bones and ethmoid labyrinth (Fig. 3-6). Such injuries are addressed in Chapter 4.

The response of the nasal framework to injury is somewhat unusual in children, and any classification system must make this distinction. While a depressed fracture of one or both nasal bones may occur with lateral blows, anterior blows frequently result in an "open-book" fracture (Fig. 3-7). This probably occurs because the nasal bones are not fused in the midline until adolescence. Open-book fractures result in a flattening of the nasal bridge. Also, the upper lateral cartilages may be detached from the under surface of the nasal bones because of the relatively loose attachment of these cartilages to bone in children. Even in severe injuries, such fractures of bone and cartilage are often unsuspected, and are not revealed until accentuated by subsequent developmental changes.

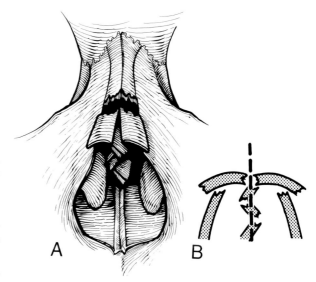

Fig. 3-7. (**A & B**) Open-book fracture seen in children.

By far the most common type of nasal fracture results from a lateral blow. In one series of 173 consecutive patients, this type of fracture constituted 66 percent (unilateral – 25 percent, bilateral – 41 percent), while those occurring as a result of force on the frontal plane made up only 13 percent.[1] In another large study 94 percent of fractures were secondary to lateral force, and 6 percent were secondary to frontal force.[5]

EVALUATION

Uncomplicated nasal fractures are those not associated with other injuries and may be evaluated and treated with relative ease. More severe fractures can test the abilities of even the most experienced maxillofacial surgeon. The cause of the injury and the direction and intensity of the force should be ascertained. Although edema of the injured nose may increase any obstructive symptoms, the patient should be asked about his ability to breathe through each side of his nose both before and after the injury. Likewise, it is important

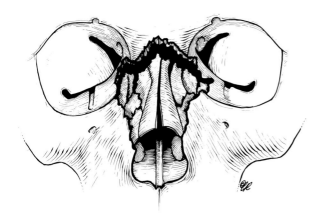

Fig. 3-6. Comminuted fracture of the nose and ethmoids.

to assess the shape of the nose before and after the injury. Patients rarely will bring photographs of themselves; but in many states, a frontal view of the patient can be found on his or her driver's license. The patient should be questioned regarding previous surgery on the nose or symptoms of prior nasal disease, especially those of allergic rhinitis.

A history can be somewhat more difficult to obtain from a child. If a child has sustained a blow to the nose and presents with epistaxis or a suggestion of deformity, it is safe to assume that the child has sustained a nasal fracture. The clinician must be especially alert to the child who cannot breathe through the nose after a nasal injury. In this case, a septal hematoma, a condition that dictates immediate intervention, must be ruled out.

Patients with nasal fractures usually have epistaxis, swelling, periorbital ecchymosis, tenderness of the nasal dorsum, and crepitus of the nasal bones. In addition an obvious nasal deformity and obstruction of the nose may be present. Nasal obstruction may be secondary to displaced bony or

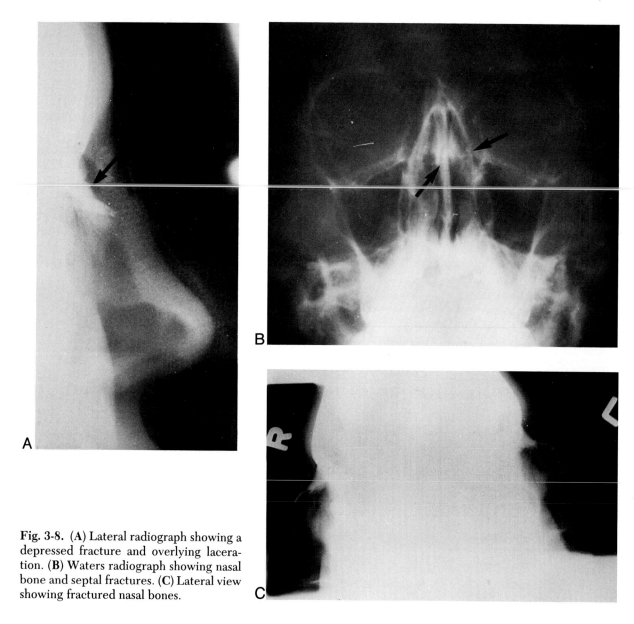

Fig. 3-8. (A) Lateral radiograph showing a depressed fracture and overlying laceration. (B) Waters radiograph showing nasal bone and septal fractures. (C) Lateral view showing fractured nasal bones.

cartilaginous structures, edema, clots, a septal hematoma, a hematoma of the external nose, or swelling of the mucosa and turbinates. Occasionally, a patient will present with subcutaneous emphysema secondary to attempted nose blowing that has forced air through the lacerated mucoperiosteum.

Examination of the patient should begin with careful observation of the nose to determine whether deviation of the nasal bones or septum and flattening or broadening of the nasal dorsum have occurred. Palpation of the fractured nose will usually confirm mobility and crepitation of the nasal bones, unless the bones are impacted. The fractured nose will invariably be tender to the touch. If the root of the nose appears depressed below the frontal bone, thorough evaluation should be made for nasoethmoid fracture. If such a fracture is suspected, evaluation of the intercanthal distance and the lacrimal system must be included. In addition, the presence of a cerebrospinal fluid (CSF) leak should be ruled out (see Chapter 4). In the adult a thorough nasal examination can be performed under local and topical anesthesia using a nasal speculum and a head light or head mirror. Evaluation of the nasal passages and nasal septum should attempt to identify mucosal tears, ecchymosis, septal hematoma, or dislocation of the septum along the floor of the nose. It is important to remember that deformities and deviations of the nasal dorsum and septum may be pre-existing.

If a child has sustained a blow to the nose associated with epistaxis or an apparent nasal deformity, then the nose should be thoroughly evaluated. In the great majority of cases, a child's nose is best evaluated and treated under general anesthesia. Because the nasal skeleton in children is more cartilaginous than bony, diagnosis of nasal fracture in a child may be more difficult to make than in an adult. The combination of traumatic edema plus the relatively small size of a child's external nose complicates the diagnosis. In addition, the overall elasticity and compliance of the structures of a child's nose will allow significant cartilaginous injuries with subsequent hematoma while bony structures remain unharmed. Thus, a minor injury in a child can result in major long-term deformities. Since the nose in most children is straight and symmetrical, any deviation following injury should be considered important.

Radiographs of the nose (Fig. 3-8) (Waters view, lateral soft tissue view, and axial view of the nasal bones) may show the fracture, but even an experienced observer may have difficulty differentiating fractures from suture lines or vascular markings. Since 10 to 47 percent of clinically apparent nasal fractures have normal-appearing radiographs, the physical examination is generally more valuable for determining the location and extent of fracture as well as for assessing adequate reduction.[1,5]

Photographs are an extremely valuable means of documenting the appearance of the nose before and after treatment. Photographs taken before the injury can aid the physician, particularly in assessing pre-existing deformities. The best photographs of the nose are obtained with a 35 mm, single lens reflex camera using a 105 mm macrolens. Ideally, these photographs should be taken with a proper backdrop and adequate lighting. Documentation should include a minimum of color slides, and 5″ × 7″ black and white photographs can be helpful in the pretreatment evaluation of the patient.[6] All photographs should be identified with the patient's name, age, diagnosis, and date.

THERAPY

Hippocrates should be considered the originator of the modern management of nasal fractures. In the fifth century b.c. he advocated closed reduction of fractures followed by selected nasal packing and the application of a plaster splint to the nasal dorsum. He considered timing to be extremely important and preferred to treat nasal fractures on the day of the accident.[7]

The objective of therapy for nasal fractures is the restoration of normal function and appearance. In nondisplaced fractures reduction may not be necessary, and symptomatic treatment and protection of the nose with tape or cast will probably suffice. If, however, a cosmetic or functional abnormality exists, intervention is required. It is generally agreed that the best chance for successful treatment of a nasal fracture is when therapy is instituted in the first 2 to 3 hours after injury before edema, hematoma, and obstruction have occurred. If a few hours have elapsed since the injury and marked swelling is present, there is no harm in waiting up to 7 to 10 days in adults before definitive management. In children rapid reduction, preferably within 5 to 7 days, is important due to early fibrosis.

Reduction of nasal fractures is best performed using optimal anesthesia, lighting, and instruments. Most fractures in adults can be reduced while the patient is awake. The combination of 4 percent topical cocaine (200 mg maximum) and locally injected 1 percent lidocaine with 1 : 100,000 epinephrine (less than 30 ml) has been found to be effective anesthesia. Subcutaneous injection over the nasal dorsum and anterior nasal spine, as well as a submucosal injection in the septum, should be performed. Regional anesthesia for the nasal dorsum should include injection in both infraorbital foramina and both supratrochlear foramina. In addition adequate monitoring, an intravenous line, and appropriate premedication should be part of the intraoperative management of these patients. As stated earlier, nasal fractures in children are best managed under general anesthesia.

Any nasal fracture that involves the nasal bones only can usually be reduced by the closed approach. However, nasal fractures that include the nasal septum usually require an open septal reduction in conjunction with closed reduction of the nasal bones. In unusual cases open access to the nasal bones themselves is required.

Closed Reduction

Following adequate topical, local, and regional anesthesia, the nose should be thoroughly cleaned of clots, hematomas, and debris. For the unilaterally depressed nasal fracture, a blunt-ended heavy instrument should be inserted under the nasal bone and the bone elevated and replaced by digital pressure. It is important to place the instrument carefully under the fracture and not too high in the nose where it might impinge on the under surface of the adjacent portion of the frontal bone, causing dam-

age to mucosa without effective reduction. Almost any blunt-ended elevator including the Boise elevator, Goldman elevator, Ash forceps, Walsham's forceps, or a periosteal elevator wrapped with petroleum gauze will be adequate. In the case of a bilateral nasal bone fracture in which the nasal pyramid has been displaced, the blunt-ended instrument can be placed under the depressed bone while external pressure is applied to the opposite nasal bone. If pressure fails to reduce the bony fracture, the presence of an incomplete or greenstick fracture should be considered. In this case, the fracture may be completed by external digital pressure. Figure 3-9 shows the result of a closed reduction of a depressed right nasal bone fracture.

Open Reduction

It has been stated that as the septum goes so goes the nose. An open reduction of the septum is indicated whenever a nasal fracture is associated with a fracture of the septum. Failure to treat the fractured or deviated septum will often result in an initial "successful" reduction followed by failure when the splints and casts are removed.

A unilateral hemitransfixion incision allows adequate exposure to the nasal septum. Following elevation of a mucoperichondrial flap, cartilage fragments can be repositioned under direct vision. A septal reconstruction rather than radical resection of the septal cartilage is advocated. After minimal resection of overriding cartilage, fragments can be secured in proper position by through and through sutures of 4-0 chromic or plain catgut. If the cartilage is buckled, it can be weakened by cross-hatching or an excision of small strips of cartilage. If the bone of the perpendicular plate or vomer is involved in the fracture, any bone that is obstructing the nasal passage can be safely removed, since it is not necessary for support of the septum.

A septal spur is the most common manifestation of a septal injury and is usually the result of dislocation of the quadrangular cartilage from the maxillary crest. After elevation of a mucoperichondrial flap, the cartilage may be repositioned under direct observation. Commonly, a strip of cartilage will have to be removed from the inferior border of the

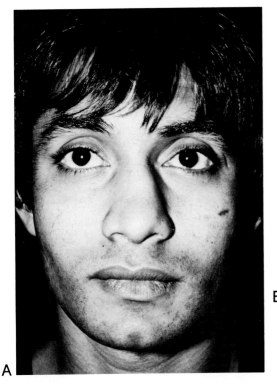

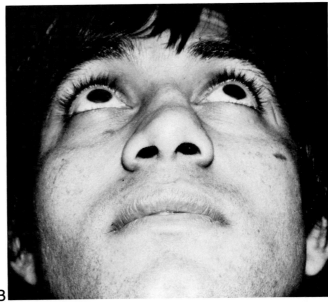

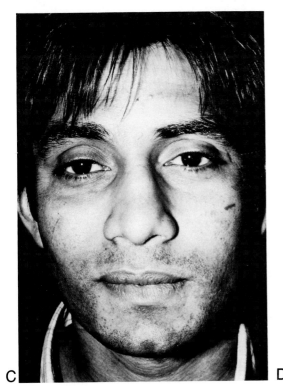

Fig. 3-9. (**A & B**) Frontal and basal views of a depressed right nasal bone fracture. (**C & D**) Postoperative view showing results of a closed reduction.

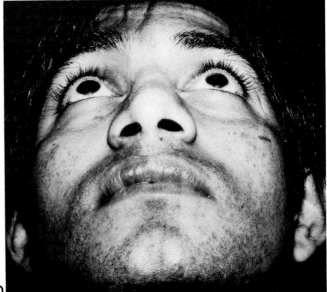

cartilage in order to successfully replace the cartilage in the groove. Deviation of the septum at the point of junction of the cartilage and ethmoid or vomer bone can be addressed by resecting the deviated bone and allowing the cartilage to return to the midline. Ideally, the end result of any septal procedure should be a midline septum that provides adequate airway and support without any packing or external splinting. If following reduction no mucosal tear is present, an incision should be placed along the inferior margin of the elevated flap to ensure adequate drainage. A running suture of 4-0 chromic or plain catgut in the horizontal plane should be placed to coapt the mucosal flaps and obliterate any dead space. A double knot can be placed at one end of the suture and a running suture can then be placed back and forth through the septum from deep in the nose to its caudal end. Placing the knot at one end prevents the suture from pulling through the septum and avoids the necessity of a tie deep in the nasal cavity. This suture eliminates dead space and prevents hematoma formation.

If closed reduction of the nasal bones with or without open reduction of the nasal septum does not result in successful reduction of a nasal fracture, then open reduction of the nasal bones must be considered. The obvious exception to this rule would be a severely comminuted fracture, since an open reduction of such a fracture may result in collapse of the nasal dorsum. Specific indications for an open reduction of the nasal dorsum include the presence of severely impacted bony fragments that cannot be reduced by closed reduction, compound fractures of the nasal dorsum with fragments present intranasally and extranasally, and the presence of an old or partially healed nasal fracture. In any case, a limited open approach is advocated. An intercartilaginous incision (between the upper and lower lateral cartilages) with elevation of the soft tissue of the nose to the pyriform aperture should be performed. Osteotomies may be necessary for impacted fractures. Any cartilaginous deviation of the supratip or tip area should be adequately reduced when the nasal bones are properly aligned.

Intranasal dressing is usually not necessary in the treatment of nasal fractures if reduction of the septum and dorsum is successful, if there is no undue hemorrhage, and if the reduced fragments main-

tain their realigned position. In a review of over 800 cases of nasal surgery, Stucker reported that less than 9 percent of cases required nasal packing.[8] If epistaxis is a problem, control can usually be provided by placement of small amounts of absorbable material such as Gelfoam or Oxycel. Intranasal support is sometimes necessary in the high dorsal area. Again, a small amount of packing high in the nose is usually adequate. Two to three layers of Telfa or half-inch strips of gauze impregnated with petroleum or antibiotic ointment can be used effectively. When tears of the intranasal mucosa are present, thin Silastic splints should be placed on either side of the nasal septum and secured to the caudal septum with a single suture of 4-0 nylon. These splints prevent synechia from forming between the septum and the lateral walls of the nose.

An external cast should be placed over the nasal dorsum following adequate reduction of the fracture. The cast stabilizes fragments, prevents subluxation of loose fragments, protects against further injury, helps maintain the reduction of fragments, and reduces the accumulation of blood and edema between the skin and underlying bony framework. A small cast is adequate, since immobilization of the nose is rarely a problem due to the minimal traction on fracture segments by the facial muscles. In fact, the tape and cast over the nasal dorsum should cover only the skin of the nose and not extend over the forehead or cheek, as facial movements in these areas will result in unwanted motion of the nose itself (Fig. 3-10). Taping of the nasal dorsum is best performed using one-half inch steristrips applied in a parallel overlapping manner from the nasofrontal region of the dorsum to the supratip area. The tape should extend laterally to include the nasal processes of the maxillary bones. Application of the tape should be firm enough to eliminate any dead space between the skin and underlying bone or cartilage. Following taping, a plaster of paris cast of six to seven layers can be placed over the tape. There is enough moisture from the plaster of paris so that saturation of the underlying steristrips will hold the plaster cast in place. Such a cast should be left in place for 5 to 7 days. Following its removal, the patient should be counseled to avoid further nasal trauma, including application of any heavy-framed glasses over the nasal dorsum.

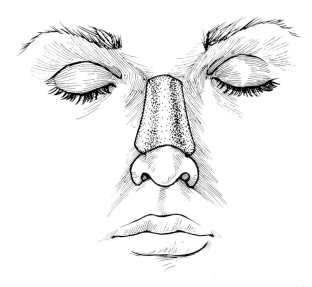

Fig. 3-10. Recommended size and shape of external cast.

Unconventional Reduction

Certain types of nasal fractures require specific treatment approaches. Compound nasal fractures involving the overlying soft tissue and skin often require the placement of small gauge wire through the fractured bones to directly reduce fragments. If the cartilage of the supratip or tip area is involved, these cartilaginous fragments should be aligned and sutured directly with absorbable suture. All lacerations of the inner lining of the nose are best treated by direct repair. Such repair will reduce the incidence of stenosis and synechia. Moderately comminuted nasal fractures are probably best treated by closed reduction of the bony fragments and an open reduction of the septum. Usually, the fragments can be maintained in proper position by an intranasal pack and an external cast. More severely comminuted nasal fractures should be treated by closed reduction, with or without the addition of lead plates. Quite commonly, however, an open approach is necessary several weeks or months following closed reduction to achieve the best cosmetic and functional result.

The application of lead plates for nasal fractures is seldom indicated. Certainly, the placement of such plates is appropriate when nasoethmoidal in-juries have occurred (see Chapter 4). Otherwise, lead plates may be utilized in severely comminuted nasal fractures. Plates should be placed over Telfa gauze on either side of the external nasal pyramid and secured by through and through nonabsorbable suture. The suture should pass through the plate, the skin of the nose, between comminuted fragments of bone, through the septum, and then through the opposite side and back. Lead plates are commonly used with high intranasal packing to properly maintain fragments in position.

External traction is rarely needed for nasal fractures. It may be indicated when nasal bones are projected backward and impacted into the interorbital space secondary to severe frontal blows. External traction allows the proper vector of force to reduce and maintain the dorsal bony fragments in proper alignment. Usually, a figure-of-eight wire is looped through the fragments of bone and attached by a rubber band or wire to an external appliance or a molded biphasic apparatus. External traction is rarely required for over 2 weeks in adults and 7 to 10 days in children.

The treatment of nasal fractures in children is somewhat different than that for adults. Proper evaluation and treatment of nasal injuries is particularly important for the normal development of the midface, since injuries at an early age may result in nasal and midfacial deformities that may not become apparent for several years. Likewise, caution must be observed in any operative approach to the nose of the child to avoid injury to growth centers known to be present in this area. Animal studies have confirmed that removal of septal cartilage and mucoperichondrium will distort the growth of the nose and midface.[9] Bernstein, however, showed that submucous resection of the septal cartilage in 6-week-old dogs did not result in an abnormal growth of the nose or midface if the mucoperichondrial flaps were left intact.[10] Likewise, other animal studies have shown that simple manipulation of the septum does not affect growth of the nose or midface.[11] Finally, osteotomies both medial and lateral do not appear to affect the growth of the midface of animals.[12] In one clinical study, 44 children, ages 8 to 12, underwent septorhinoplasties that included medial and lateral osteotomies, dissection and repositioning of the alar cartilages, and septoplasty. No alteration in nasal or facial growth was found in any of these children.[13] Nevertheless, a relatively conservative approach to nasal fractures in children usually results in satisfactory appearance and function without the need for more radical procedures.

Reduction of nasal fractures in children is best performed under general anesthesia. Closed reduction is preferred, using the combination of a blunt-ended elevator and digital pressure. The end point of reduction, however, can be difficult to appreciate, since the cartilaginous structures of a child's nose do not move easily and do not "snap" into place as do the bones in adults. Also, nasal fractures in children are frequently of the greenstick variety. Any open septal procedure in children should be done, maintaining intact mucoperichondrial flaps and resecting a minimal amount of septal cartilage. When closed reduction of the nasal dorsum is not satisfactory, a small osteotome may be used to cut the bone and properly align the fragment.

Recently, the problem of septal dislocation in newborn children has gained attention. If such an injury is present, a closed reduction in the first 1 to 2 days of life can be performed with no anesthesia. Jazbi states that this procedure can be performed with ease and that proper alignment of the septum can be determined both by appearance and by the presence of an audible click when the cartilage is properly reduced.[14]

may be undertaken. First, the patient can be placed in the sitting position and given a mild sedative. If the bleeding continues, topical application of vasoconstricting solutions and removal of clots and debris will usually succeed in stopping any bleeding. If bleeding persists, application of absorbable hemostatic material such as Gelfoam or Oxycel may be beneficial. Cauterization of bleeding points with silver nitrate or electrocautery can also be used. Packing, since it interferes with accurate fraction reduction, should be considered only if all other methods have failed to stop the bleeding.

Part of the initial exam in any patient with a nasal injury should be the search for a septal hematoma. Failure to recognize and treat this problem can be catastrophic. Once diagnosed, the hematoma should be evacuated through a hemitransfixion incision or an incision along the floor of the nasal septum on the side of the hematoma. The hematoma can then be removed by suction and a running 4-0 chromic suture placed through and through the septum to prevent recurrence. If suture is not available, a drain through the septal incision will usually suffice. If untreated, the septal hematoma may become infected, forming a septal abscess with subsequent septic necrosis of the septal cartilage. Retraction of the columnella and saddling of the middle third of the nose can result. In addition, the nasal septum may become quite thick secondary to subperichondrial fibrosis.

EARLY COMPLICATIONS

Epistaxis frequently accompanies nasal fractures, and blood loss may be greater than clinically apparent because several hundred milliliters may be swallowed by the patient. In such cases, caution must be used if general anesthesia is considered, since vomiting and aspiration can become a problem. Usually, even severe epistaxis is of short duration and ceases spontaneously. If bleeding is persistent or repeated, several conservative measures

DELAYED COMPLICATIONS

Infection of soft tissues, cartilage, or bone is a rare complication of a nasal fracture. Many clinicians advocate the use of prophylactic antibiotics in the case of nasal fractures to avoid this complication. Clinical evidence demonstrating the efficacy of this prophylaxis, however, is lacking. In a well-controlled study of over 200 patients undergoing nasal surgery in which patients were randomized into two treatment groups (one receiving antibiotics and the other receiving no antibiotics), the incidence of infection in both groups was less than 2 percent.[15] Based on this information, the prophylactic use of antibiotics for nasal fractures cannot be advocated except under specific circumstances, such as compound fractures with gross contamination of the wound and those cases where intranasal dressing is employed. In the former situation, a thorough irrigation and debridement of obviously devitalized tissue, when necessary, is probably more effective. The most significant sequelae to infections in nasal trauma are septal abscess and osteitis or osteomyelitis of the nasal bones. Fortunately, these problems are very unusual. A septal abscess can be prevented by draining septal hematomas. Osteitis of the nasal bones is a serious problem that can lead to septic necrosis of the bony structures and loss of the entire nasal skeleton. Treatment of these conditions includes drainage and debridement of all devitalized tissue. A culture of the area should be obtained and antibiotics prescribed based on culture and sensitivity results.

Synechiae or adhesions between the septum and nasal turbinates can occur if lacerations of the mucosa of the internal nose are present. Synechiae can be avoided by careful closure of lacerations and the intranasal placement of thin, soft Silastic or plastic splints. Once synechiae have formed, they are best treated by cutting the adhesive band and splinting the nasal cavity.

Another potential sequela of compound nasal fractures is webbing and stenosis of the valve area. This occurs secondary to considerable damage (often loss) of mucous membrane in the nasal vestibule area. Careful realignment and closure of lacerations in the valve area during initial management will help prevent this problem. Delayed treatment for small areas of webbing includes the use of Z-plasties in the affected mucous membrane. Extensive webbing requires grafting either with simple grafts of split thickness skin or dermis, or composite grafts of skin and subcutaneous tissue and cartilage, usually taken from the ear.

The most common late sequela of nasal fractures is delayed deformity secondary to malunion. Such malunion results in both a cosmetic and functional disorder. It can be said that virtually all traumatic deformities of the septum and external nose are a result of inattention or improper medical attention at the time of initial injury. Up to 90 percent of nasal operations performed in some practices are for correction of such traumatic deformities. Proper treatment of delayed deformities is standard septoplasty or septorhinoplasty.

SUMMARY

Fractures of the nasal skeleton are the most common and most easily treated of all facial fractures. Nevertheless, failure to recognize the injury and provide proper treatment can result in serious cosmetic and functional deformities.

REFERENCES

1. Illum P, Kristensen S, Jorgensen K, Pedersen CB: Role of fixation in the treatment of nasal fractures. Clin Otolaryngol 8:191, 1983
2. Goode RL, Spooner TR: Management of nasal fractures in children. Clin Pediatr 11:526, 1972
3. Moran WB: Nasal trauma in children. Otolaryngol Clin North Am 15:513, 1984
4. Converse JM: Surgical Treatment of Facial Injuries. 3rd Ed. Williams & Wilkins, Baltimore, 1974
5. Murray JAM, Maran AGD: The treatment of nasal injuries by manipulation. J Laryngol Otol 94:1405, 1980
6. Morello DC, Converse JM, Allen D: Making uniform photographic records in plastic surgery. Plast Reconstr Surg 59:366, 1977
7. Gahhos F, Ariyan S: Facial fractures: Hippocratic management. Head Neck Surg 6:1007, 1984
8. Stucker FJ, Ansel DG: A case against nasal packing. Laryngoscope 88:1314, 1978

9. Sarnat BG, Wexler MR: Growth of the face and jaws after resection of the septal cartilage in the rabbit. Am J Anat 118:755, 1966

10. Bernstein L: Early submucous resection of nasal septal cartilage. Arch Otolaryngol 97:273, 1973

11. Wexler MR, Sarnat BG: Rabbit snout growth after dislocation of nasal septum. Arch Otolaryngol 81:68, 1965

12. Hadley R: Nasal injuries in children. NY State J Med 1:1, 1969

13. Ortiz-Monasterio F, Olmedo A: Corrective rhinoplasty before puberty: a long term follow-up. Plast Reconstr Surg 68:381, 1981

14. Jazbi B: Subluxation of the nasal septum in the newborn: etiology, diagnosis and treatment. Otolaryngol Clin North Am 10:125, 1977

15. Weimert TA, Yoder MG: Antibiotics and nasal surgery. Laryngoscope 90:667, 1980

Naso-Orbital Fractures

4

Craig A. Foster
John E. Sherman

The fronto-naso-orbital region is the anatomic crossroad between nasal, orbital, sinus, and cranial cavities. Trauma to this region may injure contents in any or all of these cavities. The projecting nasal framework is the weakest portion of the facial skeleton and the most frequently disrupted. Force applied anteriorly can result in posterior displacement of that framework, injuring nasal, orbital, sinus, and intracranial structures.

REGIONAL ANATOMY

The medial orbital walls are very thin and weak in contrast to the heavier abutments of the nasal process of the frontal bone and frontal processes of the maxilla. This is best illustrated by transillumination of the skull (Fig. 4-1). Posterior to these thick bony abutments, the thin lacrimal bones and delicate laminae papyraceae are susceptible to trauma. The anterior and posterior ethmoidal foramina lie along the upper border of the lamina papyracea in the frontoethmoidal suture (Fig. 4-2). This suture represents the intracranial level of the cribriform plate. The anterior ethmoidal foramen transmits the nasociliary nerve and the anterior ethmoidal artery. The posterior ethmoidal nerve and vessels pass through the posterior foramen. Posterior displacement and disruption of bone may sever these vessels causing orbital hematoma.

The most posterior portion of the medial orbital wall is formed by the body of the sphenoid, through which the optic nerve exits. Skeletal disruption of this area may involve the optic nerve and lead to blindness.

Interorbital Space

The interorbital space is the area between the orbits and beneath the floor of the anterior cranial fossa at the cribriform plate (Fig. 4-3). This space contains the two ethmoid labyrinths, one on either side of the perpendicular plate of the ethmoid, and is wider anteriorly than posteriorly. The superior limit is the cribriform plate; the lateral limit is the

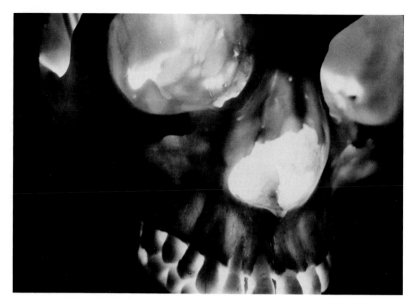

Fig. 4-1. Transillumination of the skull showing thin nasal bones surrounded by thick central abutments of the glabella and maxillofrontal processes and the very thin medial orbital wall behind the maxillofrontal abutment.

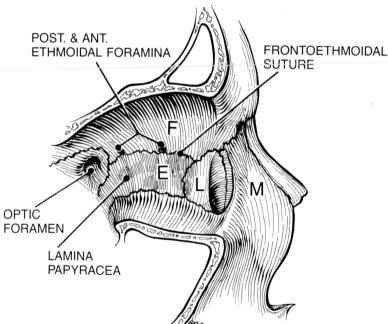

POST. & ANT.
ETHMOIDAL FORAMINA

FRONTOETHMOIDAL
SUTURE

F

E

L

M

OPTIC
FORAMEN

LAMINA
PAPYRACEA

Fig. 4-2. Bony anatomy of the medial orbital wall. F, Frontal; E, Ethmoid; L, Lacrimal; M, Maxilla.

medial orbital wall. The interorbital space is divided approximately in half by the perpendicular plate of the ethmoid and septum. Its posterior limit is the anterior face of the sphenoid. Anteriorly, it is closed by the frontal processes of the maxilla, the nasal bones, and the nasal process of the frontal bone.

The interorbital space contains the honeycomb-like ethmoid air cells, superior and middle turbinates, and perpendicular plate of the ethmoid, which forms the posterior-superior portion of the nasal septum. Any anteriorly directed force sufficient to fracture the strong anterior abutments meets little resistance posteriorly from the thin

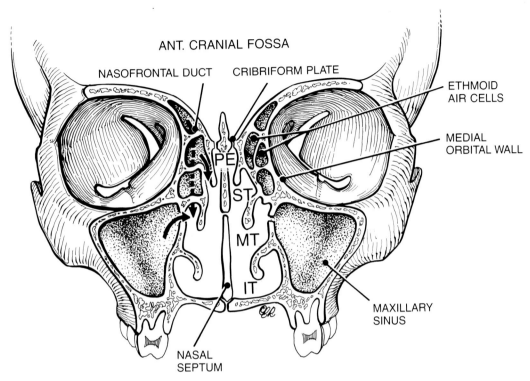

Fig. 4-3. Bony anatomy of the interorbital space and adjacent structures. PE, Perpendicular plate of the ethmoid; ST, Superior turbinate; MT, Middle turbinate; IT, Inferior turbinate.

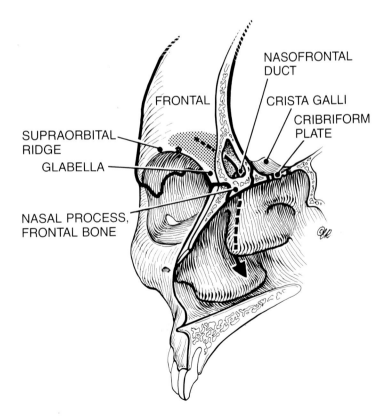

Fig. 4-4. Course of the nasofrontal duct in the lateral wall of the nose.

honeycomb of the ethmoid labyrinth. The ethmoidal sinus occupies the upper lateral wall of the nose. The maxillary sinus is lateral to the lower half of the ethmoidal sinus. The ethmoid projects about 2 mm above the level of the cribriform laterally. The sinus is pyramidal in shape, measuring 3.5 to 5 cm long and 1.5 to 2.5 cm wide. The ethmoid cells drain into the middle meatus of the nose. Embryologically, the frontal sinus is a direct extension of the ethmoid. Therefore, the nasofrontal duct courses through or drains into the anterior ethmoid and then into the middle meatus (Fig. 4-4). The roof of the interorbital space is the cribriform plate; this area is frequently involved in naso-orbital fractures. The olfactory tracts, with closely adherent dura, are often disrupted, which results in lacerated dura and cerebrospinal fluid (CSF) leakage. The brain may be penetrated by sharp, thin bone fragments which cause necrosis of brain tissue. The thin lamina papyracea is continuous with the floor of the orbit. Fractures of the medial orbital wall may extend into the floor of the orbit and cause concomitant blowout fractures.

The Frontal Bone

The frontal bone is shield shaped and consists of a vertical portion constituting the forehead and a horizontal portion forming the supraorbital ridges and the roofs of the orbital and anterior nasal cavities. Between the supraorbital margins and below the glabella, the frontal bone projects downward to join the nasal bones. The nasal process of the frontal bone lies under the nasal bones and frontal processes of the maxilla, supporting the bridge of the nose and forming strong anterior facial abutments. The horizontal portions of the frontal bone are paired, thin, triangular-shaped plates that form part of the roof of the orbit. They are separated by the ethmoid labyrinth and cribriform plate.

The Frontal Sinus

The frontal sinus varies widely in size and shape and is occasionally absent. Embryologically, the frontal sinus is an extension of the ethmoidal sinus. The sinus is generally pyramidal in shape with ante-

rior, posterior, and inferior walls. The floor or inferior wall corresponds to the roof of the orbit and cribriform plate, contains the nasofrontal ducts, and is the thinnest wall. The anterior wall is thickest and is composed of cortical and cancellous bone. The posterior wall is thinner, separates the frontal lobes from the sinus, and is composed of compact bone.

SURGICAL PATHOLOGY

The usual cause of naso-orbital fracture is an anteriorly applied force over the upper portion of the nasal bridge. The weakest point of the facial skeleton is the nasal bones, which fracture under impact loads of 30 to 80 g.[1] Force directed posteriorly drives the nasal bones through their associated abutments. Once the abutments are disrupted, little further resistance is offered by the thin matchbox-like structures of the ethmoid air cell system. Fractures involving the cribriform plate and anterior cranial fossa may cause CSF leakage and brain damage. The lacrimal drainage apparatus may be lacerated, the medial canthal tendon disrupted, and the levator palpebra avulsed or lacerated. Orbital blowout, medial maxillary fractures, or frac-

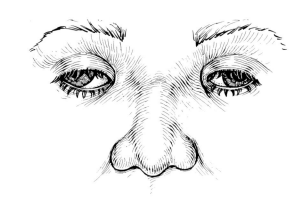

Fig. 4-5. Representation of clinical findings in a fronto-naso-orbital fracture. Note the depressed nasal root, wide intercanthal distance, partial obstruction of the medial canthal angles by epicanthal folds, and shortening of the horizontal palpebral fissures.

tures of other facial bones may occur, particularly in the middle third of the face. The frontal bone may be fractured, causing damage to the frontal sinus or nasofrontal drainage ducts.

EVALUATION

Clinical Exam

The patient presenting with fronto-orbital-nasal disruption has a characteristic appearance (Fig. 4-5). The bridge of the nose is flattened, seemingly pushed between the eyes. The medial canthal regions are swollen and ecchymotic. The Furnas traction test may indicate canthal disruption[2] (Fig. 4-6). The eyelids are edematous, and subconjunctival hemorrhages are usually present. Edema and hematoma often mask underlying skeletal disruptions. Fronto-orbito-nasal disruptions are frequently associated with orbital blowout fractures, maxillary Lefort fractures, or zygomatic fractures.

Intranasal examination may reveal septal fracture with associated septal hematoma. Palpation of the nasal bridge or glabellar regions may reveal motility or crepitation. Overlying soft tissues may often be lacerated with bursting-type injuries that expose underlying fractures.

The patient may be unconscious during examination, or history of the injury may include loss of consciousness. This is suggestive of brain injury, either direct or concussive.

Clear nasal discharge or salty postnasal drip is highly suggestive of CSF leakage. Bilateral jugular compression may cause a sudden increase in fluid escape. Chemical analysis of the drainage should reveal it to be free of mucin and to contain sugar if the leakage is CSF. Anosmia can indicate a dural tear in the ethmoidal roof or cribriform plate area.

Radiographic Evaluation

Plain skull films may reveal frontal bone or other skull fractures. Pneumoencephalos, or intracranial air, indicates direct communication between nasal and/or sinus cavities and the cranial cavity.

Sinus films show clouding of the ethmoid air cell system. The maxillary sinuses can be clear unless directly involved with a medial maxillary fracture, blowout fracture, zygoma fracture, or Lefort fracture. Lateral films show posterior displacement of the nasal root. Orbital films may show air in the orbit or lids, indicating communication with fractured sinus cavities.

Complex motion tomograms through the interorbital space are particularly useful in identifying fracture lines and indicating degree of disruption. Computed tomography (CT) scanning is invaluable for the evaluation of brain injury and injury to associated soft tissues. CT also aids in the three-dimensional evaluation of the injury, which allows a comprehensive surgical plan to be formulated. Cervical spine films must be obtained in all patients with significant head or facial trauma to rule out associated cervical spine injuries.

Classification of Fracture

Classification of nasal fractures has been suggested by Rowe and Killey,[3] Stranc,[4] and Gruss.[5] Clinically, fronto-naso-orbital fractures can be divided into two groups: telescoped and laterally spread.[6] In the first group, the nasal bones and central portions of the frontonasal processes of the maxilla are driven posteriorly as a unit. The medial canthal

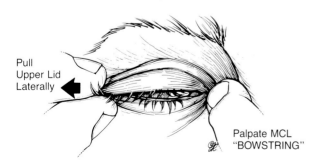

Pull
Upper Lid
Laterally

Palpate MCL
"BOWSTRING"

Fig. 4-6. Demonstration of the Furnas traction test in which the lid is pulled laterally and the medial canthal region is palpated for the "bowstring."

ligaments may have no lateral disruption or distraction. An excessively acute nasofrontal angle is characteristic (Fig. 4-7).

In the second type of injury, which is more commonly seen, the nasal bones and the facial abutments are comminuted (Fig. 4-8). The posteriorly displaced mass is not maintained as a unit, and the bony structures fragment and spread laterally. Medial canthal tendon disruption with traumatic telecanthus and lacrimal sac injury usually occur with this type of fracture. Over and above the two basic types of naso-orbital injury, other associated regional injuries may occur, depending on the character and amount of injuring force.[5]

PRINCIPLES OF INITIAL REPAIR

Ideally, fronto-naso-orbital dislocations should be totally reconstructed in one initial, well-planned surgical enterprise. All tissue elements should be managed according to precise predetermined plan. Strict adherence to the principle of restoring anatomy by reassembly of the whole unit — bones, soft tissues, and specialized structures — is the only way to control total reconstruction.

Factors adversely affecting this approach include edema masking subadjacent bone and soft tissue disruptions. Routine initial radiographs often do not give an adequate evaluation of the trauma, which leads to undetected lesions. Skin wounds in the region of injury may be hastily sutured in the emergency room before adequate direct examination. Individual components of the total injury may be treated initially at the expense of others that are usually neurologic or ophthalmologic in nature. An initial total reconstruction is technically easier to perform and prevents secondary sequelae as well as the necessity of delayed reconstruction, which is often difficult and suboptimal.

Formulation of the preoperative plan includes information from detailed physical examination and radiographs, which include specialized studies such as complex motion tomograms and CT scanning. This information is evaluated by the maxillofacial trauma surgeon in conjunction with the radiologist, neurosurgeon, and ophthalmologist. A three-dimensional analysis of the trauma and planned reconstruction are important in detecting lesions and anticipating problems likely to be encountered during surgery. The guiding principle is piece by piece reassembly of the craniofacial fractures with rigid self-blocking internal fixation.[5-9] This internal fixation is most often achieved by interosseous fragment wire fixation and proceeds as outlined below.

Orbital Rim Reconstruction

The orbital rim is used to support and initiate orbital and nasal reconstruction, starting laterally from stable bones, such as the frontal bone, orbital rim, or maxilla. If any of these are fractured, reduction must begin with the next stable lateral or superior bony structure. Various incisions utilized for approach to these fractures are illustrated (Fig. 4-9). Adequate exposure is essential for these repairs.[5,10,11] Reduction and immobilization proceed medially towards the nose. Transnasal wiring, with or without medial canthal tendons, and wiring to the frontal bone superiorly complete orbital rim reconstruction. Occasionally, excessive fragmentation precludes direct fragment-to-fragment wiring. In such instances, a single well-contoured bone graft may be wired to stable medial and lateral elements to complete orbital rim reconstruction (Fig. 4-10).

Orbital Wall Reconstruction

Reconstruction of fractured orbital walls usually requires placement of a rigid supporting structure to substitute for thin, fragmented bone. Autogenous bone grafts are recommended for orbital wall reconstruction.[5,7-9] Iliac crest, rib, or calvarial bone[12] are the most frequently used donor sites.

The lateral orbital wall is usually reduced when the fracture is reduced. The orbital floor is often

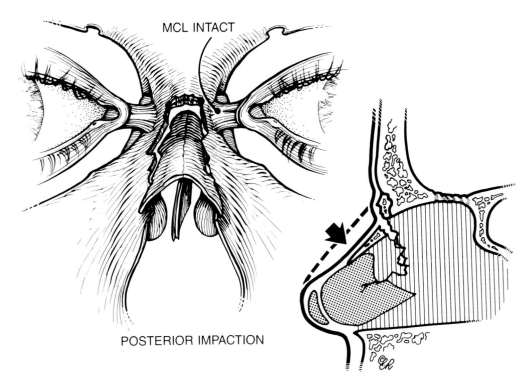

Fig. 4-7. Representation of the posterior impaction type of fracture. The medial canthal tendons are intact.

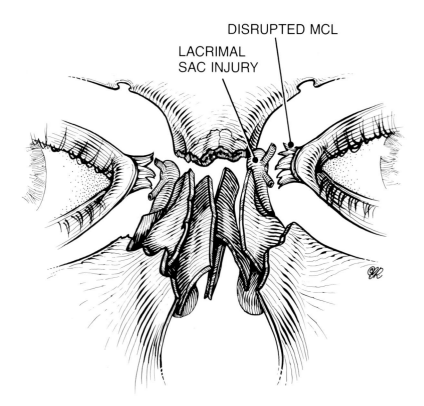

Fig. 4-8. The more usual type of injury has extensive bony disruption with lateral spread and avulsion of medial canthal tendons.

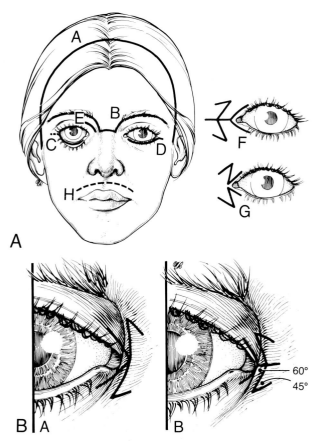

A

B

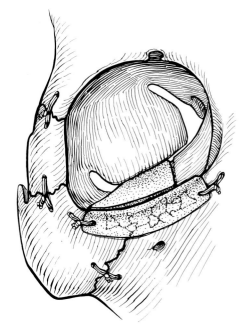

Fig. 4-10. Use of a small contoured split rib graft to reconstruct a comminuted orbital rim. Note also a bone graft in the orbital floor.

Fig. 4-9. (A) Representation of the various types of incisions utilized for exposure of a fracture. A, Bicoronal; B, Brow or open sky; C, Transconjunctival with lateral canthal extension; D, Subciliary; E, Upper lid or Lynch; F, Mustardé; G, Converse double Z-plasty; H, Buccal transoral. (B) Incisions for correction of epicanthal folding: A, Converse double Z-plasty and B, Mustardé "jumping man" for which angles are represented.

involved with a blowout fracture. All herniated orbital contents are reduced. The infraorbital nerve is inspected, and all impinging bone fragments are released. The orbital floor is reconstructed by placing a well-fitted and well-shaped bone graft so that it rests on stable surfaces. Small disruptions of the orbital floor may be supported by a sheet of Gel film (see clinical cases, Figures 4-14 to 4-33). Occasionally, the orbital floor may be reduced and supported from below. Access is gained with a Caldwell-Luc approach and the floor supported by packing (see Chapter 5). The packing is removed in

4 to 6 weeks via a nasal antral window, which is placed at the time of repair. Orbital mobility is assessed intraoperatively by forced duction testing. The medial wall, in these fractures, is almost always crushed, with entrapment of the medial rectus muscle. The medial rectus muscle is released and motility again assessed by forced duction. Careful exploration of the medial canthal tendon and lacrimal drainage apparatus identifies any injury to these structures. A medial bone graft may be used to reconstruct this wall and a transnasal canthoplasty used to transfix the graft (Fig. 4-11).

Septonasal Reconstruction

The direct or transnasal wiring of the comminuted abutments gives a stable foundation for reduction of nasal bones. The nasal bones may be repositioned and maintained with an external dressing, directly wired, or reconstructed with onlay bone grafting.[8,13] The nasal septum is inspected for hematoma and fracture dislocation. Hematomas are drained via incisions in the mucoperichondrium, and fracture dislocations are reduced. Intranasal stents of Silastic sheeting are placed and secured with a suture placed anteriorly in the membranous septum. These stents support the reduced septum and prevent synechia formation. A nasal packing completes internal stenting.

Soft Tissue Injuries

Following stable reduction or grafting of bone fractures, soft tissue injuries may be approached. The medial canthal tendons are often displaced. If the tendons are still attached to an adequate bone anchor, reduction and fixation of bone fragments will suffice. If the tendon is torn or the bone inadequate, canthoplasty is necessary. Adequate exposure with identification of the tendon and lacrimal drainage apparatus is essential. The tendons are anchored by transnasal passage of #30 or #28 stainless steel wire. A bone graft may be incorporated in the transnasal wiring for support and reconstruction of the medial wall. The canthi and transnasal canthoplasty should be carefully positioned to avoid overcorrection and to counter eyelid tension that pulls laterally and anteriorly. The lateral canthal tendon is most often reduced by reconstruction of the orbital rim. If it has been avulsed, a canthoplasty anchoring the tendon to holes drilled in the orbital rim is necessary.

The lacrimal drainage apparatus may be damaged and should be evaluated by direct inspection, catheterization, and dye injection. Impinging bone fragments are released. Canalicular and sac lacerations are repaired with fine suture, and catheter stents are maintained for 2 to 3 months. Dacryocystorhinostomy, conjunctivorhinostomy, and/or Jones tube insertion may be indicated in cases with extensive damage to the drainage apparatus. Such damage is best dealt with initially because secondary reconstruction may endanger the canthoplasty. Lacrimal drainage repair or reconstruction should be completed after passing canthoplasty wires and prior to tightening these wires. Where extensive damage to the lacrimal drainage apparatus is not apparent by direct examination, observation and,

if necessary, delayed repair are recommended.[5]

Medial canthal region reconstruction is completed by ensuring close juxtaposition of skin and subcutaneous tissue to bone on either side of the nose. This is accomplished by passing a second set of transnasal wires. The holes for these wires are placed just anterior to the anterior lacrimal crest. The wires are passed through kidney-shaped acrylic or lead plates, padded with Telfa, and twisted snugly but not tightly (Fig. 4-12). These

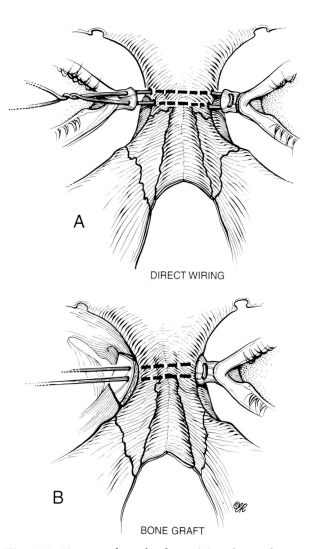

Fig. 4-11. Transnasal canthoplasty, (**A**) without a bone graft and (**B**) with a bone graft to reconstruct the medial orbital wall.

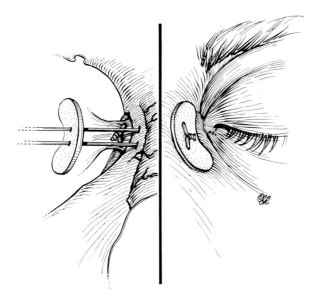

Fig. 4-12. Transnasal wiring of lead or acrylic plates superficial to the canthoplasty. The plates prevent lateral traction, hematoma, and scar formation and provide a better contour in this area.

plates prevent lateral traction in the area as well as hematoma formation and excessive scar tissue. They are removed after 2 weeks.

Globe injuries require the attention of the ophthalmologist. Globe damage is not rare in these injuries, with a reported incidence of 10 to 40 percent.[14] A thorough exam by an ophthalmologist is essential. Globe injuries are managed after orbital bone reconstitution but prior to tightening canthoplasty wires. If enucleation is indicated, an orbital conformer should be placed immediately to maintain socket space for prosthetic rehabilitation.

Frontal and Anterior Basicranial Injuries

If significant frontal skull injury, posterior frontal sinus injury, roof of orbit injury, or cribriform plate disruption is present, then combined neurosurgical and maxillofacial intervention is indicated. These injuries can be expected to be more significant than indicated on tomograms or CT scanning.

The best approach is via a bicoronal scalp incision combined with a bifrontal bone flap. This approach also allows access to orbital and nasal fractures. An intact frontal bar should be left to support the lower facial skeleton. Retraction of the frontal lobes allows direct evaluation of injuries to the base of skull, brain, and dura. Basicranial injuries are repaired in three layers[7] (Fig. 4-13). After debridement of necrotic brain and small bone fragments, dural tears are sutured and reinforced with an overlay pericranial patch. Pericranium is harvested from the temporoparietal region through the bicoronal incision. In the frontoethmoid region, nasal mucosa is carefully repaired, everting the edges into the nose. Cancellous bone grafts bridge bone gaps in the basicranium, separating cranial and facial cavities. Resection of the crista galli, which is oftened fractured, facilitates placement of bone grafts.

If the posterior wall of the frontal sinus is extensively disrupted, it should be resected and all sinus mucosa removed. The nasofrontal ducts should be obliterated with bone grafts or fascial plugs, and the frontal lobes allowed to come forward and cranialize the frontal sinus.

The frontal bar is repaired by reassembly of fragments or bone grafts. The bone flap is repositioned. If this piece is fractured, or if there is a defect, bone grafting with intergraft wire osteosynthesis to create a stable monobloc is necessary. Split calvarial bone grafts may be used to reconstitute larger frontal bone defects.[12,15] Trephination holes are filled with cancellous chips or bone dust to avoid frontal depressions.

To complete the reconstruction, remaining soft tissues are repaired in layers by standard plastic surgical techniques.

SUMMARY OF PRINCIPLES OF INITIAL RECONSTRUCTION

The recommended sequence in the evaluation and treatment of fronto-orbito-nasal disruption may be summarized as follows:

1. Clinical and radiographic examination with three-dimensional evaluation of all injuries and formulation of a surgical plan.
2. Bicoronal approach with bifrontal craniotomy, if necessary, for evaluation and repair of basi-cranium, frontal sinus, and forehead.
3. Reconstruction of orbital rim in a lateral to medial progression.
4. Reconstruction of orbital walls.
5. Lacrimal drainage reconstruction, if there is obvious direct disruption.
6. Medial canthoplasty.

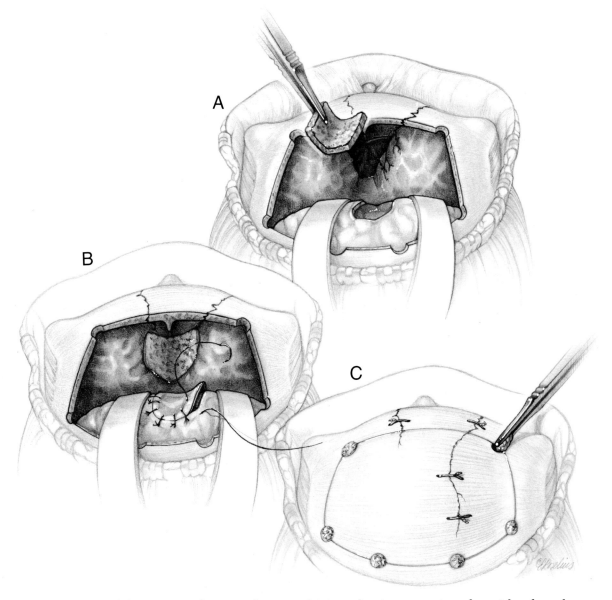

Fig. 4-13. (**A**) Exposure of anterior basicranial injury showing separation of cranial and nasal cavities with a contoured bone graft. (**B**) Repair and/or reinforcement of the dura with a pericranial patch. (**C**) Replacement of the bifrontal craniotomy bone flap and filling of trephine holes with bone dust.

7. Septonasal reconstruction.
8. Placement of lead or acrylic plates.
9. Closure of soft tissue.

Figures 4-14 and 4-28 illustrate an example of acute reconstruction of a comminuted fronto-orbito-nasal fracture. Figures 4-29 to 4-33 illustrate a second case of acute reconstruction of a posteriorly displaced fracture.

PRINCIPLES OF DELAYED REPAIR

Although the ideal approach is one-stage initial reconstruction, the surgeon is often faced with complications or sequelae resulting from incomplete or improper initial management. Newer techniques of craniofacial reconstruction, described by Tessier,[16-18] allow one-stage delayed reconstruction of residual deformities.

Once again, this reconstruction revolves around careful clinical and radiographic evaluation coupled with three-dimensional analysis of deformities to accurately plan surgery.

In evaluating deformities for secondary reconstruction three types of lesions are identified: loss of bone, malunion of bony parts, and scarring and malposition of soft parts. Surgical correction for each is specific.

Loss of Bone

Loss of bone occurs from trauma, infection, and loss of periosteum from multiple procedures that lead to devitalized bone and bone resorption. Principles in restoration of bone include: separation of cranial cavities from facial and sinus cavities, reconstitution of orbital and nasal walls, restoration of contour, and protection for vital structures, such as the brain.[19] A bicoronal incision with bifrontal craniotomy allows access to the anterior cranial base and upper facial skeleton. Brain and dural re-

pair with closure of CSF leaks, separation of cranial and sinus cavities by bone grafting, and fronto-or-bito-nasal reconstruction can be performed.

Malunion of Bony Parts

Malunions are the result of inadequate or delayed reduction of fractures. To restore function and contour, malunited bones should be refractured and repositioned so that anatomy is restored. If there is bone loss or gaps after osteotomy, bone grafts will be needed for stabilization of the repositioned parts. After mobilization and repositioning, solid fixation is absolutely necessary to maintain reduction.

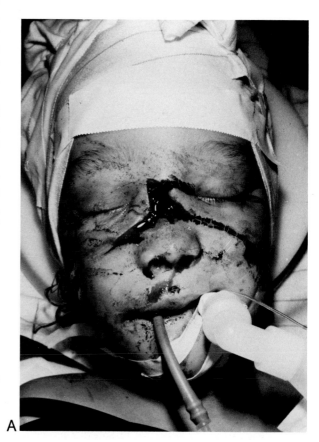

A

Fig. 4-14. (A) Nine-year-old male with laceration over the nasal dorsum and glabellar regions that was sustained in a motor vehicle accident. *(Figure continues.)*

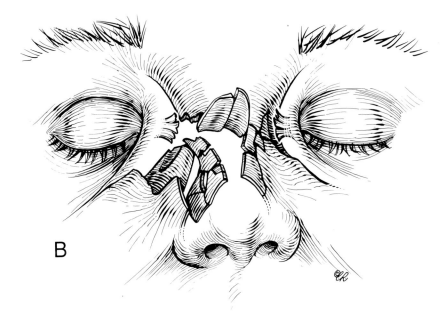

Fig. 4-14 *(Continued).* **(B)** Schematic representation of the bony disruption.

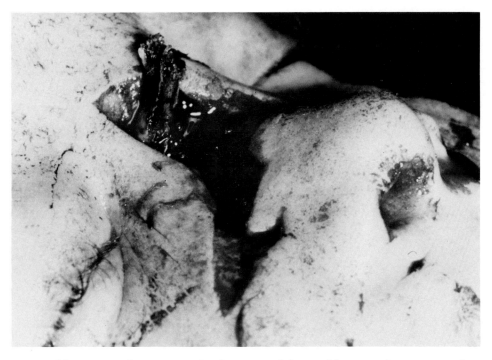

Fig. 4-15. Oblique view showing retrodisplacement of the nasal bones with superior avulsion of the root of the nose and glabella.

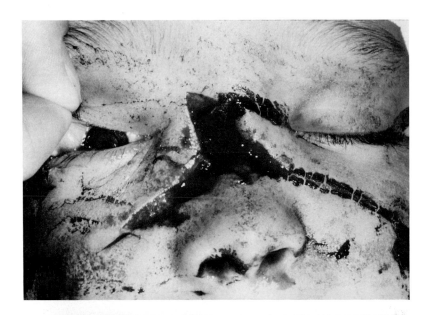

Fig. 4-16. Furnas traction test of this patient shows disruption of both medial canthal tendons.

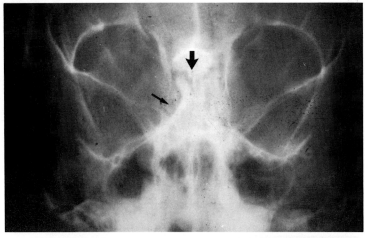

Fig. 4-17. Waters radiograph showing right medial maxillary fracture (small arrow) with naso-orbital disruption at the level of the cribriform plate (large arrow).

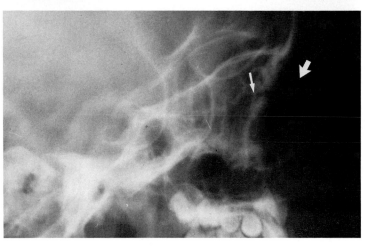

Fig. 4-18. Lateral radiograph showing a fracture of the perpendicular plate of the ethmoid at the cribriform plate (small arrow) and the superiorly displaced root of the nose (large arrow).

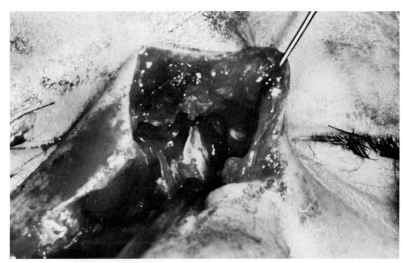

Fig. 4-19. Direct examination at the site of injury reveals total disruption of bony and soft tissue elements of the fronto-naso-orbital region.

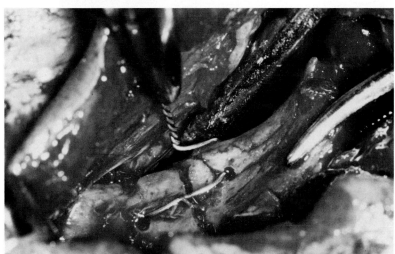

Fig. 4-20. Working laterally to medially, from stable to unstable elements, the right medial maxillary fracture is reduced and stabilized.

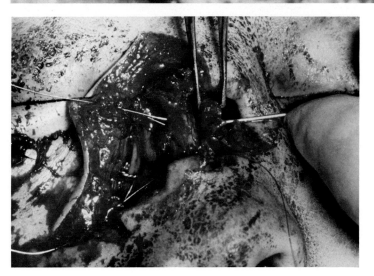

Fig. 4-21. The mattress wire is placed through a spinal needle passed through the drilled holes.

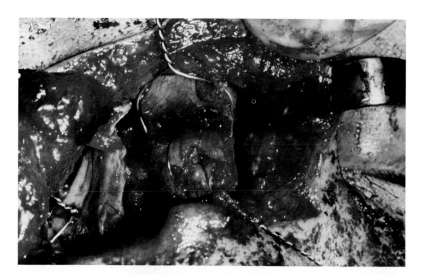

Fig. 4-22. Nasal bones are reduced and stabilized by the lower mattress wire. The superiorly displaced root of the nose and glabella have been reduced and stabilized by the superior wire. Note the wire fixation of the right medial maxillary fracture and the avulsed right medial canthal tendon.

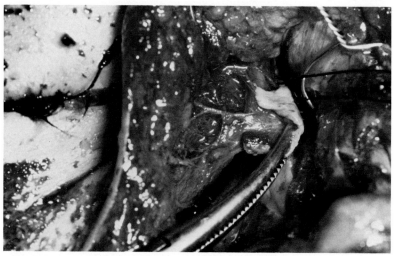

Fig. 4-23. Both canthal tendons are avulsed. This shows direct identification of the right medial canthal ligament. Note the 4-0 silk suture placed earlier for identification.

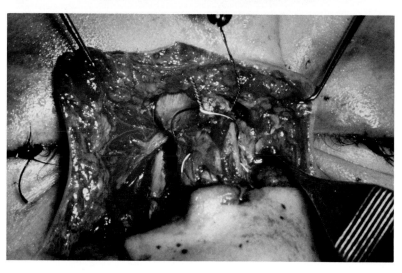

Fig. 4-24. Following transnasal canthoplasty with a #30 stainless steel wire, careful adjustment of the tension is necessary for accurate repositioning of the ligaments.

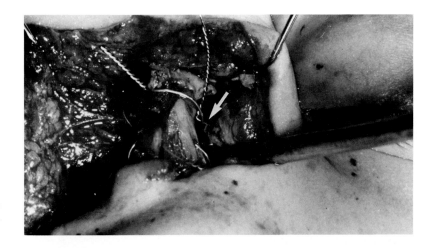

Fig. 4-25. View showing wire through the left canthal tendon, emphasizing accurate repositioning. Note that the wire is not too tight (arrow) so as to avoid overcorrection.

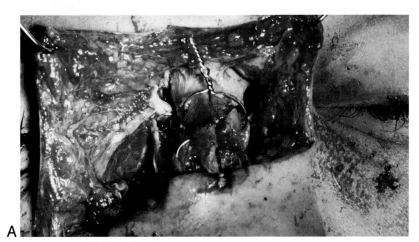

A

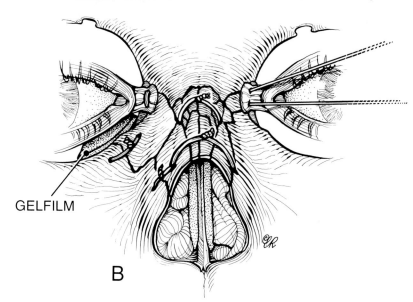

GELFILM

B

Fig. 4-26. (A) Completion of the bony reconstruction and canthal repositioning. (B) Schematic representation of the reconstruction.

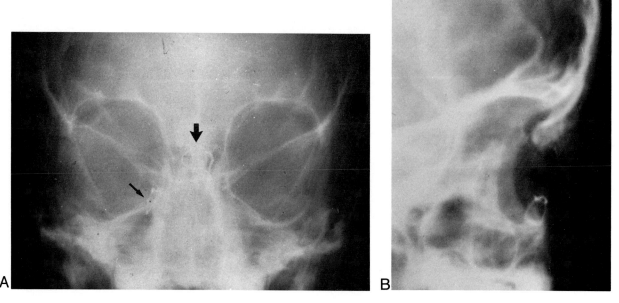

Fig. 4-27. Postoperative radiographs. **(A)** Caldwell view demonstrating medial maxillary (small arrow) and glabellar (large arrow) reduction wires. **(B)** Lateral view showing reduction of glabella and nasal bone mass.

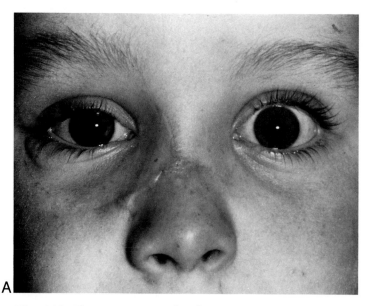

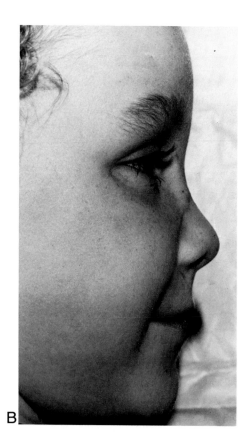

Fig. 4-28. The patient 9 weeks after surgery. **(A)** Full-face view showing nasal scarring. The ptosis of the right upper lid resolved spontaneously. **(B)** Lateral view *(Figure continues.)*

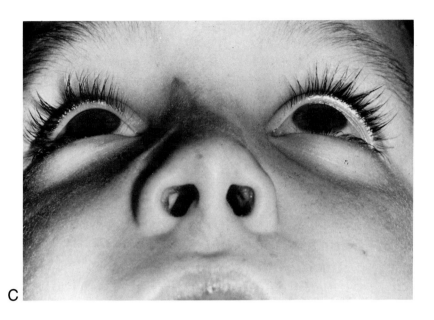

Fig. 4-28 *(Continued).* **(C)** Basal view demonstrating adequate reduction of the nasal dorsum.

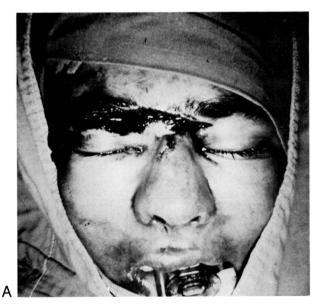

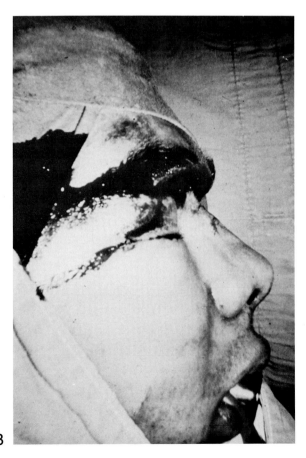

Fig. 4-29. **(A)** Frontal and **(B)** lateral views of a posteriorly displaced fracture in a 20-year-old male involved in a motor vehicle accident. The patient was struck high on the glabellar region.

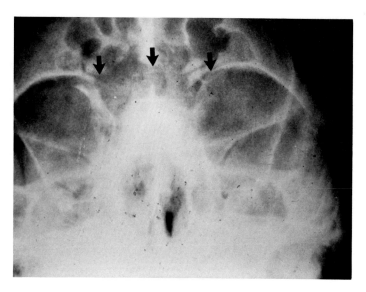

Fig. 4-30. Waters radiograph shows disruption (arrows) of the nasal root and superior medial orbital walls. Note however that the medial orbital walls are intact.

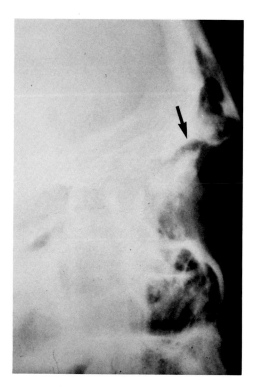

Fig. 4-31. Lateral view demonstrating retrodisplacement of the nasal sinus and perpendicular plate of the ethmoid at the level of the cribriform plate.

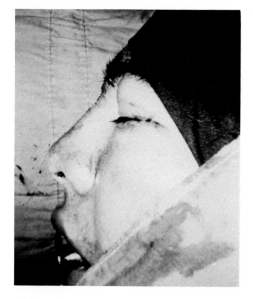

Fig. 4-32. Immediate postoperative lateral view demonstrating the reduction of the nasal bones and glabella and the reestablishment of the nasofrontal angle.

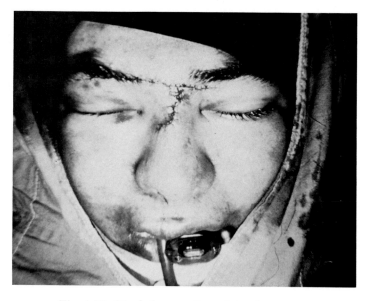

Fig. 4-33. Final closure of overlying laceration.

Malposition and Scarring of Soft Tissue

Most commonly, these deformities occur around the eyelids and medial canthal regions and are accompanied by post-traumatic telecanthus and lacrimal drainage dysfunction. Delayed reconstruction of traumatic telecanthus involves four separate surgical steps.[6,13,20–22]

Correction of cutaneous scarring or epicanthal folds. The double opposing Z-plasty of Converse[21] and the Mustardé[23] rectangular flap procedures are effective for this correction.

Restoration of bone contour in the medial canthal and nasal regions. This involves removal of malpositioned overlapped bone fragments and scar tissue in the medial canthal region,[6] as these tissues occupy space necessary to reposition and anchor the medial canthus. Nasal recontouring usually involves osteotomies and/or bone grafting.[11]

Restoration of lacrimal drainage. Dacryocystorhinostomy or conjunctivorhinostomy with tube insertion may be necessary to restore tear drainage (see Chapter 6).

Medial canthoplasty. The medical canthoplasty is performed with transnasal wiring or unilateral intranasal button anchorage. The medial canthal tendon is carefully dissected from surrounding scar tissues. If it has been destroyed, the tarsal plates are identified and used for anchoring. Complete mobilization of the soft tissues of the orbit by circumferential dissection of the orbital rim and walls with lateral cantholysis is necessary for adequate repositioning of the medial canthus. Burr holes in the medial orbital wall are placed posteriorly and superiorly to the anatomic position of the canthus to overcorrect the deformity. The canthus or tarsal plates are fixed by transnasal wiring or unilateral button wire fixation.[6,13,21]

Post-traumatic ptosis may result from disruption of the levator palpebra superioris, nerve injury, or direct muscle injury. In many instances, post-traumatic ptosis resolves with time, if the muscle has not been avulsed or lacerated. If levator function is adequate, reinsertion or shortening of the muscle will improve persistant ptosis.

SUMMARY OF DELAYED RECONSTRUCTION

Salient points to be stressed in delayed reconstruction are (1) the need for fastidious dural repair with suturing and pericranial grafting, (2) separation of cranial and facial cavities by bone grafting, (3) cranialization of the frontal sinuses with obliteration of nasofrontal ducts, if indicated, (4) orbital, frontal, and nasal bony reconstruction via osteotomies and bone grafts with solid monobloc fixation, (5) repositioning of misplaced soft tissue elements, particularly the medial canthus, (6) restoration of lacrimal drainage, and (7) scar revision.[19] Figures 4-34 to 4-46 illustrate an example of post-traumatic medial canthal deformity.

CONCLUSION

The fronto-orbito-nasal region represents, in a compact area, the anatomic confluence of many vitally important structures. Trauma to this area may injure contents of the cranial, orbital, sinus, and nasal cavities. These injuries are rarely immediately life threatening. The close cooperation and combined efforts of the maxillofacial surgeon, neurosurgeon, opthalmologist, and radiologist are essential for optimum treatment. Clinical and radiographic studies with a three-dimensional spatial analysis of the combined injuries are necessary for preoperative planning. Initial total reconstruction with rehabilitation of all lesions is the recommended treatment of these injuries. Inadequate initial evaluation and treatment with persistent deformity require similar preoperative analysis and planning. Delayed one-stage reconstruction of all persistent lesions is possible with modern craniofacial technique.

Complications associated with fronto-orbito-nasal fractures revolve around injury to regional

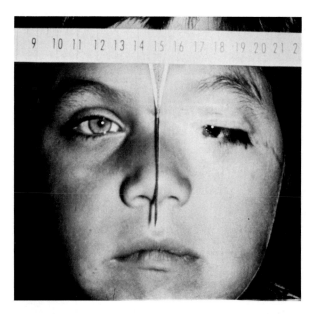

Fig. 4-34. Post-traumatic telecanthus and ptosis in a 10-year-old male. There had been three previous attempts at canthoplasty.

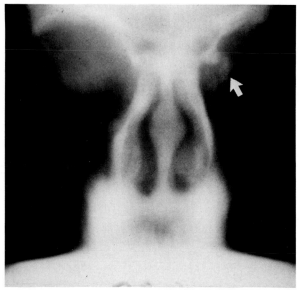

Fig. 4-35. Tomography revealing bony exostosis from malpositioned, overlapped bone fragments.

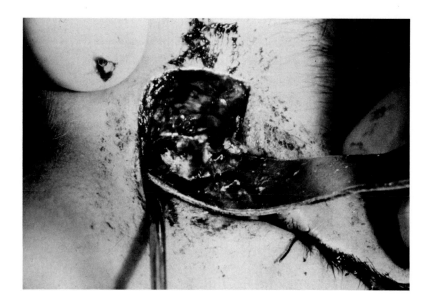

Fig. 4-36. The bone fragment is removed.

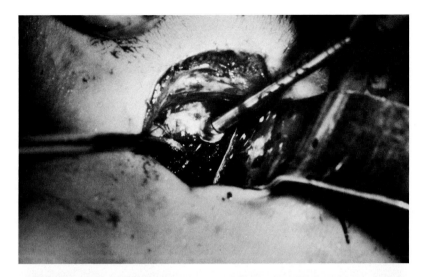

Fig. 4-37. Utilizing a rotary burr, the medial orbital wall is further reduced and contoured to create a space in which to reposition the canthus.

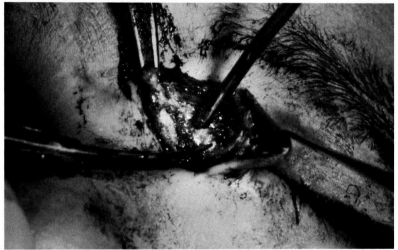

A

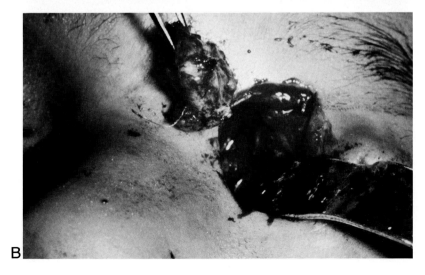

B

Fig. 4-38. (A) Scar tissues destroying and replacing the medial canthus are exposed and (B) removed to further create space for canthal repositioning. Note the wire that is present from a previous canthoplasty.

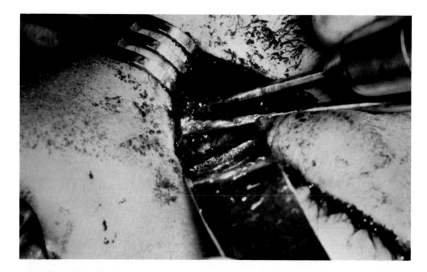

Fig. 4-39. Drill holes are placed through the recontoured medial wall into the nasal cavity at the desired position of the canthus.

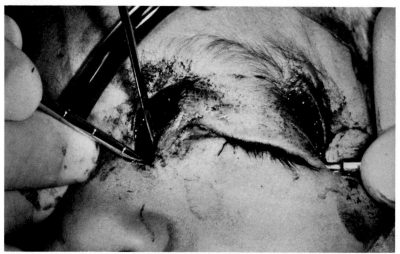

Fig. 4-40. Through medial and lateral incisions, complete subperiosteal degloving of the soft tissues of the orbital cavity is performed in conjunction with lysis of the lateral canthal ligament.

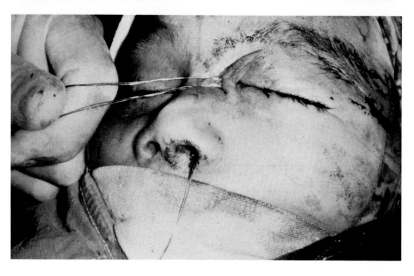

Fig. 4-41. Canthoplasty wires have been secured to the tarsal plates and the intranasal pullout wire (see Fig. 4-44).

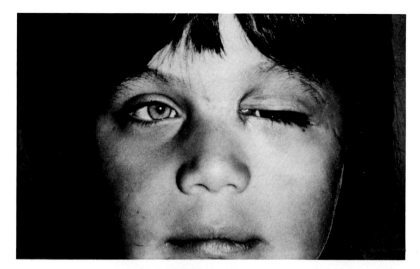

Fig. 4-42. Early postoperative view showing canthal repositioning and persistent ptosis.

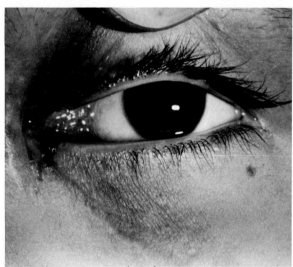

Fig. 4-43. Close-up view of repositioned canthus. Partial resection of the caruncle and ptosis correction were performed later.

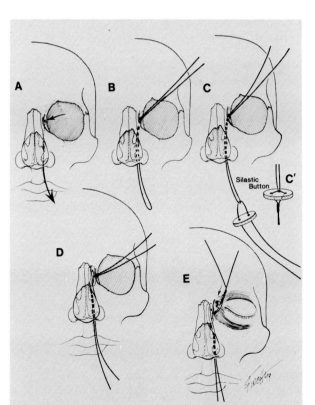

Fig. 4-44. Schematic drawing illustrating the technique of unilateral canthoplasty with an intranasal plastic button and pullout wire. (Duvall HA, Foster CF, Lyons DP, Letson RD: Medial canthoplasty, early and delayed repair. Laryngoscope 91:173, 1981.)

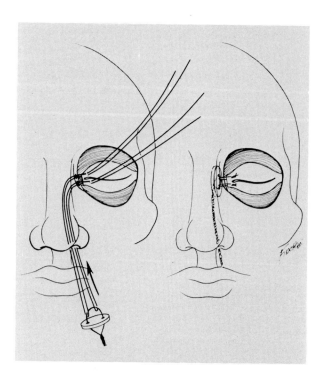

Fig. 4-45. Schematic drawing illustrating the anchoring of the tarsal plates when the canthal ligament is destroyed, as in the case presented. (Duvall HA, Foster CF, Lyons DP, Letson RD: Medial canthoplasty, early and delayed repair. Larynogoscope 91:173, 1981.)

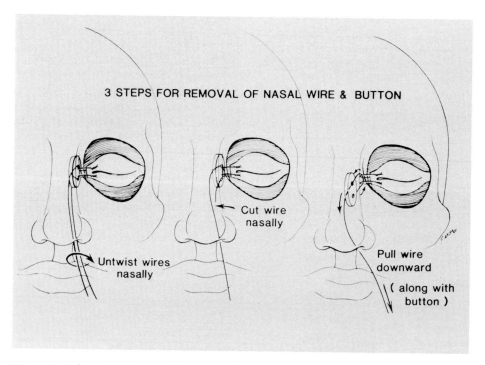

3 STEPS FOR REMOVAL OF NASAL WIRE & BUTTON

Untwist wires nasally

Cut wire nasally

Pull wire downward

(along with button)

Fig. 4-46. Schematic drawing illustrating the steps for removal of the plastic button and pullout wires after adequate healing of the canthoplasty. (Duvall HA, Foster CF, Lyons DP, Letson RD: Medial canthoplasty, early and delayed repair. Laryngoscope 91:173, 1981.)

vital structures. These include the brain and meninges, sinuses, orbits and adnexa, lacrimal drainage system, nose and respiratory system, and cosmetic-expressive systems. Most complications ensue from inadequate initial diagnosis, resulting in undetected lesions and incomplete reconstruction.

REFERENCES

1. Swearingingen JJ: Tolerances of the human face to crash impact. Federal Aviation Agency, Oklahoma City, 1965
2. Furnas DW, Bircoll MH: Eyelash traction test to determine if the medial canthal ligament is detached. Plast Reconstr Surg 52:315, 1973
3. Rowe NL, Killey HC: Fractures of the facial skeleton. Williams & Wilkins, Baltimore, 1956
4. Stranc MF, Robertson GA: Classification of internal injuries of the nasal skeleton. Ann Plast Surg 2:468, 1979
5. Gruss JS: Naso-ethmoid-orbital fractures: Classification and role of primary bone grafting. Plast Reconstr Surg 75(3):303, 1985
6. Duvall AJ, Foster CA, Lyons DP, Letson RD: Medial Canthoplasty: Early and delayed repair. Laryngoscope 91:173, 1981
7. Merville LC, Real JP: Fronto-orbito nasal dislocations. Initial total reconstruction. Scand J Plast Reconstr Surg 15:287, 1981
8. Gruss JS, Fronto-naso-orbital trauma. Clin Plast Surg 9:577, 1982
9. Manson PN, Crawley WA, Yaremchuk MJ, et al: Midface fractures: Advantages of immediate extended open reduction and bone grafting. Plast Reconstr Surg 76:1, 1985
10. Converse, JM, Hogan VM: Open-sky approach for reduction of naso-orbital fractures: Case report. Plast Reconstr Surg 46:396, 1970
11. Converse JM, Firman F, Wood-Smith D, et al: Conjunctival approach in orbital fractures. Plast Reconstr Surg 52:656, 1973
12. Tessier P: Autogenous bone grafts taken from the calvarium for facial and cranial applications. Clin Plast Surg 9(4)531, 1982
13. Converse JM, Smith B, Wood-Smith D: Deformities of the mid-face resulting from malunited orbital and naso-orbital fractures. Clin Plast Surg 2:107, 1975
14. Jabaley MD, Lerman M, Sanders HJ: Ocular injuries in orbital fractures: A review of 119 cases. Plast Reconstr Surg 56:410, 1975
15. Psillakis JM, Nocchi VL, Zanini SA: Repair of large defects of frontal bone with free graft of outer table of parietal bone. Plast Reconstr Surg 64:827, 1979
16. Tessier P, Hervouet F, Delbut JP: Dislocations orbito-nasals. p. 96. In Troutman RC, Converse JM, Smith B (eds): Plastic and Reconstructive Surgery of Eye and Adenexa. Butterworth, Washington D.C., 1962
17. Tessier P: Total osteotomy of the middle third of the face for faciostenosis or for sequelae of LeFort 111 fracture. Plast Reconstr Surg 48:553, 1971
18. Tessier P, Rougier F, Hervouet F, et al: Chirurgie Plastique Orbito-palpebrale. Masson, Paris, 1977
19. Merville LC, Derome P, deSaint-Jarre G: Fronto-orbito-nasal dislocations: Secondary treatment of sequelae. Scand J Plast Reconstr Surg 15:299, 1981
20. Converse JM, Smith B: Naso-orbital fractures. Trans Am Acad Ophthal Otolaryngol 67:622, 1963
21. Converse JM, Smith B: Naso-orbital fractures and traumatic deformities of the medial canthus. Plast Reconstr Surg 38:147, 1966
22. Mathog RH, Bauer W: Post traumatic pseudo hypertelorism (Telecanthus). Arch Otolaryngol 105:81, 1979
23. Mustardé JC: Plastic Surgery in Infancy and Childhood. p. 251. Churchill Livingstone, Edinburgh, 1971

Orbital Fractures

5

Glenn W. Jelks
Gregory La Trenta

The type and severity of orbital fracture depends on the magnitude and direction of force applied to the orbital area. Orbital trauma often involves injury to the highly specialized tissues of the eyelids, lacrimal apparatus, and intraorbital contents (see Chapter 6). Fractures of the orbital bones may occur independently but are usually associated with other facial bone fractures. Orbital fractures may involve only the bone within the orbital cavity with no disruption of the orbital rims. These fractures are known as pure orbital fractures and usually involve the inferior or medial walls. More commonly orbital fractures involve both the orbital rims and walls to produce more complex bony disruptions (e.g., trimalar, LeFort II, LeFort III, nasoethmoidal, and panfacial fractures).

The main goal in treating the patient with an orbital injury is to restore normal function and appearance. Although early treatment is important in minimizing any cosmetic and functional disability, orbital fractures are rarely surgical emergencies. Appropriate ancillary clinical and radiological studies should be performed to assist the surgeon in analysis of the injuries. Combining this information with a firm foundation in anatomy allows the surgeon to obtain more accurate reconstructions while minimizing complications.

ANATOMICAL CONSIDERATIONS

The Bony Orbit

The ocular globes reside in two symmetrical bony cavities on either side of the nose. Seven bones of the cranial and facial skeleton contribute to form each orbit. The frontal, ethmoid, sphenoid, maxilla, zygoma, lacrimal, and palatine bones combine to give the orbital cavity the shape of a quadrangular pyramid with its base directed forward, outward, and slightly downward. The widest orbital diameter is actually located approximately 1 cm within the orbital rims. The optic foramen lies on a medial and slightly superior plane in the apex of the orbit. In children the orbital floor is situated at a lower level in relation to the inferior orbital rim owing to lack of maxillary sinus development. As the anterior two thirds of the orbital cavity joins the posterior one third, it takes the shape of a triangular pyramid where the optic nerve and origins of the extraocular muscles reside.

The average adult dimensions of the orbit are listed in Table 5-1. The adult orbit is usually slightly wider than it is high, and depth can vary

Table 5-1. Average Orbital Dimensions

Orbital width	40 mm
Orbital height	35 mm
Depth	45–55 mm
Extraorbital width	100 mm
Interorbital width	25 mm
Orbital volume	30 cc
Ocular globe volume	7 cc

depending upon the method of measurement from orbital rim to optic foramen. The extraorbital width is the distance between the lateral margins of the orbits, and the interorbital width is the distance between the medial orbital walls.

Figure 5-1 depicts the geometry of the orbits. The nasomalar angle, or the angle from the base of the nasal bone to the lateral orbital rims, is approximately 145°. Recognition of this anatomic relationship of the lateral orbital rim and the more anteriorly positioned vertical axis of the globe is very helpful in the surgical correction of late post-traumatic enophthalmos.[1] The angle between the lateral walls of the orbits is 90°, and the angle be-

tween the medial and lateral wall of each orbit is 45°. The medial orbital walls are roughly parallel. The orbital axes diverge by 45°, and there is a disparity of approximately 22° between the orbital and visual axes.

Orbital Rims

The superior orbital rim is formed by the frontal bone. The supraorbital notch lies 25 mm lateral to the midline of the glabella on the margin of the orbit. In approximately 25 percent of orbits, this notch is a true bony canal 5 to 15 mm long. The supraorbital artery and nerves pass through this opening. The supratrochlear vessels and nerves cross the rim just medial to the supraorbital notch or canal. About 5 mm behind the superior-medial aspect of the orbit is the trochlear fossa, a small circular pit in the bone to which attaches the cartilaginous pulley for the superior oblique tendon. The two supraorbital rims join at the midline to form the glabella.

The frontozygomatic suture joins the zygomatic process of the frontal bone superiorly and the anterior-superior portion of the zygoma inferiorly to constitute the lateral orbital rim. Ten millimeters inferior to the frontozygomatic sutures and 2 mm within the lateral orbital cavity lies the lateral orbital tubercle of Whitnall. Attached to this tubercle are the lateral canthal tendon, the check ligament of the lateral rectus muscle, the suspensory ligament of Lockwood, and the lateral extension of the aponeurosis of the levator muscle. These combined attachments are known as the lateral retinaculum of Hesser. It is important to recognize these anatomic relationships in performing orbital explorations or repairs in this region (Fig. 5-2).

The inferior orbital rim is composed of the zygoma laterally and the superior portion of the maxilla medially. The zygomaticomaxillary suture joins these two bones in the middle of the rim. The infraorbital canal lies 10 mm inferior to the most medial extent of this suture. The infraorbital artery and nerve exit this canal (Fig. 5-2).

The medial orbital rim is composed of the frontal process of the maxilla and the anterior lacrimal crest. The superior nasal orbital margin is continu-

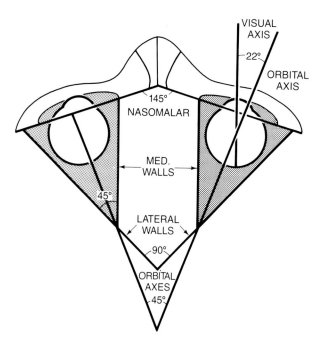

Fig. 5-1. Geometry of the orbits. (Modified from Eggers HM: Functional anatomy of the extraocular muscles. In Duane TD, Jaeger EA (eds): Biomedical Foundation of Ophthalmology, Harper & Row, New York, 1982.)

ous with the posterior lacrimal crest, and the inferior nasal orbital margin is continuous with the anterior lacrimal crest. This discontinuity forms the lacrimal fossa for the lacrimal sac (Fig. 5-2).

Orbital Walls

The roof of the orbit is approximately triangular in shape with the base placed anteriorly. It is composed mainly of the orbital plate of the frontal bone, but posteriorly it receives a minor contribution from the lesser wing of the sphenoid. The fossa for the orbital portion of the lacrimal gland is a depression situated along the anterior and lateral aspects of the roof under the zygomatic process of the frontal bone. The anterior portion of the roof can be pneumatized by an extension of either the frontal or ethmoid sinus air cells. The roof separates the orbit from the anterior cranial fossa and may be as thin as 1 mm. Posteriorly the roof of the orbit terminates at the optic canal (Fig. 5-2).

The lateral wall is formed by the orbital plate of the greater wing of the sphenoid and the orbital portion of the zygoma. The superior orbital fissure separates the roof from the lateral wall of the orbit. This fissure also separates the greater and lesser wings of the sphenoid; cranial nerves III, IV, V (frontal, lacrimal, and nasociliary branches of the ophthalmic division), and VI pass through the superior orbital fissure into the orbit. The superior oph-

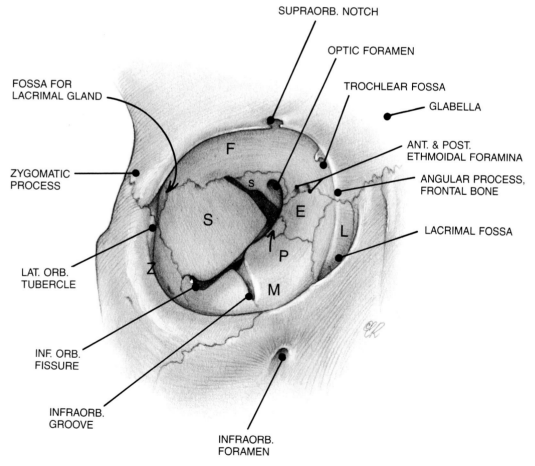

Fig. 5-2. The right orbit viewed along its axis. The orbital rims and walls can be best visualized in this orientation. F, Frontal; E, Ethmoid; L, Lacriminal; M, Maxilla; P, Palatine; Z, Zygoma; S, Sphenoid (greater wing); s, Sphenoid (lesser wing).

the orbital branch of the middle men-
, and sympathetic fibers from the
nus plexus also pass through this fis-
eral orbital wall is related to the tem-
ontaining the temporalis muscle anteriorly. Posteriorly the lateral wall separates the
orbit from the temporal lobe of the brain within the
middle cranial fossa.

The inferior orbital fissure is between the floor
and lateral wall of the orbit, and communicates
with the infratemporal fossa. The maxillary division
of cranial nerve V, the infraorbital artery, the zygomatic nerve, branches of the sphenopalatine ganglion, and branches from the inferior ophthalmic
vein pass through the inferior fissure (Fig. 5-2).

The floor of the orbit is also the roof of the maxillary sinus. It is composed of the thin orbital plate of
the maxilla medial to the infraorbital groove, the
zygomatic bone anterolaterally, and the orbital
process of the palatine bone that forms a triangular
area posteriorly. The floor is traversed by the infraorbital groove, which is converted to a canal
more anteriorly. Within the canal is the infraorbital
nerve, infraorbital artery, and occasionally a vein.
From the more posterior aspect of the canal, the
dental canals descend and carry the middle superior alveolar nerves to the molar and bicuspid teeth
of the upper jaw. More anteriorly, the anterior-superior alveolar nerves, terminal branches of the
maxillary division of cranial nerve V, pass to the
canine and incisor teeth.

In the posterior portion of the orbital floor, there
is an area of very thin bone that represents the
weakest portion of the orbit. This area is continuous with the medial wall and lamina papyracea of
the ethmoids. The inferior oblique muscle originates from the medial aspect of the orbital floor just
lateral to the opening of the nasolacrimal canal and
just behind the orbital rim (Fig. 5-2).

The medial wall is composed of the orbital plate
(lamina papyracea) of the ethmoids centrally, the
angular process of the frontal bone anterosuperi-
orly, and the lacrimal bone anteroinferiorly. Anterior and posterior ethmoidal foramina are usually
present within the frontoethmoidal suture. The anterior ethmoidal foramen contains the anterior
ethmoidal artery and the anterior ethmoidal
branch of the nasociliary nerve. The posterior eth-

moidal foramen allows passage of the posterior
ethmoidal artery and the sphenoethmoidal branch
of the nasociliary nerve.

ETIOLOGY AND CLASSIFICATION

Orbital fractures have been estimated to occur in
17 percent of facial fractures.[2] According to Garrett, orbital and ocular damage occur in 10 percent
of head injuries sustained in motor vehicle accidents in the United States.[3] A 10-year analysis of
orbital blowout fractures by Converse et al., revealed that over 50 percent of such fractures resulted from automobile accidents. Other causes
were fists, elbows, wooden planks, snowballs,
shoes, and table edges.[4]

When the face strikes the dashboard in automobile accidents, the thick orbital rim is displaced
posteriorly transmitting the force to the orbital
contents. This often results in a combined orbital
rim and floor fracture or an impure blowout fracture. Any orbital floor fracture associated with an
adjacent facial bone fracture is by convention defined as an impure blowout fracture.[5]

In a pure blowout fracture, a sudden increase in
intraorbital pressure from a force applied to the
soft tissues of the orbit results solely in an orbital
wall fracture.[6,7] According to Emery et al., the most
common cause of a pure blowout fracture is the
human fist,[8] but Converse et al.[4] list more than 20
other causes. Furthermore, a pure blowout fracture often occurs through a specific portion of the
floor of the orbit.[4]

Fractures of the medial wall have a similar etiology and may also be associated with nasoethmoidal
fractures. Medial wall fractures are associated with
orbital floor blowout fractures in an incidence from
5 to 50 percent.[9–11]

Lateral orbital wall fractures occur with fractures of the zygoma. The weakest point of the lateral orbital rim is located at the frontozygomatic

suture. The weakest portion of the lateral orbital wall is the thin zygomatic plate articulating with the greater wing of the sphenoid and separating the orbit from the temporal fossa. Fractures of the lateral wall of the orbit involve fractures of the zygomatic bone exclusive of the zygomatic process.

Orbital roof fractures are rare, reported by Dodick et al. in only two cases.[11] LaGrange in 1918 showed that the thin medial portion of the orbital roof when fractured is displaced posteriorly into the superior orbital fissure and optic foramen.[12] Orbital roof fractures usually occur in severe trauma with supraorbital rim, frontal bone, and naso-orbital fractures. Rare cases of penetrating injury[13] and anterior cranial fossa blow-in fractures have been noted.[14]

Supraorbital rim fractures have been estimated to occur in 5 percent of patients suffering fractures of the facial bones.[2] These can occur independently or with naso-orbital and glabellar fractures. The usual mechanism is severe direct trauma to the supraorbital arch.

PATHOPHYSIOLOGY

Pfeiffer in 1943 presented 120 cases of orbital wall fractures with their characteristic radiographic findings.[15] In this series he described a mechanism whereby a blow to the eye may cause an orbital wall fracture. Experimental proof came with the classic experiment of Smith and Regan in 1957.[16] Using a single human cadaver and a hurling ball simulating trauma, a pure orbital floor blowout fracture was produced. By 1960 the generally accepted concept of the mechanism for a blowout fracture was increased intraorbital pressure caused by a nonpenetrating object greater than 5 cm in diameter. This resulted in a fracture of the thin portion of the orbital floor and frequently of the medial wall with entrapment of the inferior rectus muscle, medial rectus muscle, and surrounding orbital tissues.[6,7] Kazanjian and Converse offered two theories: (1)

backward displacement of the strong bone of the orbital rim that resulted in comminution of the thin bone into multiple small pieces, or (2) increased internal orbital pressure caused by a blow to the soft tissue of the orbit thereby producing fracture of the weak area without affecting the more resistant orbital rim.[17]

Despite numerous large series appearing in the literature documenting a 14 to 40 percent incidence of serious ocular complications of orbital blowout fracture,[4,8,18–24] controversy over the cause of a blowout fracture persists. One of the reasons for such controversy has been that the amount of intraorbital pressure sufficient to cause a blowout fracture would result in an inordinate amount of intraocular injury. Tajima and Fujino, using dried human skulls, epoxy eye models, a 120-g brass weight, and high-speed cameras, noted a buckling force transmitted to the orbital floor with the application of force to the infraorbital margin.[25–27] A two-point blowout fracture of the orbital floor was noted when the weight was dropped from a height of 20 cm, whereas force applied to the eyeball alone produced only a linear floor fracture. No orbital rim fractures were noted. Fujino concluded that trauma to the infraorbital rim with or without a transmitted rise in intraorbital pressure occurs more commonly with objects greater than 5 cm in diameter. The transmitted buckling force was a more plausible explanation for a pure blowout fracture.

EVALUATION

History

A history of facial impact to the dashboard, windshield, or steering wheel in a motor vehicle accident, a blow to the naso-orbital area in an altercation, or facial injury during a sporting event should alert the physician to the possibility of orbital frac-

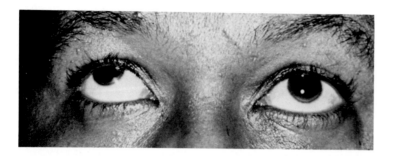

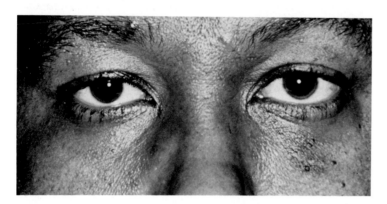

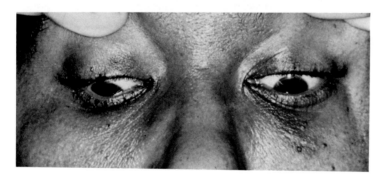

Fig. 5-3. Disparity in the ocular globe position is apparent when the patient looks upward. Diplopia is present in the upgaze position.

ture. Blowout fractures are more frequent on the left side because most individuals are right-handed, and many blowout fractures are caused by human fist. One should be suspicious with a patient who has a "black eye" and complains of visual difficulty. Ophthalmological consultation is essential for a thorough evaluation.

Clinical Exam

King in 1944 recognized the triad of signs and symptoms of the classic "blowout" fracture: diplo-pia, enophthalmos, and infraorbital nerve hypoesthesia.[28]

In Putterman's series, diplopia was present in 72 percent of patients, 54 percent in the functional position, 18 percent in the extreme position, and 28 percent combined.[29] This has been attributed to vertical muscle imbalance due to damage to the nerve supply of muscles or herniation and entrapment of the inferior rectus muscle, inferior oblique muscle, suspensory ligament of Lockwood, periorbita, or intermuscular fascial expansion. The inferior rectus and the inferior oblique connect intimately at the point where the oblique crosses beneath the rectus; disturbances of both muscles are often noted. If the fracture is lateral to the infraorbital groove or canal, the inferior rectus and oblique may not be involved. Therefore, location of the fracture often determines signs and symptoms.

The inferior division of cranial nerve III innervates inferior rectus and inferior oblique muscles. The nerve to the inferior rectus passes along the upper aspect of the muscle to enter at the junction of the posterior and middle thirds. The nerve to the inferior oblique passes along the lateral aspect of the inferior rectus muscle entering more distally. The inferior oblique nerve is more vulnerable to injury than the inferior rectus nerve. It is important to establish diplopia in the primary position or in any extreme of ocular gaze. Most commonly diplopia is elicited when the patient looks upward. The ocular position discrepancy is best evaluated with this maneuver (Fig. 5-3).

Entrapment can be demonstrated by the reduction of upward ocular excursion utilizing the forced duction test.[30] After placement of a few drops of topical anesthetic solution into the conjunctival sac, the ocular globe is grasped with forceps at the insertion of the inferior rectus 7 mm from the limbus and moved superiorly. This test helps document mechanical entrapment as a cause for the patient's diplopia. Unfortunately, the forced duction test may appear positive under local anesthesia and be negative under general anesthesia. Thus this maneuver is not an infallible test of entrapment. More sophisticated electromyographic studies of saccadic velocities may help differentiate muscle entrapment from nerve damage.[4]

Enophthalmos was noted by Emery et al. in 14 percent of their 159 patients. This sign is often masked by pseudoproptosis secondary to hemorrhage and edema in soft tissues; however, an increased upper lid sulcus deformity may be immediately noted in extensive blowout fractures. True exophthalmos may rarely be noted in the presence of a post-traumatic arteriovenous communication between the internal carotid artery and the cavernous sinus.[4] Enophthalmos has mainly been attributed to escape of periorbital fat into the maxillary and/or ethmoid sinus. Late post-traumatic enophthalmos may be caused by orbital fat displacement from the muscle cone, shortening and fibrosis of injured extraocular muscles, and an increased orbital volume.[4]

Infraorbital nerve hypoesthesia was noted in 21 percent of Putterman's series.[29] This finding suggests a central floor fracture with either neuropraxia or transection of the infraorbital nerve.[4] Absence of infraorbital nerve hypoesthesia implies that the fracture may be lateral, medial, or posterior to the infraorbital groove or canal. Other signs and symptoms are lid ecchymosis, epiphora, cyclotropia, periorbital emphysema,[31] and even mediastinal emphysema.[32]

Tethering of the medial rectus muscle, persistence of enophthalmos, and lack of full abduction following adequate treatment of an orbital floor fracture strongly suggest medial orbital wall fracture and entrapment within the ethmoid sinus.[33] Prasad believes medial rectus entrapment to be less likely because of the anatomic matrix of the ethmoid bone and sinus.[34] Other findings with medial wall fracture may be horizontal diplopia with restricted abduction, enophthalmos on abduction, a narrowed palpebral fissure, and increasing post-injury enophthalmos.[11,35-38]

Lateral orbital wall fractures are suggested by frontozygomatic dysjunction and downward displacement of the lateral orbital floor. Ectropion of the lower lid and downward displacement of the lateral canthus may also be noted.

Orbital roof fractures usually are part of severe craniofacial injuries. The trochlea of the superior oblique muscle may be displaced resulting in vertical diplopia.[39] Orbital soft tissue entrapment into the frontal sinus and persistent globe displacement have been noted.[40] Fractures at the supraorbital ridge are usually evident by a bony depression. If the causative impact is great, concomitant glabellar and naso-orbital fractures as well as brain injury may occur.

Roentgenographic Evaluation

Plain anterior-posterior roentgenograms may be interpreted as suspicious for orbital floor fracture when clouding of the maxillary sinus is present. A Waters view is essential, and in orbital floor fractures the double line of the orbital rim may not be

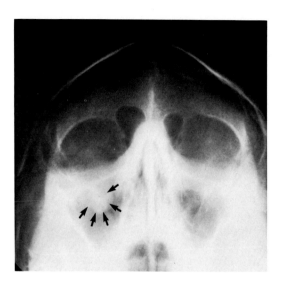

Fig. 5-4. Waters view showing right orbital floor fracture with orbital contents (arrows) within the maxillary sinus.

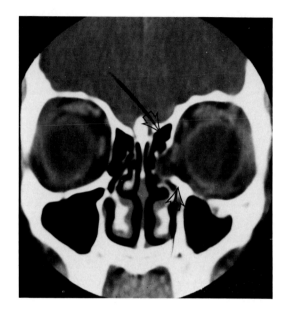

Fig. 5-6. Coronal CT scan showing left orbital floor and medial wall fracture. The orbital contents (arrows) are visualized within the ethmoids.   →

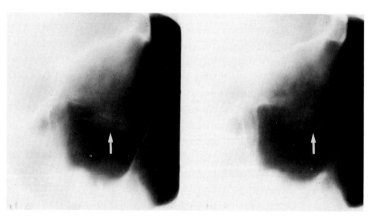

Fig. 5-5. Lateral tomogram showing orbital floor fracture with orbital contents (arrows) prolapsed into maxillary sinus.

present, fragmentation and depression of the floor may be noted, and the orbital contents may even be seen within the maxillary sinus (Fig. 5-4).[41] In medial wall fractures clouding of the ethmoid sinus, the presence of air within the orbit, and medial displacement of fragments of the medial orbital wall have been noted.

Polytomography with hypocycloidal movement has been advocated in all difficult cases and is essential for lateral wall, orbital roof, and supraorbital rim fractures. Tomograms are positive in 72 to 80 percent of cases[42] with a false-positive rate of 14 percent.[43] Surgical intervention therefore should not be undertaken on radiological signs alone (Fig. 5-5).

Axial and coronal CT scans are the most accurate means of study for orbital floor blowout fractures[44,45] and medial orbital blowout factures (Fig. 5-6).[46,47] In a recent experiment with eight human cadaver models and induced orbital blowout fractures, Hammarschlag et al.[48] found that coronal and sagittal CT scans provided overall improved diagnosis over plain radiographs and AP tomograms. Anatomical correlation was used in all cases.

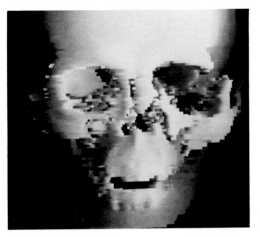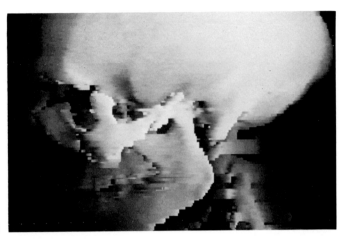

B

Fig. 5-7. (A) Reformatted CT scan providing three-dimensional visualization of a left zygoma, complex fracture with orbital floor, and lateral wall disruptions. Note the significant inferior-lateral displacement of the fracture fragment. (B) Left lateral view showing position of zygoma fractures in relation to craniofacial skeleton.

CT is superb at displaying anterior ethmoid clouding in ethmoid sinus fractures,[49] orbital trauma associated with orbital fractures,[50] and frontal sinus fractures.[51] A recent review of CT in orbital fractures has been expertly detailed by Kassel et al.[49] Computer graphic conversion of standard information into a three-dimensional representation of the bony deformity has recently become available. This is especially helpful in evaluating impure or complex orbital fractures (Fig. 5-7).

hyphema, corneal abrasion and laceration, and angle chamber recession or disruption. Posterior chamber complications include iridodialysis, iris sphincter rupture, ciliary body rupture, and lens subluxation or dislocation. Globe complications include vitreous hemorrhage, choroidal rupture, retinal detachment, commotio retinae, retrobulbar hemorrhage, scleral laceration, optic nerve contusion, hematoma, and laceration (Table 5-2) (see Chapter 6).

Special Studies

As previously mentioned, the short course of the nerve to the inferior rectus renders it less vulnerable to injury in orbital floor fractures than the nerve to the inferior oblique. Some authors have found this fact useful and employ electromyographic studies (EMG) to determine whether nerve conduction has been interrupted or whether muscle entrapment is the primary injury.[4]

In the seven largest series of orbital floor fractures comprising 720 patients, a 14 to 40 percent incidence of serious ocular complications has been documented.[4,8,18–24] These ocular complications make it essential that complete ophthalmologic examination be performed in all cases of periorbital trauma. Anterior chamber complications include

THERAPY

Nonoperative Versus Operative

The nonoperative approach to blowout fractures was popularized by Putterman et al.[29] in 1974 and Helveston in 1976.[52] This approach was advocated after six cases of postoperative loss of vision were noted in a series of 72 patients treated for blowout fractures.[53] A 50 percent incidence of persistent diplopia and 14 percent incidence of persistent enophthalmos after surgical repair were reported in

Table 5-2. Ocular Injuries

	No. of Patients	Blowout Fractures	Serious Eye Injury (%)	Eye Displacement into Maxillary Sinus	Ruptured Displaced Eye	Blindness	Epiphora
Jabaley[23]	119	22	29		7		
Emery[8]	159	159	35	2			
Fradkin[19]	53	53	40				
Liebsohn[22]	119	119	32		4		
McCoy[18]	855	138	15		32	28[a]	6
Milauskas[24]	84	84	14	1	3	3	2
Converse[2]	145	145	31	1		5[b]	

[a] Optic nerve injury
[b] Visual impairment

49 patients in another series.[8] Putterman studied 57 patients with pure blowout fractures which were treated nonoperatively. Initially, 68 percent of patients had diplopia. With nonoperative management the incidence of residual diplopia in 15° excursion of gaze was only 4 percent in patients studied retrospectively and prospectively. Residual diplopia in extreme positions of gaze was 25 percent in those patients retrospectively studied and 27 percent in those prospectively studied. Residual enophthalmos occurred in 65 percent of the retrospective group and 36 percent of the prospective group. These authors advocated that no patient with a pure blowout fracture should be operated upon immediately, but rather should be kept under observation for 4 to 6 months. Soft tissue edema, hemorrhage, inferior rectus, and inferior oblique nerve damage rather than bony entrapment were felt to be the primary causes of restricted ocular motility in the acute and subacute periods. Delayed motility problems were believed to be the result of fibrosis, which was just as likely to occur in surgically treated patients as in those nonsurgically treated.

Considerable experience with delayed treatment in 50 patients reported by Converse et al.[4] yielded persistent diplopia in 40 percent and persistent enophthalmos in 22 percent of patients 1 year after surgery. Their limited success with these 50 patients led to their objection to nonoperative treatment of blowout fractures, since the sequelae were far more complicated to correct at a later date than if a well-timed primary surgical repair had been performed.[54]

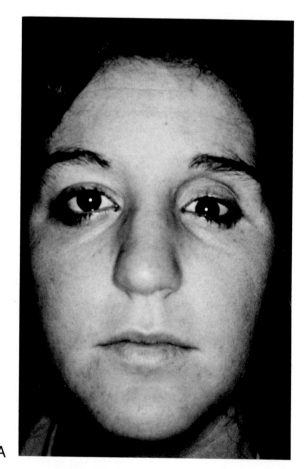

A

Fig. 5-8. (A) Patient with left orbital blowout fracture manifesting enophthalmos and high-lid sulcus deformities. *(Figure continues.)*

in Orbital Blowout Fractures

Vitreous Hemorrhage/Hyphema	Eye Muscle Imbalance	Angle Recession/Glaucoma	Dislocated Lens	Commotio Retinae	Traumatic Cataract	Corneal Injury	Retinal Contusion/Detachment
2		2				5	2
2/10		0/2	1		1	3	2/1
.3/2				11	4		2
10/5	5	4	1	12	2	6	13
	4	2					
1/1		1/1	1	1	1		1
	43						

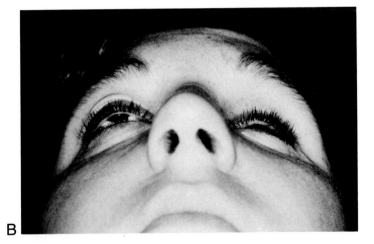

B

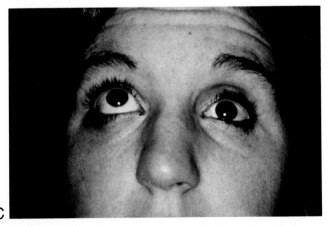

C

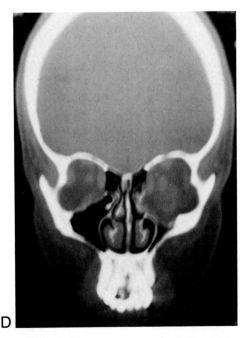

D

Fig. 5-8 *(Continued)*. **(B)** The degree of enophthalmos is best appreciated from a "worm's eye" view. **(C)** Entrapment of the inferior orbital structures is suggested when failure of eye elevation occurs. This is confirmed with a forced duction test. **(D)** CT scan demonstrating left medial wall and floor fractures with associated prolapse of orbital tissues.

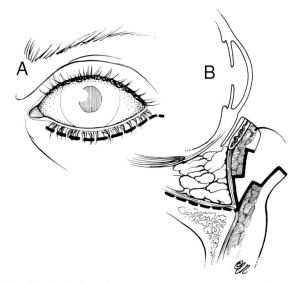

Fig. 5-9. (A) The subciliary approach to the orbit places the incision just below the lower lid lashes. (B) Cross-sectional view demonstrates a "stepped" approach to the inferior orbital rim.

SURGICAL CORRECTION

Indications

The present trend is for delayed operative repair at 10 to 14 days if the patient shows no signs of improvement, or if there are worsening signs and symptoms. Indications include persistence of enophthalmos, restriction of ocular motility, a positive forced duction test, and radiographic evidence of significant fractures[54] (Fig. 5-8). Complete dehiscence of the orbital floor and medial wall with entrapment fractures are indications for operative intervention.[8,54] Close collaboration with ophthalmologists is imperative for appropriate treatment of any associated ocular injuries. Primary operative treatment for lateral wall, orbital roof, and supraorbital rim fractures has been strongly advocated.[55]

Surgical Approaches to the Orbit

Subciliary

In the subciliary approach the incision is placed 2 to 3 mm below the lower lid margin. The skin is undermined over the pretarsal orbicularis muscle. The preseptal portion of the orbicularis is then incised until the septum is reached. Dissection is continued to the rim of the orbit. The maxillary periosteum is sharply incised, providing access to the inferior orbital floor (Fig. 5-9).

This incision gives direct access to the floor and in most cases, leaves an inconspicuous scar (Fig. 5-10). Careful closure should be performed to avoid vertical shortening of the lower lid with eversion of the lower lid margin. In one series the incidence of lower lid ectropion was 42 percent.[56]

Transconjunctival

After everting the lower lid, an incision through the conjunctiva at the lower border of the tarsus is performed. A lateral canthotomy and canthal release can be added if more exposure is required[57] (Fig. 5-11). Dissection anterior to the orbital septum is then carried to the periosteum of the inferior orbital rim, which is incised and elevated. If performed carefully, the orbit can be explored without the extrusion of retroseptal orbital fat (Fig. 5-12). With the transconjunctival approach the medial orbit can be better visualized, and inadvertant injury to the proximal lacrimal system is also less likely. Lower lid retraction or cicatricial deformity can be prevented by incorporating lower lid horizontal shortening and lateral canthal suspension at the time of closure (Fig. 5-13).

Infralid

The infralid approach involves making an incision over the inferior orbital rim in the malar area. When compared to conjunctival-lateral canthotomy and subciliary incisions, this incision provided rapid access, adequate exposure, and acceptable scars in a recent randomized prospective study.[56,58] Disadvantages include healing with cicatrix formation that results in a retracted scar, persistent lid edema, and vertical shortening of the lower lid.[56,58]

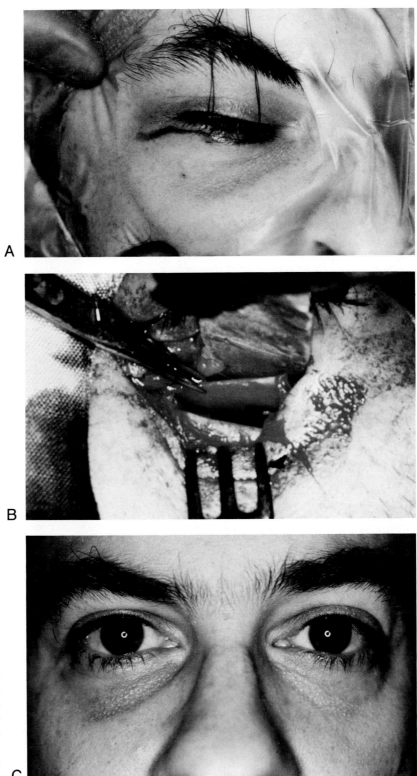

Fig. 5-10. (A) Patient being prepared for a right subciliary approach to the orbit. Note the lid traction sutures and the ink marking the proposed skin incision. **(B)** An iliac bone graft is inserted by way of a subciliary incision to reconstruct the orbital floor defect. **(C)** Patient 4 months after surgery, with inconspicuous scar.

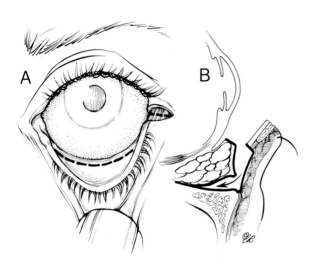

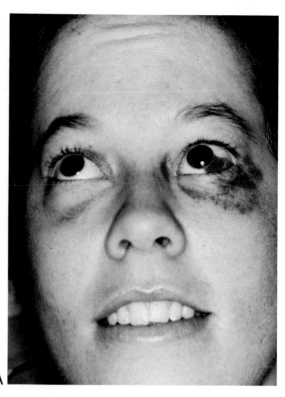

Fig. 5-11. (A) Schematic representation of lateral canthotomy, lateral canthalysis, and subtarsal transconjunctival incisions. **(B)** Cross-sectional view demonstrating the anterior septal approach to the inferior orbital rim.

Fig. 5-12. (A) Patient 3 days after left orbital injury. Note that elevation of the left globe is moderately limited, with resultant subjective diplopia. **(B)** A Waters view suggests a left orbital floor fracture with prolapse of orbital contents into the maxillary sinus. **(C)** A coronal CT scan demonstrates dehiscence in the left orbital floor, prolapse of orbital contents, and fluid in the maxillary sinus.

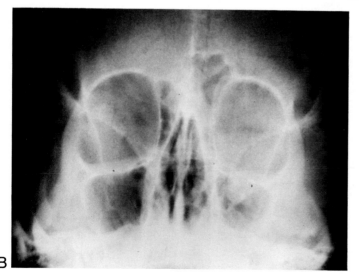

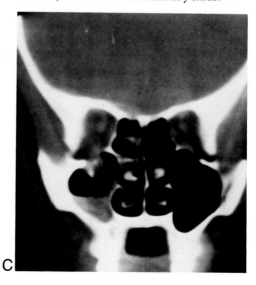

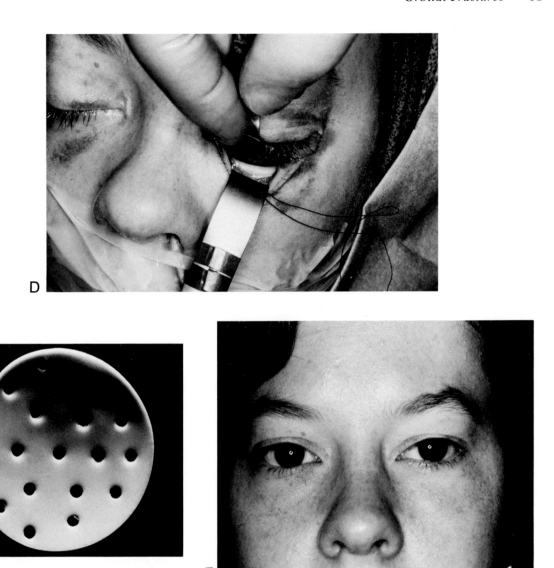

Fig. 5-12 *(Continued)*. **(D)** Discrete bony dehiscence of the orbital floor was found after repositioning of the orbital contents by way of a lateral canthal release and transconjunctival approach. **(E)** A perforated Teflon sheet was placed over the bony defect and affixed to the inferior orbital rim. **(F)** Patient 6 months after surgery. Note the good position of the lid and globe and the inconspicuous lateral canthal scar.

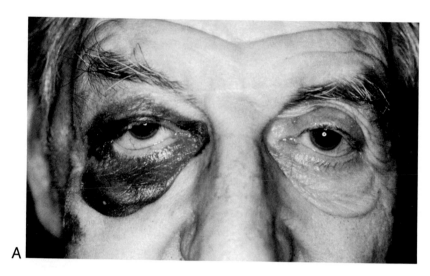

A

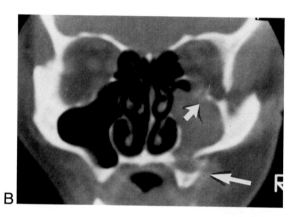

B

Fig. 5-13. **(A)** Patient 5 days after right orbital trauma. Depression of the right zygomatic arch and inferior displacement of the malar region are apparent. **(B)** A CT scan shows an orbital floor fracture, inferior and medial rotation of the zygoma, and a lateral maxillary wall fracture. **(C)** The surgical approach by way of a lateral canthal release and transconjunctival incision allowed osteosynthesis of fractures and placement of an iliac bone graft on the defects in the medial wall and floor of the orbit. *(Figure continues.)*

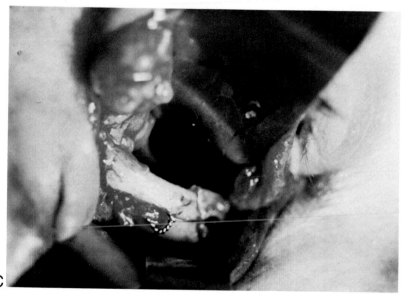

C

Direct Conjunctival

Popularized by Tenzel and Miller,[59] the direct conjunctival approach involves a direct fornix incision with a retroseptal approach to the orbital rim. Exposure is facilitated by a Desmarres retractor on the lower lid. Because this approach penetrates the orbital septum and fat, exposure is somewhat limited, and it is best suited for exploration of small blowout fractures. There is no external scar, and lower lid retraction is rare.

Caldwell-Luc

The Caldwell-Luc approach allows reduction and correction of fractures of the zygomatic complex and orbital floor by an approach through the maxillary antrum. Access into the antrum is obtained by incision through the buccal mucosa overlying the canine fossa of the maxilla. The periosteum is stripped and the antrum entered using bone drills or biting forceps. Prolapsed orbital tissue and bone

Fig. 5-13 *(Continued)*. **(D)** Patient 4 months after surgery. A right lower lid horizontal shortening and lateral canthal repositioning was performed at the time of the original orbital surgery.

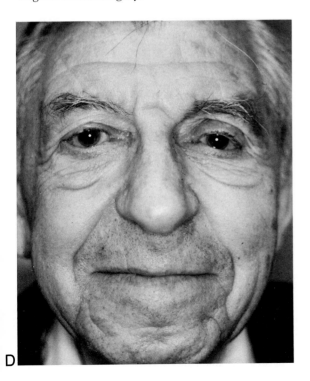

D

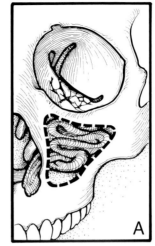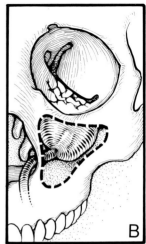

Fig. 5-14. **(A)** The Caldwell-Luc approach to the orbit allows access to the maxillary sinus (dotted lines). Elevation of bone fragments and orbital structures must be carefully performed and may be held in position with gauze packing or **(B)** a balloon catheter, which is brought out through an antrostomy.

fragments are elevated into position and held in place with packing or an intra-antral balloon catheter (Fig. 5-14). A nasoantrostomy below the inferior turbinate is performed, and the packing or catheter is brought out through the nose. The packing is left in place for 10 to 21 days. It has been advocated that the Caldwell-Luc approach should be combined with a transcutaneous or tansconjunctival eyelid approach for large comminuted floor fractures, with or without an associated zygoma fracture.[59,60] Reduction of the fracture should be observed from above and below to avoid damage to the globe from bone fragments or overreduction of the fracture. Complications which have been reported with this approach include maxillary sinusitis,[61] failure to correct extraocular motility problems,[8,62] postoperative entrapment of previously free extraocular muscles,[62] and central retinal artery and optic nerve compromise.[63,64] In treating 77 cases of orbital floor fracture, Goldman and Hessburg reported a 9 to 10 percent postoperative persistence of enophthalmos and diplopia in extreme gaze with the Caldwell-Luc antral packing method, as opposed to 14 to 16 percent postoperative persistence with prosthetic floor implant procedures.[61]

The Caldwell-Luc approach provides direct access to the maxillary antrum, and in a case of traumatic displacement of the ocular globe into this space, it allows excellent exposure and control during the repositioning of the globe (Fig. 5-15).

Orbital Reconstruction

After the orbital rim is encountered, subperiosteal elevation is extended posteriorly until the fracture is identified. Elevation of the orbital contents by careful manipulation is performed, using two retractors. Restoration of orbital floor continuity is required except in small fractures where entrapped structures can be freed and no floor defect noted. Floor reconstruction should restore orbital volume, seal off the maxillary sinus, and provide a smooth surface over which the globe and its fascia can glide. This is performed by inserting autograft or allograft material.

Autografts

For large comminuted and contaminated defects of the orbital floor, autogenous bone is considered the best substance for reconstruction. Converse et

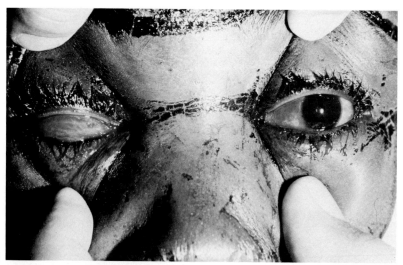

A

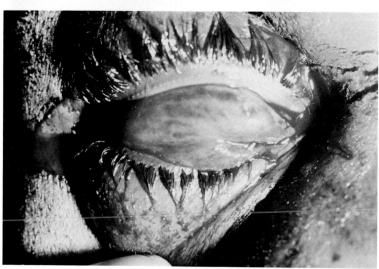

B

Fig. 5-15. (A) A forced opening of the right eyelid revealing the absence of the ocular globe. (B) Close-up view of the forced eyelid opening. *(Figure continues.)*

al.[55] recommend iliac bone grafts in adults and split rib grafts for extremely large defects in children (see Chapter 7). Other sources used for grafts are anterior maxillary bone (Fig. 5-16), the perpendicular plate of the ethmoid, and septal cartilage.[55,56] Split-thickness calvarial bone (see Chapter 7) could also be used.

Allografts

If a fracture results in a moderate-sized defect, an inorganic material such as Supramid, Silastic, Teflon, Marlex, or cranioplast can be used to fill it. Browning and Walter[65] have reported successful use of alloplasts in 75 patients with orbital floor fractures, with only one case of acute and one case of chronic infection. However, extrusion or migration of the implanted material is always a potential problem.

Children

The maxillary sinus is small in the young child and the floor of the orbit is concave, dipping behind the rim of the orbit. Despite the small size of the maxillary sinus, blowout of the orbital contents occurs by the same mechanism as in the adult, and restoration of orbital continuity by similar methods is recom-

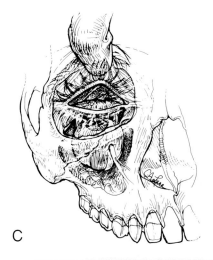

C

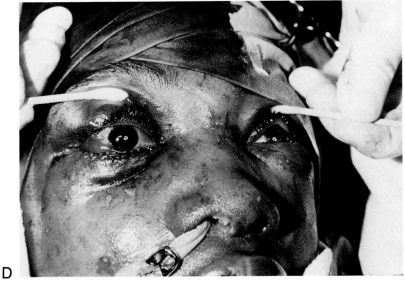

Fig. 5-15 *(Continued)*. **(C)** A schematic drawing demonstrates the traumatic displacement of the right globe into the maxillary sinus through a large floor and medial wall fracture. **(D)** An intraoperative photograph shows an adequate ocular position following a Caldwell-Luc approach with Iodoform gauze packing.

D

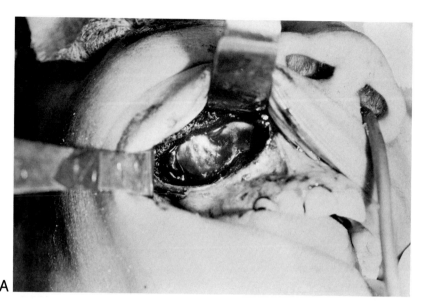

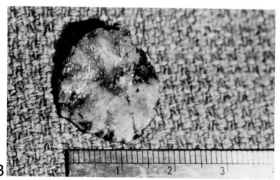

Fig. 5-16. Anterior wall graft. (A) The anterior maxilla is exposed for the harvesting of a graft in a case of pure blowout fracture. (B) Harvested graft. (C) The graft is placed to reconstruct the floor of the orbit.

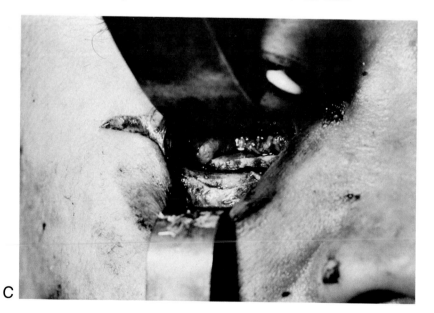

mended. Comminuted fragments should be carefully reconstructed at an earlier time post-injury, as they consolidate more rapidly in the child than in the adult.

comminuted, a thin iliac bone graft to restore contour is often required.[55] Detailed treatment of associated frontal sinus fractures is covered in Chapter 2.

OTHER FRACTURES OF THE ORBIT

Medial Wall

The medial orbital wall can be exposed by two approaches: the medially extended inferior rim route,[66] or the medial orbital Lynch approach over the anterior lacrimal crest.[67] Meticulous dissection to identify and preserve the medial canthal tendon is imperative.[66] After releasing the entrapped tissue, an autograft or allograft implant is positioned to restore the medial orbital wall continuity.[55]

Lateral Wall

Fractures of the lateral wall can be severe, causing frontozygomatic disjunction and displacement of the lateral portion of the orbital floor. A bicoronal flap for exposure, direct interosseous fragment wiring, and bone grafting to restore orbital framework are usually indicated.[55]

A direct incision over the superior lateral rim is used to repair dislocation of the frontozygomatic suture with direct fragment wiring.

Orbital Roof/Supraorbital Rim

Fractures of the orbital roof usually occur with supraorbital rim and frontal bone fractures. Therefore, a combined craniofacial approach is often required. The orbital roof is usually repaired with a bone graft after the anterior fossa is exposed and any necessary neurosurgical repairs performed.[55]

Isolated roof and arch fractures can be approached via an eyebrow incision slanted to parallel the direction of the hair follicles in the brow. If the anterior wall of the frontal sinus is severely

COMPLICATIONS

Hematoma and Blindness

Hemorrhage with an expanding hematoma can occur following repair of medial wall fractures when bleeding from the anterior and posterior ethmoidal arteries or the sinus mucosa is not controlled. Usually an orbital hemorrhage originates from the branches of the infraorbital artery or veins and resolves spontaneously. If the bleeding is severe and associated with pain, proptosis, and visual loss, orbital decompression may be necessary. If detected early, suture removal with exploration and evacuation of any hematoma is required.[55] Formal optic nerve decompression is rarely needed. Nicholson and Guzak[53] reported six cases of blindness in their series of 72 blowout fractures. They also reported another two cases upon review of the literature through 1971. Lederman in 1981 reported another five cases of blindness following orbital blowout fractures.[68] Miller et al.[69] reported a patient with a midfacial fracture who on the fourth day of observation lost visual acuity in the affected eye, which was followed by permanent optic nerve atrophy. This observation highlights the fact that blindness occurs in orbital trauma, usually from a compressive or vascular compromise of the optic nerve. Traumatic optic canal fractures may cause direct optic nerve compression or actual transection. It is generally agreed that immediate post-traumatic visual loss is not likely to recover and represents an irreversible optic nerve injury. Vision that progressively becomes worse following an injury is often favorably improved with high-dose steroid administration with or without optic nerve decompression.[70,71]

Infection

Maxillary sinusitis or infection around an implanted autograft or allograft rarely occurs and is usually controlled by appropriate antibiotic therapy. Drainage of an abscess and removal of implanted material may be required.

Extrusion of Implant

In a report of 99 cases of orbital floor reconstruction with alloplastic implants, Browning[72] noted four acute infections and three implant extrusions. Extrusions usually occurred with an associated chronic low-grade infection. Also noted were three cases of hypertropia, one case of scleral show, one case of severe allergic reaction, and two cases of self-limited orbital hemorrhage. Kroll and Wolpen[67] also noted nine cases of extrusion of synthetic implants. Six cases of visual loss reported by Nicholson and Guzak were thought to be caused either by direct optic nerve trauma or by pressure resulting from poor placement of silicone sheeting implants.[53] A case of implant migration causing lacrimal sac obstruction and dacryocystitis has also been reported.[73]

Improved results with alloplastic implants have been obtained by using an anteriorly notched tongue to prevent extrusion,[55] reapproximating periosteum over the implant,[8] anchoring the implant to bone with sutures,[74] smoothing the edges of the implant,[55] and inserting Marlex mesh implants to encourage fibrous ingrowth.[67]

Infraorbital Nerve Anesthesia or Neuralgia

Pressure on the infraorbital nerve from bone fragments in the infraorbital canal or from the alloplastic implant or autograft must be avoided. Anesthesia, hypesthesia, or panesthesia may occur from all or part of the infraorbital nerve distribution. Return of sensation may occur as late as 1 year after treatment.[55] Rarely an infraorbital neuralgia with severe pain may occur. This requires nerve decompression and neurolysis.[7]

Persistent Diplopia

It is important to distinguish diplopia in the primary field of gaze versus that occuring only in the extremes of gaze. It is also necessary to distinguish the etiology of the diplopia. A neuromuscular etiology may require up to 6 months to show any resolution. Corrective extraocular muscle surgery should be considered after this period of time. In a report of 20 patients with persistent diplopia, Harley[75] reported that inferior rectus and inferior oblique muscles entrapped in a blowout fracture for longer than 2 months failed to function even after fracture repair. Converse et al.[55] noted the most frequent cause of persistent postoperative diplopia was failure to free entrapped tissue at the primary surgical intervention. Harley recommends orbital exploration to release entrapped orbital contents. If diplopia persists longer than 3 months following the orbital release, corrective extraocular muscle surgery is recommended. In his 20 cases, 3 were corrected completely, and 17 cases were able to achieve fusion in primary and reading positions.

Ectropion or Vertical Lid Retraction

Lower lid malpositions ranging from scleral show to frank ectropion may occur. This usually results from a scar contracture of the orbital septum to the lid structures. Reconstruction requires a lysis of the adhesions and repositioning of the eyelid.

Persistent Enophthalmos

Despite adequate reduction of orbital fractures, enophthalmos may develop. Several etiologies have been postulated, but orbital fat displacement from the muscle cone, fat atrophy, and persistently increased orbital volume best explain the condition.

If surgical intervention is delayed more than 2 months, the mobilization of tissue is restricted by scar and early fibrous union of the fracture fragments. Late correction of post-traumatic enophthalmos requires determination of whether the globe will be easily displaced anteriorly; this is accomplished by the forced forward-traction test, which consists of grasping the insertions of the medial and lateral recti muscles on the globe and applying an anteriorly directed force. If the globe is easily displaced, correction of the enophthalmos is more predictable.

Late correction of enophthalmos requires complete periosteal release of any adhesions, insertion of iliac bone grafts, and in some cases selected orbital marginal osteotomies.[1] Iliac bone is harvested, appropriately shaped, and inserted into the orbital cavity to elevate and anteriorly project the globe.[76] A lateral wall medial displacement has been shown to decrease orbital volume and assist in correction of the enophthalmos.[1] Additional bone grafts can be placed in the medial orbit via a medial canthal incision. Bone grafts in the posterior-superior and lateral orbit may be placed through a lateral canthal or eyebrow incision. An attempt should be made to place graft material behind the equator of the globe in an effort to project it into an overcorrected position.

Extensive loss of the bony orbital floor with disruption of the inferior fascial support system and Lockwood's suspensory ligament can result in an inferiorly displaced globe. This is termed ocular hypotropia and must be differentiated from orbital dystopia resulting from bony malalignment. Correction of ocular hypotropia entails appropriately placed orbital floor bone grafts and fascial suspension at the lateral canthus. Orbital dystopia requires selected osteotomies and movement of the orbit with its contents.

REFERENCES

1. Kawamoto HK Jr: Late posttraumatic enophthalmos: A correctable deformity. Plast Reconstr Surg 69:423, 1980
2. Schultz RC: Supraorbital and glabellar fractures. Plast Reconstr Surg 45:227, 1970
3. Garrett JW: Ocular-orbital Injuries in Automobile Accidents. Bull, No. 4 Automotive Crash Injury Research of the Cornell Aeronautical Laboratory, Inc. Buffalo, NY, 1963
4. Converse JM, Smith B, Obear MF, Wood-Smith D: Orbital blowout fractures: A ten year study. Plast Reconstr Surg 39:20, 1967
5. Cramer LM, Tooze FM, Lerman S: Blowout fractures of the orbit. Br J Plast Surg 18:171, 1965
6. Converse JM, Smith B: Enophthalmos and diplopia in fracture of the orbital floor. Br J Plast Surg 9:265, 1957
7. Converse JM, Smith B: Blowout fracture of the floor of the orbital. Trans Am Acad Ophthalmol Otol 64:676, 1960
8. Emery JM, von Noorden GK, Schlernitzaver DA: Orbital floor fractures: Long term follow-up of cases with and without surgical repair. Trans Am Acad Ophthalmol Otol 75:802, 1971
9. Gould HR, Titus O: Internal orbital fractures: The value of laminography in diagnosis. Am J Roent 97:618, 1966
10. Jones DE, Evans JNG: Blowout fractures of the orbit: An investigation into their anatomical basis. J Laryng 81:1109, 1967
11. Dodick MM, Galin MA, Lilleton JT, Sod LM: Concomitant medial wall fracture and blowout fractures of the orbital. Arch
12. LaGrange F: De l'anaPlerose orbitaire. Bull Acad Natl Med Paris 80:64, 1918
13. Zismor T, Noyek AM: Orbital trauma. p. 551. In Potts DG (ed): Radiology of the Skull and Brain. C.V. Mosby, St. Louis, 1971
14. Sato O, Kamitani H, Kokunai T: Blow-in fracture of both orbital roofs caused by shear strain of the skull. J Neurosurg 49:734, 1978
15. Pfeiffer RL: Traumatic enophthalmos. Am J Ophthalmol 30:718, 1943
16. Smith B, Regan WF Jr: Blowout fracture of the orbit: Mechanism and correction of internal orbital fracture. Am J Ophthalmol 44:733, 1957
17. Kazanjian VH, Converse JM: The Surgical Treatment of Facial Injuries. Williams & Wilkins, Baltimore, 1959
18. McCoy FJ, Chendlen RA, Magnan CG, Moore JR: An analysis of facial fractures and their complications. Plast Reconstr Surg 29:381, 1962
19. Fradkin AH: Orbital floor fractures and ocular complications. Am J Ophthalmol 72:699, 1971
20. Miller GR, Tenzel RR: Ocular complications of midfacial fractures. Plast Reconstr Surg 39:37, 1967
21. Herzzov V: Signs, therapy and follow-up of cases with pure blowout fractures of the orbit. Albrecht Von Grates Arch Klin Ophthalmol 196(2):143, 1975
22. Leibsohn J, Burton TC, Scott WE: Orbital floor fractures: A retrospective study. Ann Ophthalmol

8:1057, 1976

23. Jabaley MD, Lerman M, Saunders H: Ocular injury in orbital fractures: A review of 119 cases. Plast Reconstr Surg 56:410, 1975

24. Milauskas AT, Fueger GF: Serious ocular complications associated with blowout fractures of the orbit. Am J Ophthalmol 62:670, 1966

25. Tajima S, Fujino T, Oshiro T: Mechanism of orbital blowout fractures. I. Stress coat test. Keio J Med 23:71, 1974

26. Fujino T: Mechanism of orbital blowout fractures. II. Analysis by high speed camera in two dimensional eye models. Keio J Med 23:115, 1974

27. Fujino T: Experimental blowout fracture of the orbit. Plast Reconstr Surg 54:81, 1974

28. King EF: Disease of the orbit and sphenoidal sinus fractures of the orbit. Tans Ophthalmol Soc UK 64:134, 1977

29. Putterman AM: New surgical management of blowout fractures of the orbital floor. Am S Ophthalmol 77:212, 1974

30. Hoffman WB: Injuries to the zygomatic and maxillary bones. Otol Clin North Am 2:303, 1969

31. DeMan K, Wingaarde R: Downward displacement of the eye resulting from orbital emphyema. J Maxillofac Surg 8:152, 1980

32. Habal MB, Beart R, Murray JF: Fractures of the orbital floor. Am J Surg 123:606, 1972

33. Rougier MJ: Resultants fonctinonels due traitement chirurgical des paralysies oculaires secondaires aux tramatismes de la face. Bull Soc Ophthalmol Fr 65:502, 1965

34. Prasad SS: Blowout fracture of the medial wall of the orbit. p. 23. In Bleeker GM (ed): Second International Symposium on Orbital Disorders. Vol. 14. Karger, Stockholm, 1975

35. Edwards WC, Ridley RW: Blowout fracture of the medial orbital wall. Am J Ophthalmol 65:248, 1968

36. Rumelt MD, Ernst JT: Isolated blowout fracture of the medial wall of the orbit with medial rectus entrapment. Am J Ophthalmol 73:451, 1972

37. Leone CR Jr, Lloyd WC III, Rylander G: Surgical repair of medial wall fractures. Am J Ophthalmol 97:349, 1984

38. Davidson TM, Oleson RM, Nahum AM: Medial orbital wall fracture with rectus entrapment. Arch Otolaryngol 101:33, 1975

39. McClurg FL, Swanson PJ: An orbital roof fracture causing diplopia. Arch Otolaryngol 102:497, 1976

40. Curtin HD, Wolf P, Schramn V: Orbital root blowout fractures. AJR 139:969, 1982

41. Zismor T, Smith B, Fasano C, Converse JM: Roentgen diagnosis of blowout fractures of the orbit. Am J Roentgenol 87:1009, 1962

42. Fueger GF, Milauskas AT, Britton W: Roentgenological evaluation of the orbital blowout injuries. Am J Roentgenol 97:614, 1966

43. Crickelair G, Rein J, Potter G: A critical look at blowout fractures. Plast Reconstr Surg 49:374, 1972

44. Grove AS Jr, Tadmor R, New PF, Momore KS: Orbital fracture evaluation by coronal computed tomography. Am J Ophthalmol 85:679, 1978

45. Yamamoto Y, Sakusai M, Asari S: Towne and semisagittal CT in the evaluation of blowout fracture of the orbit. J CAT 2:306, 1983

46. Zilkha A: CT of blowout fracture of the medial orbital wall. AJNR 2:427, 1981

47. Grove AS: Orbital trauma and CT. Ophthalmology 87:403, 1980

48. Hammerschlag SB, Hughes S, O'Reiley GV, et al: Blowout fracture of the orbit: A comparison of CT and conventional radiography with anatomic correlation. Radiology 143:487, 1982

49. Kassel EE, Noyek AM, Cooper PW: CT in facial trauma. J Otolaryngol 12:10, 1983

50. Grove AS Jr: Orbital trauma evaluation by CT. Int Ophthalmol Clin 22:133, 1982

51. Noyek AM, Kassel EE: CT in frontal sinus fractures. Arch Otolaryngol 108:378, 1982

52. Helveston EM: The relationship of extraocular muscle problems to orbital floor fractures: Early and late management. Trans Am Acad Ophthalmol Otol 63:660, 1976

53. Nicholson H, Guzak SV: Visual loss complication repair of orbital floor fractures. Arch Ophthalmol 86:369, 1971

54. Converse JM, Smith B: On the treatment of blowout fractures of the orbit. Plast Reconstr Surg 62:100, 1978

55. Converse JM: Reconstructive Plastic Surgery. Vol. II. W.B. Saunders, Philadelphia, 1977

56. Wray, RC, Holtmann B, Ribando JM, et al: A comparison of conjunctival and subciliary inciliary incisions for orbital fractures. Br J Plast Surg 30:142, 1977

57. Converse JM, Firmin F, Wood-Smith D, Friedland JA: The conjunctival approach in orbital fractures. Plast Reconstr Surg 52:656, 1973

58. Holtmann B, Wray RC, Lilthe A: A randomized comparison of four incisions for orbital fracture. Plast Reconstr Surg 67:731, 1973

59. Tenzel RR, Miller GR: Orbital fracture repair, conjunctival approach. Am J Ophthalmol 71:1141, 1971

60. Aeillo LM, Myers E: Blowout Fractures of the Orbi-

tal Floor. Arch Otolaryngol 82:638, 1965

61. Abrahams JW, Dodd RW: A combined procedure of early surgical management. Arch Ophthalmol 68:169, 1962

62. Goldman RJ, Hessburg PC: Appraisal of surgical correction in 130 cases of orbital floor fracture. Am J Ophthalmol 76:152, 1973

63. Butler MR, Morledge D, Holt GD: A system of surgical approaches to orbital floor fractures. Trans Am Ophthalmol Soc O 75:519, 1971

64. Nicholson DH, Guzak SV: Visual loss complicating repair of orbital floor fractures. Arch Ophthalmol 86:369, 1971

65. Mandel M: Orbital floor blowout fractures, reconstruction using autogenous maxillary wall bone grafts. Am J Surg 130:590, 1975

66. Smith B, Putterman A: Fixation of orbital floor implants. Arch Ophthalmol 83:598, 1970

67. Kroll M, Wolpen J: Orbital blowout fractures. Am J Ophthalmol 64:1169, 1967

68. Lederman IR: Loss of vision associated with surgical treatment of zygomatic-orbital floor fracture. Plast Reconst Surg 68:94, 1981

69. Harley RD: Surgical management of persistent diplopia in blowout fractures of the orbit. Ann Ophthalmol 7:1621, 1975

70. Kennerdell JS, Amsbaugh GA, Myers EN: Transantral-ethmoidal decompression of optic canal fracture. Arch Ophthalmol 94:1040, 1976

71. Anderson RL, Panje WR, Gross CE: Optic nerve blindness following blunt forehead trauma. Ophthalmology 89:445, 1982

72. Browning CW, Walker RV: The use of alloplastics in 75 cases of orbital floor reconstruction. Am J Ophthalmol 60:684, 1964

73. Gozum E: Blowout fracture of the orbit. p. 477. In symposium on Maxillofacial Trauma. Otolaryngol Clin North Am 9:317, 1976

74. Kohn R, Romano PE, Puklin JE: Lacrimal obstruction after migration of orbital floor implant. Am J Ophthalmol 82:934, 1976

75. Mathog R: Reconstruction of the orbit following trauma. p. 585. In Symposium on Trauma to the Head and Neck. Otolaryngol Clin North Am 16:471, 1983

76. Mustardé JC: Repair/Reconstruction in the Orbital Region. Williams & Wilkins, Baltimore, 1971

SUGGESTED READINGS

Bloem JJ, Meulen JC, Ramselaar JM: Orbital roof fractures. Mod Probl Ophthalmol 14:510, 1975

Browning CW: Alloplast material in orbital repair. Am J Ophthalmol 63:955, 1967

Converse JM, Cole JG, Smith B: Late treatment of blowout fracture of the orbit. Plast Reconstr Surg 28:183, 1961

Dortzbach RK: Orbital floor fractures. Ophthalmic Plast Reconstr Surg 1:149, 1985

Dulley B, Fells P: Long-term follow-up of orbital blow-out fracture with and without surgery. Mod Probl Ophthalmol 14:467, 1975

Margarone JE: Lateral orbital rim fracture: An usual case. J Am Dent Assoc 105:657, 1982

Miller GR: Blindness developing a few days after a midfacial fracture. Plast Reconstr Surg 42:387, 1968

Mustardé JC, Jones LT, Callahan A: Ophthalmic Plastic Surgery. p. 190. Aesculapius, Birmingham, AL, 1970

Newmark H, Kant N, Duerksen R, Pribram HW: Orbital floor fracture: An unusual complication. Neurosurgery 12(5):555, 1983

Smith B, Griffiths JD: Optic atrophy following Caldwell-Luc procedure. Arch Ophthalmol 86:15, 1971

Strane MF, Gustavson EH: Primary treatment of fractures of the orbital roof. Proc R Soc Lon 66:303, 1973

Wilkens RB, Havins WE: Current treatment of blow-out fractures. Ophthalmology 89:464, 1982

Orbital Adnexal Injuries

6

Richard Dean Lisman
Henry M. Spinelli

In an increasingly mobile and violent society, orbital adnexal trauma is commonly encountered by surgeons treating midfacial injuries. In general, trauma to the orbital region can be classified as blunt trauma or penetrating injuries. Each of these two groups can be further subdivided into injuries sustained by (1) objects of greater dimension than the horizontal aperture of the orbit, which cause adnexal injury and (2) objects that easily fit into the horizontal orbital dimension, which cause globe injury.

ANATOMY

The anatomy of the orbit must be briefly reviewed to elucidate the pathophysiology and treatment of blunt injuries to the globe (see Chapter 5). The orbit is made up of seven bones (Fig. 6-1) with the bony abutments of the external orbital aperture comprised of four firm bones: (1) the supraorbital arch and nasal spine of the frontal bone superiorly,

(2) the zygomatic process of the frontal bone and frontal process of the zygoma laterally, (3) the zygoma and maxilla inferiorly, and (4) the frontal process of the maxilla and nasal bones medially. The medial wall is made up of a complex arrangement of fragile bones including the lacrimal bone and thin lamina papyracea of the ethmoid. The floor of the orbit consists of maxillary, sphenoid, and ethmoid bones. An object such as a fist or ball of greater dimension than the vertical or horizontal diameter of the orbit will rarely fracture the orbital rim, unless the rim is struck obliquely or directly with extreme force (Fig. 6-2). Instead, forces are transmitted upon the globe back into the orbital apex pushing orbital fat and connective tissue septa away from the globe. The thinnest margins of the orbit, the orbital floor and medial wall, are first to "blow out." Blunt injuries sustained with objects of greater diameter than the orbital rim will produce orbital fractures. Injuries received with objects of lesser diameter than the horizontal orbital aperture can create globe, lid, and lacrimal injuries (Fig. 6-3).

A red eye that presents after trauma may indicate a number of common ocular abnormalities. A simple corneal abrasion will produce conjunctival injection and require pressure patching of the in-

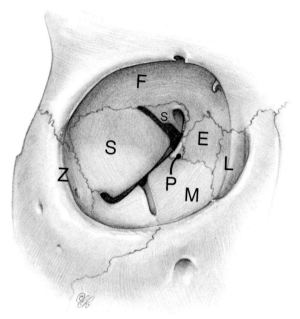

Fig. 6-1. The seven bones of the orbit. F, Frontal; S, Sphenoid (greater wing); s, Sphenoid (lesser wing); E, Ethmoid; L, Lacrimal; P. Palatine; M, Maxilla; Z, Zygoma.

(Fig. 6-4).

Ciliary injection, characterized by perilimbal vascular engorgement, may be indicative of traumatic iritis (Fig. 6-5). This is diagnosed by slit-lamp examination revealing inflammatory cells and flare within the anterior chamber of the eye. Iritis must be treated with topical dilitation of the pupil and topical corticosteroids. The globe must be inspected for obvious conjunctival or scleral tears. An equatorial or posterior globe rupture not obvious on superficial examination may present with low or absent intraocular pressure. After blunt trauma, intraocular pressures of the involved and uninvolved globes must be compared, and the globe with a lowered intraocular pressure should be suspected of having an equatorial or posterior globe rupture.

A hyphema (Fig. 6-6), or hemorrhage into the anterior chamber, usually results from microscopic tears in either the iris or ciliary body. This is a common and very serious complication of an ocular contusion. A hyphema may be small and imperceptible without a slit-lamp, or large and grossly apparent. A patient who presents with a hyphema should be admitted to the hospital and aggressively treated.

Blunt trauma with objects of a size smaller than the external orbital dimensions can cause shearing or disinsertion of the levator aponeurosis (Fig. 6-7). Following blunt or penetrating trauma, a levator aponeurosis disinsertion or dehiscence should be suspected if an obvious superficial lid

volved lid to allow the cornea to heal. If the lids are immobilized so that blinking is eliminated, the corneal epithelium will grow from the margins of the corneal defect to fill the abraded site within 24 to 48 hours, depending on the size of the abrasion

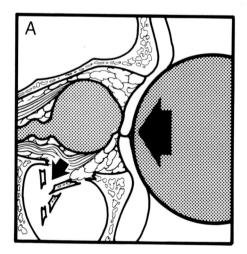

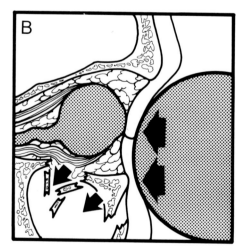

Fig. 6-2. Objects of greater diameter than the horizontal dimension of the orbit usually produce fractures, not globe trauma. (**A**) Pure blowout fracture. (**B**) Impure blowout fracture.

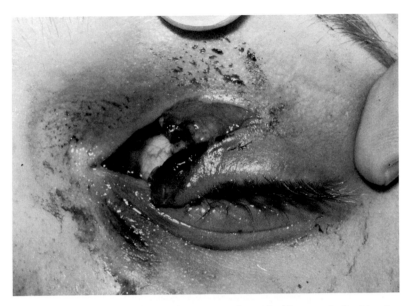

Fig. 6-3. Canalicular and eyelid laceration from the blunt end of a ski pole. This patient also sustained traumatic iritis due to the contusion.

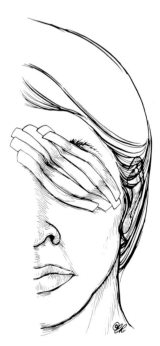

Fig. 6-4. Treatment of a corneal abrasion. Eyelid immobilization by pressure patching. The corneal epithelium regenerates within 24 to 48 hours if the upper lid is immobilized.

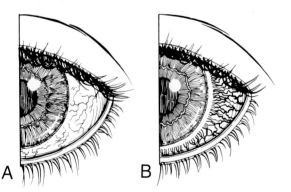

Fig. 6-5. **(A)** Conjunctival injection seen after any globe irritation or conjunctivitis. **(B)** Ciliary injection noted with a corneal abrasion or iritis.

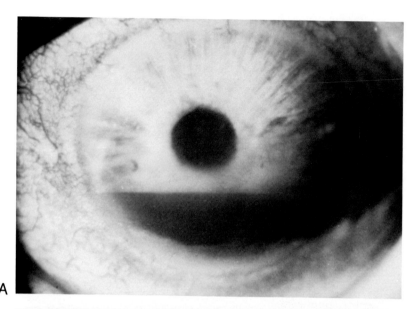

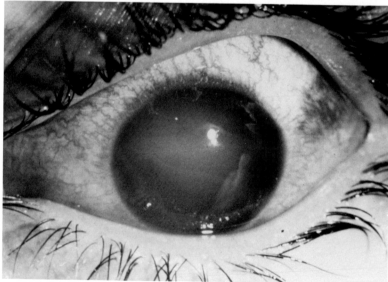

Fig. 6-6. Traumatic hyphema following blunt globe injury. (A) A 25 percent hyphema. (B) A total (100 percent) hyphema.

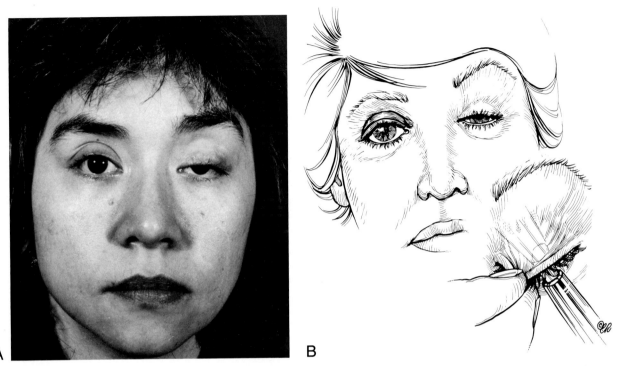

A   B

Fig. 6-7. (A) Ptosis created by a levator dehiscence or disinsertion. The eyelid crease is absent, and (B) the eyelid may be more easily transilluminated than the unaffected upper eyelid.

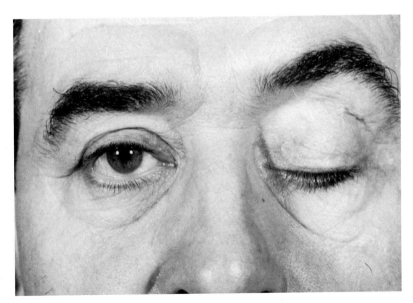

Fig. 6-8. Levator dehiscence secondary to a horizontal eyelid laceration above the eyelid margin.

laceration is not noted, with the eyelid remaining ptotic following resolution of edema. Penetrating injuries to the lid at any level above the lid margin are likely to tear the levator aponeurosis and/or levator muscle. Lacerations that are small or vertical rarely create blepharoptosis. Lacerations that are large and/or horizontal are likely to cause levator disinsertion with ptosis (Fig. 6-8). Finally, trauma in the naso-orbital region of the eyelids may involve the lacrimal excretory system. Blunt trauma without laceration may temporarily interrupt the action of the orbicularis muscle. The orbicularis aids in tear outflow through the lacrimal pump mechanism. Trauma or lacerations of the punctal and/or canalicular system may complicate blunt or penetrating injuries to the medial orbit (Fig. 6-9).

EVALUATION OF THE PATIENT FOLLOWING TRAUMA

Knowledge of the type of injury sustained can prove extremely helpful to the physician in subsequent treatment. History of the size of the object that struck the globe, the direction of the blow, and any history of penetrating injury are important. An ophthalmic exam consisting of visual acuity, pupillary function, extraocular motility, slit-lamp exami-

nation of the globe, and examination of the posterior pole, vitreous, and retina by indirect ophthalmoscopy are mandatory.

Closed head trauma with or without associated orbital trauma may produce neuro-ophthalmologic findings. Pupillary size, shape, symmetry, and both direct and consensual light reflexes should be noted. In order to have intact pupillomotor function, both pupils must constrict equally and symmetrically when light is directed into either eye. For example, direct or indirect trauma to the right optic nerve may interrupt afferent input from the right, and as a result, light shone into the left pupil may create both left and right pupillary constriction; when light is immediately switched to the right rather than the left eye, the right pupil dilates to its baseline size. This demonstrates a right afferent pupillary defect or Marcus-Gunn pupil (Fig. 6-10). Decreased visual acuity associated with a Marcus-Gunn pupil may be seen when a fracture through the apex of the orbit causes optic nerve compression from bone or from hemorrhage into the optic nerve sheath. Extraocular motion should be tested in all fields of gaze (Fig. 6-11). Paralysis or limited range of motion of the globe suggests damage to the extraocular muscles or their nerve supply.

Blowout fractures of the orbit, particularly floor fractures, may create muscle entrapment and thereby limit globe movement (Fig. 6-12) (see Fig. 7-13; also Fig. 5-4). Enophthalmos, a second sign of orbital floor fracture (Fig. 6-13), may be masked by some degree of proptosis due to edema or hemorrhage. Rarely, trauma to the orbit may damage structures that pass through the superior orbital fissure, producing any combination of motor and sensory findings (superior orbital fissure syndrome). These structures include cranial nerves III, IV, V, and VI and the superior ophthalmic vein. Painful ophthalmoplegia and pupillomotor dys-

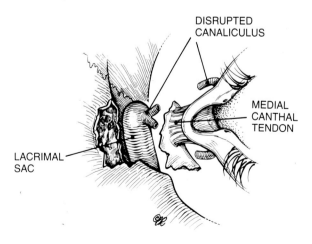

DISRUPTED CANALICULUS

MEDIAL CANTHAL TENDON

LACRIMAL SAC

Fig. 6-9. Medial canthal trauma may sever all or part of the canalicular system and medial canthal tendon. Direct trauma can sever the canaliculi, or bony fractures can displace the system. The lacrimal sac is usually uninvolved because it is protected by the canthal tendon, but any degree of trauma can fracture the bony nasolacrimal canal, creating an outflow obstruction that is noted late after trauma.

AFFECTED   UNAFFECTED

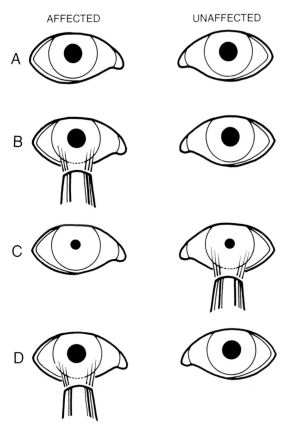

Fig. 6-10. A right afferent pupillary defect (Marcus-Gunn pupil). The light is moved from pupil to pupil (**A–D**), allowing enough time to note the functioning consensual reflex from the uninvolved eye. This is viewed as a "dilatation" of the involved pupil under direct light stimulation. The dilatation is apparent following consensual constriction of the uninvolved eye.

function are the most likely findings.

When assessing trauma to the orbital adnexa, the level of the upper lid, degree of levator function, and presence or absence of a lid crease should be determined (Fig. 6-14). This can be performed by measuring the dimensions of the palpebral fissures on both the involved and uninvolved eye in primary position as well as in upgaze and downgaze. An eyelid with an absent eyelid crease is to be suspected of having a levator disinsertion. An eyelid with minimal levator function is to be suspected of having a complete levator muscle rupture or disinsertion. The levels and presence or absence of lid creases must be compared and recorded. Post-traumatic edema or hematoma formation will create temporary ptosis (Fig. 6-15). Minimal eyelid ptosis presenting with a good eyelid crease may resolve with the clearing of edema and creation of a fibrous scar within the levator; if so, the eyelid usually becomes elevated within 2 to 6 weeks after the initial trauma. Lid lacerations not involving the lid margin may involve the levator muscle or the levator aponeurosis. In these cases the levator will fibrose and even the most ptotic of lids will elevate a few millimeters with time, if conservative treatment is followed. Isolated, direct trauma to the medial and lateral canthal tendons is rare. More commonly, a trimalar or tripod fracture of the orbit will

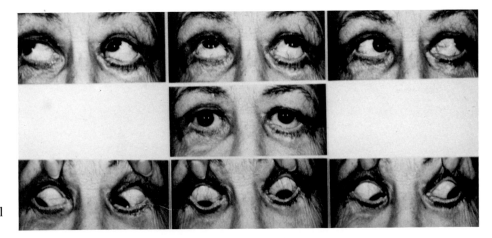

Fig. 6-11. Cardinal fields of gaze.

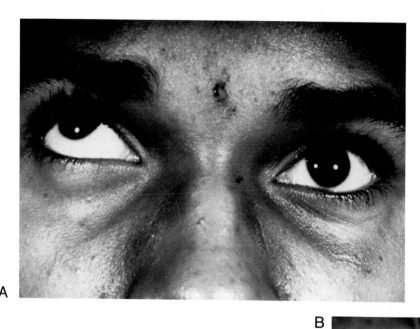

A

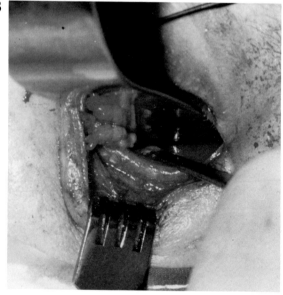

B

Fig. 6-12. (A) Limitation of upward gaze after trauma to the left orbit. (B) Entrapment of inferior orbital contents and the inferior rectus muscle following orbital blowout fracture.

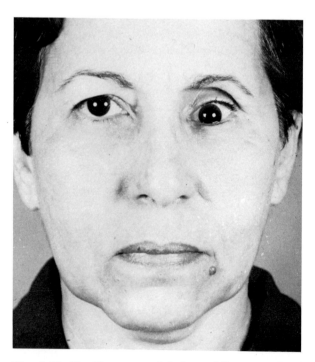

Fig. 6-13. Significant enophthalmos following orbital floor fracture.

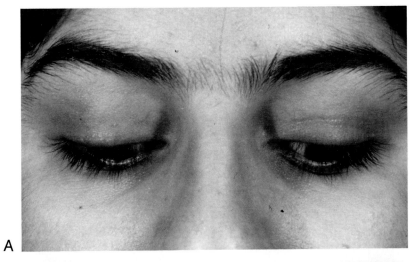

A

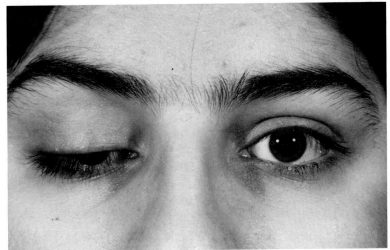

B

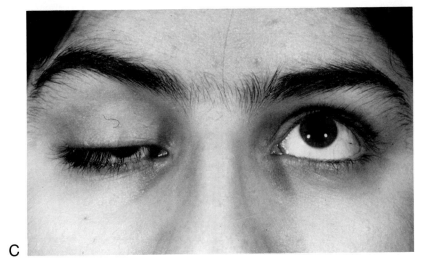

Fig. 6-14. With a millimeter rule, the degree of levator function is measured as eyelid excursion from extreme downgaze to extreme upgaze. In this case, the function is poor, only 2 to 3 mm. (**A**) Downward gaze. (**B**) Straight gaze. (**C**) Upward gaze.

C

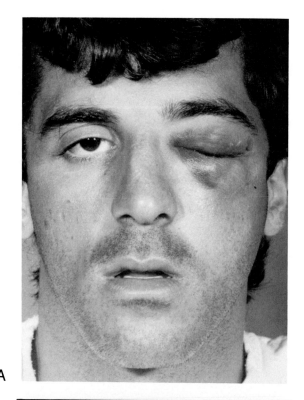

A

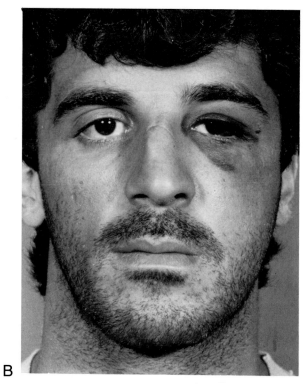

B

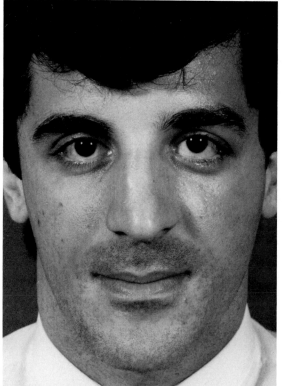

C

Fig. 6-15. (**A**) Ptosis of the upper eyelid due to edema and ecchymosis following an orbital blowout fracture. (**B&C**) Within 2 weeks, the ptosis and ecchymosis have completely resolved.

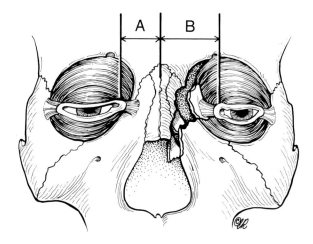

Fig. 6-16. The presence of traumatic telecanthus is determined by measuring from the midline of the nose to the inner canthal angle. If the injury is old, the bony overgrowth must be removed prior to replacing the medial canthal structures by transnasal wiring or canthoplasty (see Chapter 4).

Fig. 6-17. Five layers of upper eyelid anatomy: skin, orbicularis muscle, levator aponeurosis, Müller's muscle, and tarsus and conjunctiva.

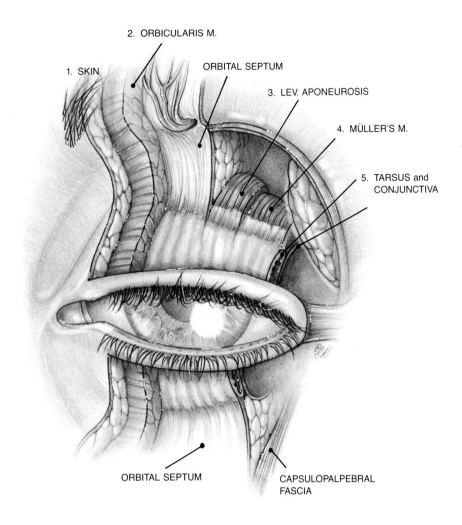

2. ORBICULARIS M.

1. SKIN

ORBITAL SEPTUM

3. LEV. APONEUROSIS

4. MÜLLER'S M.

5. TARSUS and CONJUNCTIVA

ORBITAL SEPTUM

CAPSULOPALPEBRAL FASCIA

Fig. 6-18. The orbicularis oculi muscle is divided into three parts: pretarsal, preseptal, and orbital. The tarsi join medially to create the medial canthal tendon. The pretarsal and preseptal muscles divide into superficial and deep heads, which envelop the lacrimal sac. This lacrimal diaphragm is known as the lacrimal pump. When contracted, the lacrimal pump propels tears down the nasolacrimal duct.

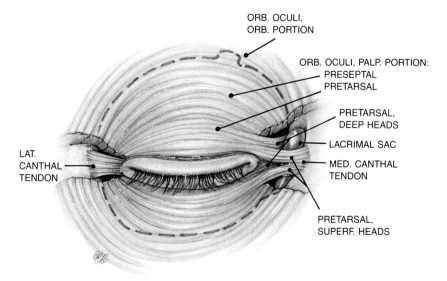

ORB. OCULI, ORB. PORTION

ORB. OCULI, PALP. PORTION:
PRESEPTAL
PRETARSAL

PRETARSAL, DEEP HEADS

LACRIMAL SAC

MED. CANTHAL TENDON

LAT. CANTHAL TENDON

PRETARSAL, SUPERF. HEADS

displace the lateral canthal tendon inferiorly (see Chapter 7). Naso-orbital fractures that sever or displace the medial canthal tendon create traumatic telecanthus (Fig. 6-16) (see Chapter 4).

Clinically the eyelid is divided into five layers from anterior to posterior: (1) skin, (2) orbicularis muscle and submuscular fascia (protractors of the eyelid), (3) levator muscle and its aponeurosis (retractors of the eyelid), (4) Müller's muscle, and (5) tarsus and conjunctiva (Fig. 6-17). The lower eyelid is analogous to the upper except that the levator complex is replaced by the capsulopalpebral fascia, which is an extension off the inferior rectus muscle. This occupies an analogous position to the levator aponeurosis of the upper eyelid.

The orbicularis muscle of both upper and lower eyelids is divided into orbital and palpebral portions. The palpebral portion is further subdivided into pretarsal and preseptal orbicularis (Fig. 6-18). The pretarsal orbicularis of both upper and lower eyelids divides medially into a superficial and deep head. The deep head of the pretarsal orbicularis inserts on the posterior lacrimal crest. The superficial heads unite to form the medial canthal tendon, which is a firm fibrous structure inserting anteriorly on the anterior lacrimal crest. The preseptal muscle also divides into superficial and deep heads,

with the deep head inserting into the posterior lacrimal fascia. The complex of pretarsal and preseptal muscles, with both superficial and deep heads enveloping the lacrimal sac, creates a lacrimal pump mechanism. Laterally, the tarsi of both upper and lower eyelids join to form the lateral canthal tendon, which inserts on the lateral orbital tubercle just within the lateral orbital rim. The tarsi of both upper and lower eyelids are located distally and are composed of dense connective tissue. The tarsus of the upper eyelid is approximately 10 mm in height, while the tarsus of the lower eyelid is only 5 to 6 mm in height. A 3-mm strip of tarsus in both upper and lower eyelids is all that is necessary to maintain the integrity of the eyelid margins and direct the eyelids and their lashes in the proper directions (Fig. 6-19). When tarsus is traumatically avulsed from the upper eyelid near or at the lid margin, entropion and trichiasis may result, especially if the posterior lamella of the lower eyelid is absent (Fig. 6-20).

The lacrimal system is composed of punctal ampullae within upper and lower eyelids that drain into the vertical 2-mm portion of the canalicular system. Each canaliculus then turns medially for 6 mm to unite and form a common canaliculus (Fig. 6-21). In approximately 90 percent of cases, the

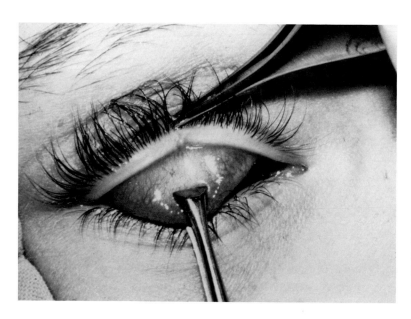

Fig. 6-19. The tarsus of the upper eyelid averages 10 mm in height; only 3 to 4 mm are required to maintain the integrity of the upper eyelid and properly direct the lashes away from the cornea.

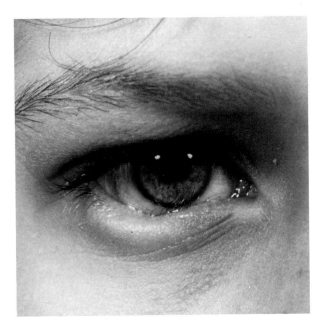

Fig. 6-20. Trichiasis and entropion of the lower eyelid are seen following a chemical burn to the posterior lamella of the lid and the subsequent shortening of tarsus and conjunctiva.

common canaliculus empties into the lacrimal sac at one juncture only. Approximately 10 percent of the population are without a common canaliculus, and in these individuals both upper and lower canaliculi enter separately into the lacrimal sac. The dome of the lacrimal sac rises over the medial canthal tendon but is collapsed except during eyelid closure. When the eyelids are open, both puncta ampullae are dilated and tears are directed along the lacus lacrimalis toward the open punctum. The pretarsal orbicularis contracts with blinking, resulting in a shortened horizontal canaliculus and tears being pumped toward the lacrimal sac (Fig. 6-22). The deep heads of the pretarsal and preseptal muscles open the lacrimal sac on eyelid closure, and a negative pressure is created within the lacrimal sac that draws the tears toward the sac. This cycle continues during eyelid opening when tears within the sac are forced down through the nasolacrimal duct. The lacrimal sac is approximately 10 mm in length. The dome of the sac is collapsed above the medial canthal tendon and is 3 to 4 mm in length. The fundus of the sac is 6 to 8 mm and the nasolacrimal duct is 10 to 12 mm in length. The duct opens 5 mm inferiorly to the vault of the anterior end of inferonasal meatus and approximately 35 mm from the entrance to the nares (Fig. 6-21).

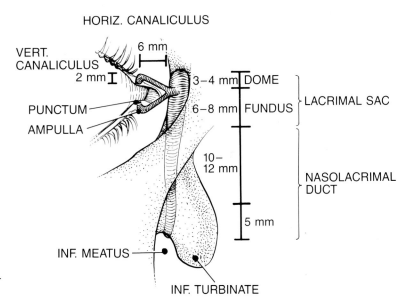

Fig. 6-21. Anatomy of the canalicular lacrimal outflow system.

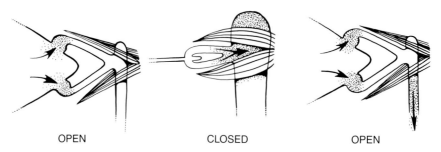

Fig. 6-22. Tears fall into the open punctal system and are propelled toward the sac by negative sac pressure. The sac collapses when the eyelids open and fills with tears that are propelled down the nasolacrimal duct by the lacrimal pump (contraction of superficial and deep heads of the pretarsal and preseptal muscles).

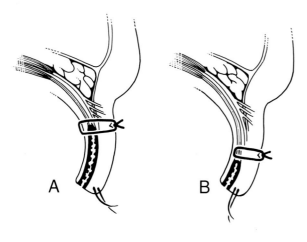

Fig. 6-23. **(A)** The eyelid fold can be recreated with a controlled scar in lacerations paralleling the lid margin. Skin edges are sutured to deep eyelid tissue by a through-and-through chromic mattress suture superior to the tarsal margin. **(B)** Alternatively, silk sutures running from the anterior eyelid surface may be used to secure skin to deep tissue. If the sutures are placed on the superior edge of tarsus, a fulcrum effect is created, rotating the eyelashes away from the cornea. If the lashes are not rotated following a through-and-through eyelid incision, ptotic lashes will produce an unsatisfactory result.

TREATMENT

Globe Injuries

The most common globe injury that results from either blunt or penetrating trauma is corneal abrasion. A defect in corneal epithelium will cause ciliary injection of the conjunctiva, epiphora, foreign body sensation, and rhinorrhea secondary to excess tearing. Treatment of corneal abrasions includes the installation of topical antibiotics and pressure patching of the globe (see Fig. 6-4). The immobilization of the upper eyelid allows the corneal epithelium from the surrounding area to migrate and fill the gap caused by the injury.

Traumatic Iritis and Hyphema

The aqueous humor flows from the posterior to the anterior chamber of the eye and is normally devoid of cells and protein. Blunt or penetrating trauma to the globe causes injury to the anterior uveal tract, with increased vascular permeability and leakage of inflammatory cells and protein into the aqueous humor. Under slit-lamp examination this leakage appears as free-floating cells within the aqueous humor, and a flare is created by the slit-lamp beam traveling through liquid having a protein concentration approximating that of blood. Treatment requires dilitation of the pupil. This enables the iris to move and prevents the formation of inflammatory adhesions between the iris and lens or iris and cornea. The inflammation may be quieted with topical steroids and antibiotics. The intraocular pressure in a globe with traumatic iritis can be found to be low, normal, or high. Significantly elevated intra-ocular pressures must be treated with ocular antihypertensive medications.

A patient with a "significant" hyphema should be hospitalized and kept at strict bed rest with his head elevated 30° to 45° to facilitate settling of the hyphema inferiorly. Bilateral eye patches and heavy sedation are sometimes recommended to assure immobility. Topical and systemic steroids, mydriatics, and ocular antihypertensive agents should be administered. Some authors recommend the use of oral antifibrinolytic agents in conjunction with the above regimen. Most hyphemas clear within 5 to 6 days; however, 25 percent of all hyphemas recur within 3 to 5 days of the initial hemorrhage. Complications related to hyphemas include corneal bloodstaining, formation of iris adhesions, and optic atrophy from transient episodes of markedly elevated intraocular pressure. The prognosis for an uncomplicated hyphema is related to the size of the initial hemorrhage. Approximately 80 percent of patients with hyphemas filling less than one-third of the anterior chamber achieve good visual acuity, while only 35 percent of those with total hyphemas obtain good visual acuity.

Corneal or Scleral Lacerations

This is an ophthalmic emergency that requires direct repair of corneal or scleral tissue. Blunt trauma great enough to create a scleral laceration should alert the surgeon to the possibility of lens dislocation, vitreous detachment, or even a retinal tear or detachment. The repair of these complications is beyond the scope of this discussion.

Eyelid Injuries

Simple Lacerations

Eyelid lacerations parallel to the lid margin of upper and lower eyelids are primarily closed. If the punctal and canalicular systems are uninvolved, deep lacerations to the lower lid can also be primarily closed. Deep sutures are not used because the orbital septum may inadvertently be sutured

and a line of tension between the sutures and the orbital septum may create a cicatricial ectropion after the wound heals. To avoid the occasional ectropion, deep sutures are not placed in the lower eyelid. Horizontal, partial- or full-thickness lacerations to the upper eyelid must be explored for damage to the levator aponeurosis. After the levator aponeurosis is identified, it should be sutured directly. The skin is closed and an eyelid fold recreated by suturing skin on either side of the laceration to deep tissue (Fig. 6-23). The eyelid fold is established where the skin is imbricated by its anchor to deep tissue.

Marginal Lacerations

Marginal lacerations of the eyelid require precise closure to eliminate cosmetic deformities. An important but simple rule is to suture identical tissue or structures on either side of the defect. The most common structures that are easily identifiable (from anterior to posterior) are the lashline, the meibomian gland orifices, and the grey line (Fig. 6-24). Three sutures are placed in the lid margin; one suture realigns the lashline and the anterior surface of the laceration, the second realigns the meibomian gland orifices denoting the superior tarsal border, and a third realigns the grey line and the posterior surface of the laceration. The three interrupted marginal sutures are aligned and 5-0 absorbable sutures are placed deeply to close the tarsal border. The only deep sutures placed in an eyelid are to close a tarsal defect; a notch or defect will result if a marginal lid laceration is repaired without closure of such a defect. A slight eversion of the lid margin must be attained after marginal lacerations are sutured. A subtle concavity in the line of repair will occur with wound contraction if the eyelid margin is not slightly overcorrected. This overcorrection will flatten within 3 to 4 weeks, resulting in a smooth lid contour. The ends of the three 6-0 silk transmarginal sutures must be left long and taped or sutured to the skin surface to avoid abrasive contact with the cornea.

Traumatic colobomas from full-thickness loss of tissue in the upper or lower eyelid can be repaired by one of several methods. In the elderly, in whom there is a significant amount of eyelid laxity, the margins of the eyelid coloboma may be trimmed and direct closure performed, as in a marginal lac-

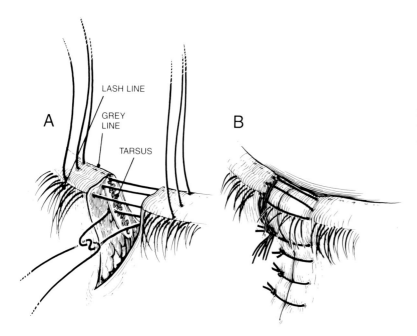

LASH LINE

GREY LINE

TARSUS

A

B

Fig. 6-24. **(A)** Marginal lacerations are repaired by aligning similar tissue on each side of the incision. The lash line, grey line, and meibomian gland orifices are classically used to align the lid margin. **(B)** Sutures must be secured inferiorly to prevent corneal irritation, and the tarsus must be closed.

Fig. 6-25. **(A)** Lower eyelid defects that cannot be closed directly are approximated by **(B)** releasing the inferior crus of the lateral canthal tendon. **(C)** Only skin sutures are needed in the lateral canthus; no deeper sutures for the aligning of the lateral commisure are required.

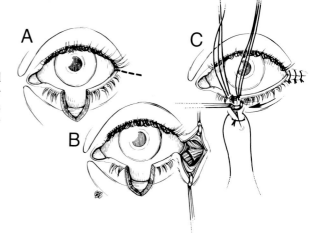

A

B

C

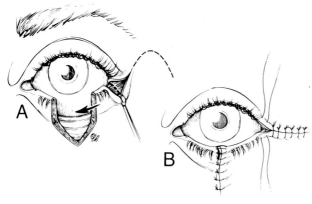

A

B

Fig. 6-26. The Tenzel semicircular flap can close eyelid defects up to 60 percent. **(A)** The inferior crus of the lateral canthal tendon must be cut, with an incision into the lateral temporal region, to create a flap. **(B)** If the radius of the flap is not long enough, the lateral portion of the eyelid will pull inferiorly with resultant scleral show.

eration, without loss of tissue. In cases where there is minimal lid laxity or a significant defect of the upper or lower eyelid, tissue must be mobilized in order to close the defect without tension. This often can be accomplished by a lateral canthotomy and release of the inferior and/or superior crus of the lateral canthal tendon, allowing advancement of marginal eyelid tissue (Fig. 6-25). A lateral canthotomy with crus release can provide 4 to 5 mm of tissue. However, a semicircular flap described by Tenzel should be performed for primary closure of upper or lower eyelid defects of greater dimensions (Fig. 6-26).

Traumatic colobomas of the eyelid due to dog or human bites can often be repaired with retrieved lost tissue which can be sutured into place as autogenous composite grafts (Fig. 6-27).

Lacerations with Large Lower Lid Defects

A two-stage procedure is often required to repair a tissue loss of greater than 60 percent in either eyelid. A Tenzel procedure is not preferred. The first stage involves a tarsoconjunctival advancement

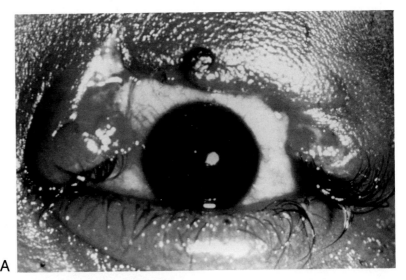

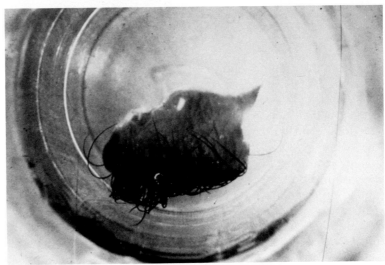

Fig. 7-27. (A & B) A human bite taken of the eyelid can be directly replaced as a composite graft. *(Figure continues.)*

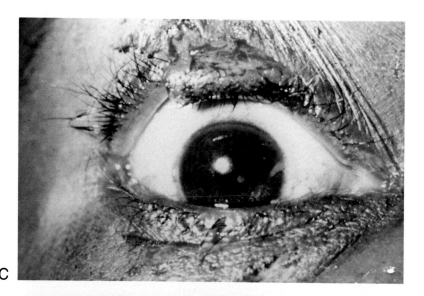

C

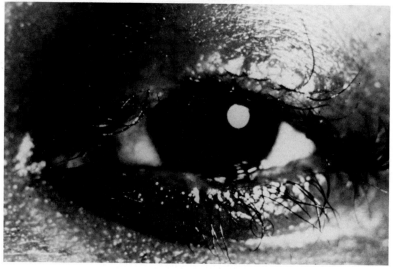

D

Fig. 6-27 *(Continued).* **(C)** Preoperative view and **(D)** postoperative view 4 weeks after trauma. The patient was given antibiotic coverage for anaerobic flora which normally reside in the mouth.

flap from the upper eyelid to fill the defect in the posterior lamella of the lower lid. The upper eyelid is everted, and the superior 6 to 7 mm of tarsus are incised and advanced inferiorly with a flap of conjunctiva to fill the posterior lamella of the lower eyelid defect (Fig. 6-28). The distal 3 to 4 mm margin of tarsus must be left intact to maintain proper eyelash position in the upper lid. The anterior lamella is provided by a split-thickness skin graft placed over the tarsoconjunctival flap. This flap can be opened within 3 to 4 weeks. Excess skin must be trimmed from the upper eyelid to allow a smooth conjunctival surface to remain on the pos-

terior aspect of the upper eyelid donor site. The lid margin of the lower eyelid is allowed to granulate following the second stage. Cautery should not be applied to the margin of the lower eyelid, since it will create a defect in an otherwise smoothly contoured eyelid margin.

Large Defects of the Upper Eyelid

A two-stage procedure is necessary to repair upper lid defects of 60 percent or greater, as in the lower eyelid. A Cutler-Beard flap is developed in the lower eyelid by performing a transverse blepharo-

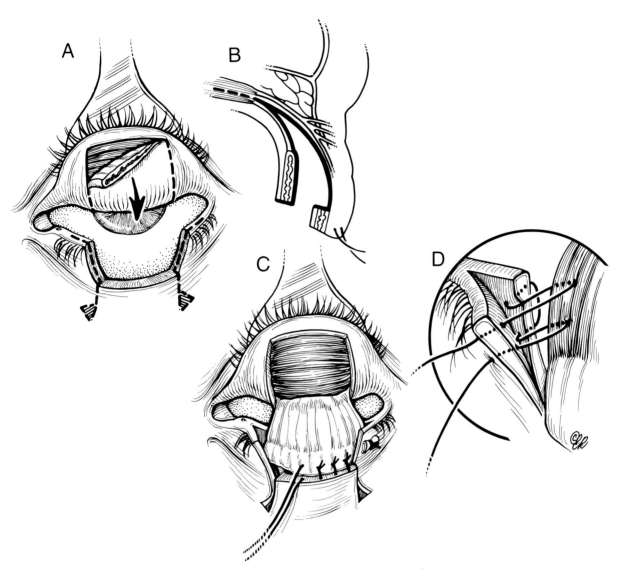

Fig. 6-28. Hughes procedure for lower lid defects. **(A)** Approximately 3 to 4 mm of tarsus are left at the margin of the upper eyelid, and a flap of tarsus and conjunctiva is dissected up to the superior fornix. This flap should be devoid of Müller's muscle, if possible. The extent of the flap is marked out to approximate the size of the lower eyelid defect. **(B)** A sagittal section shows the 3 to 4 mm rim of tarsus left intact in the upper eyelid. The dissection is carried up to the superior fornix to prevent future eyelid retraction. **(C)** The tarsoconjunctival flap is sutured into the defect of the lower eyelid. A tongue-in-groove is created at the margins of the lower eyelid defect and sutured to the tarsoconjunctival flap to produce the uniform and integral lid margin. **(D)** The conjunctival portion of the tarsoconjunctival flap is sutured between two flaps of tarsus remaining at the margins of the lower lid defect. The margins of the advancement flap are held in position by 6-0 silk sutures tied over bolsters. *(Figure continues.)*

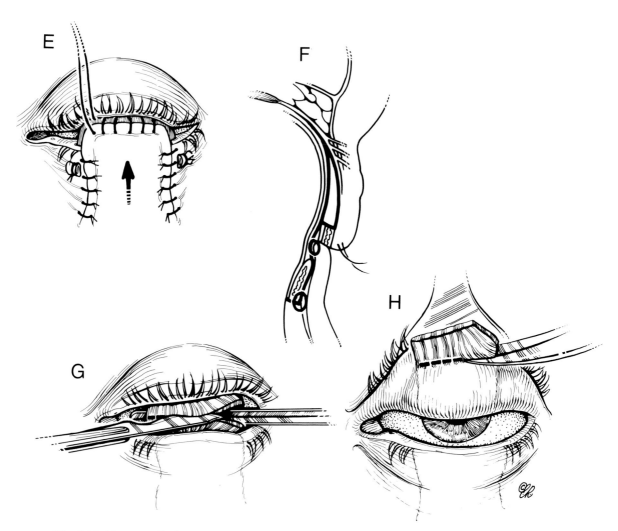

Fig. 6-28 *(Continued).* **(E)** Following the placement of the tarsoconjunctival flap from the upper eyelid to the lower eyelid defect, a free skin graft or advancement of tissue from the surrounding area can be placed to fill the anterior lamella. It is important to overcorrect this anterior skin placement. The skin graft or transposition graft should be placed high onto the conjunctival surface superior to the pre-existing lid margin to allow for shrinking. **(F)** A sagittal section shows the united posterior lamella of the upper and lower eyelids. The lash line and anterior lamella is left unsutured and in its normal position. **(G)** A groove director is placed behind the tarsoconjunctival flap to facilitate its incision. The lower eyelid is incised straight across and slightly higher than the desired position. The lower eyelid will fall with gravity and time. **(H)** The upper eyelid is everted on a Desmarres retractor, and the posterior surface is cleaned of excess skin and/or muscle. No sutures are placed on the lid margin or posterior surface; these are left to granulate.

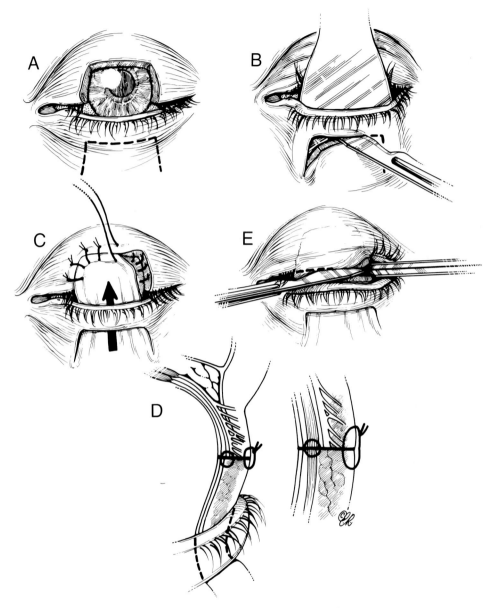

Fig. 6-29. Cutler-Beard procedure for upper eyelid defects. **(A)** A defect in the upper eyelid is created, and the advancement flap of the lower lid is marked to correspond to this defect. A bridge of 2 to 3 mm of the lower lid margin is left intact to maintain the integrity of the lash line and the marginal vessels. **(B)** A bone plate is placed behind the lower lid to facilitate dissection of the advancement flap. The globe is thereby protected and the incision is not beveled through the lower eyelid. **(C)** The advancement flap is placed beneath the bridge and sutured into the defect. Deep sutures are placed between the edges of the remaining levator aponeurosis of the upper eyelid and deep tissue of the advancement flap. **(D)** A sagittal section shows these deeper sutures through the levator aponeurosis of the upper eyelid stump and deep tissue of the lower lid. An enlargement of this critical area shows a direct skin closure and the levator aponeurosis of the upper eyelid approximated to the posterior one-third of the advancement flap. **(E)** A groove director is placed beneath the advancement flap, and this is cut straight across with a Bard-Parker scalpel. It is important not to sacrifice tissue in the upper eyelid because this will cause a coloboma, and lid lag or lagophthalmos will ensue. It may be necessary to restore the lower lid margin to repair a cicatricial ectropion.

tomy 3 to 4 mm below the lid margin (Fig. 6-29). The marginal artery, which lies within the first 3 mm of the lid, is spared. Tissue is advanced from the lower eyelid and cheek underneath the bridge flap to fill the defect of the upper eyelid coloboma. The conjunctiva of the upper lid is sutured to the conjunctiva of the advancement flap and fragments of the levator aponeurosis are joined to the orbicularis of the advancement flap with absorbable sutures. The skin is closed separately and a tarsorrhaphy performed. At the second stage of repair, the advancement flap is opened, after 3 to 6 weeks of immobilization. The inferior of the portion of the marginal bridge of the lower eyelid is denuded and sutured to the upper edge of the skin flap. The upper eyelid is trimmed and allowed to reepithelialize.

Lacrimal and Canalicular Injuries

Avulsion of the medial canthus is often complicated by transection of the upper or lower canaliculus. Direct and severe trauma to the naso-orbital region may fragment and fracture the bony nasolacrimal duct, which is often not recognized at the time of initial presentation (see Chapter 4). Canalicular injuries are treated immediately; however, nasolacrimal duct fractures can be repaired later. Examination of medial canthal injuries under the slit-lamp may show the ends of a severed canaliculus. The temporal end of a lacerated canaliculus is often easily found by placing irrigating fluid in the punctum. The medial end of a lacerated canaliculus is usually quite difficult to locate, and magnification with an operating microscope is frequently

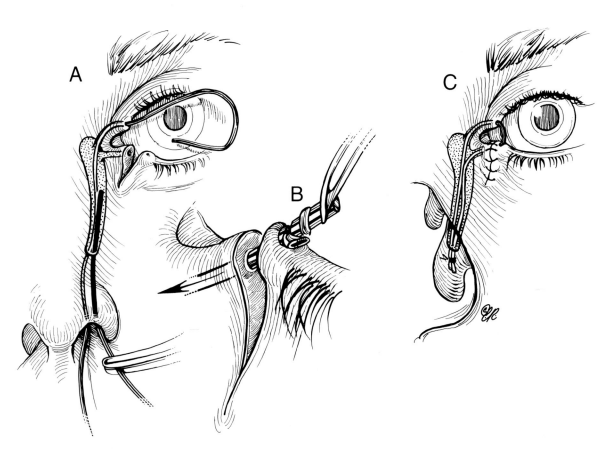

Fig. 6-30. Repair of canalicular lacerations is aided by silicone intubation. (**A–C**) Both involved and uninvolved canaliculi are intubated and secured under the inferior turbinate. Deeper sutures around the laceration approximate lacerated ends around the silicone tube.

helpful. After trauma, a severed canaliculus retracts deeply into the medial canthal tissue and must be located in the operating room. It is easier to locate the medial portion of a lacerated canaliculus within a few hours after trauma. Once the tissues have become edematous and hemorrhagic, identification of the retracted stump of a canaliculus is usually not possible.

Many methods have been described for repairing canalicular lacerations. One of the less complex methods requires passing silicone tubing swaged onto a metal stent (Crawford tubes) through the canalicular system (Fig. 6-30). One end of the tubing is passed through the uninvolved punctal system and down through the nasolacrimal duct to exit under the inferior meatus. The opposite end of the tubing is then passed through the punctum of the involved canaliculus and out the lacerated canaliculus site. Irrigation of clear fluid (saline) through the uninvolved canaliculus can often expedite location of the lacerated and contracted medial portion of the transected canaliculus by revealing the origin of a fluid stream from the medial cut end. Should this fail, fluid may be placed in the medial canthus and air injected through the uninvolved canaliculus. The bubbles of air that eminate from the severed end often help in locating this structure. Once the cut end is found, the nasolacrimal tubing is again passed through both cut ends of the canaliculus and down through the nasolacrimal duct. It is not always necessary to directly suture the ends of a severed canaliculus; although if the canaliculi are easily found, 10-0 or 9-0 Nylon suture placed under microscopic visualization may promote their apposition. By suturing deep tissues toward the canaliculus, which is properly intubated with silicone tubing, the lacerated edges usually align themselves. The lacerated edges granulate, and the tubing prevents granulation tissue from obstructing the outflow system.

A pigtail probe has been advocated for the repair of canalicular lacerations without intubation of the entire nasolacrimal system. This probe is cumbersome, and as a result, trauma to the uninvolved canaliculus is common. Less optimal procedures for the repair of a lacerated canaliculus include placement of a Viers (metal) rod or single piece of silicone through the severed canaliculus, placement of silicone tube looped between the involved and uninvolved canalicular systems without nasolacrimal duct intubation, or even direct suturing of the canaliculus. Placement of silicone tubing throughout the lacrimal system, when possible, is preferred.

The volume of tear outflow attributed to the upper and lower canalicular systems varies according to authors. Some have labeled the lower canaliculus the dominant outflow tract, attributing 70 to 80 percent of drainage through this network, while others believe that the upper and lower systems are equal contributors to tear outflow. Since tear production diminishes with age (Fig. 6-31), the surgeon may feel confident in not repairing a transected upper canaliculus in an elderly patient, especially if one believes this to be the minor outflow system (Fig. 6-32). However, attempts should be made to repair lacerations to the upper or lower canaliculus in a young patient. Nasolacrimal tubing is left in place at least 4 to 6 months. The tubes are solid so tears cannot flow through them. Tears are tracked around the tubing, and tear flow continues by capillary action. Postoperatively some patients have epiphora. This is due to the obstruction of the tear outflow system by the nasolacrimal tubing in

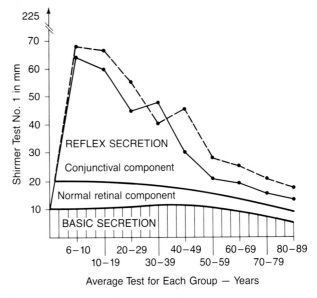

Fig. 6-31. Graph showing the diminishing tear production as women (----) and men (—) grow older, from age 6 to 89. (Redrawn from Jones L, Wobig J: Surgery of the Eyelids and Lacrimal System. Aesculapius, Birmingham, AL, 1976.)

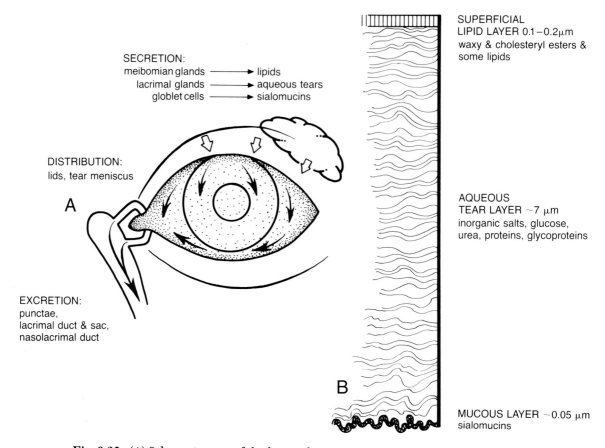

SECRETION:
meibomian glands ⟶ lipids
lacrimal glands ⟶ aqueous tears
globlet cells ⟶ sialomucins

DISTRIBUTION:
lids, tear meniscus

A

EXCRETION:
punctae,
lacrimal duct & sac,
nasolacrimal duct

SUPERFICIAL
LIPID LAYER 0.1–0.2μm
waxy & cholesteryl esters &
some lipids

AQUEOUS
TEAR LAYER ~7 μm
inorganic salts, glucose,
urea, proteins, glycoproteins

B

MUCOUS LAYER ~0.05 μm
sialomucins

Fig. 6-32. (A) Schematic view of the lacrimal apparatus. (B) Structure of the tear film.

patients with small diameter canaliculi and nasolacrimal ducts. It must be made clear to these patients that this is a temporary situation, and once the tubes are removed in 4 to 6 months the nasolacrimal system should be patent. The tubes should be left in even longer, up to 12 months, if epiphora is not exhibited during this time. It is not necessary to suture the tubing to the nasal mucosa. The tubes are simply tied together with 6-0 silk and left short under the inferior turbinate where they exit. The nasolacrimal tubes will strike the inferior end of the nares and create irritation if they are not left short.

A dacryocystorhinostomy (DCR) may be performed if a young patient presents with a severe laceration of the lower canaliculus or upper and lower canaliculi and the severed ends cannot be found. In this case, the nasolacrimal tubing is passed through the punctum, through the distal end of the canaliculus, and into the junction of the

lacrimal sac and nasal mucosa. This allows the intact temporal end of the lacerated canaliculus to be stretched towards the osteotomy. The granulation proceeds around the tubing, hopefully leaving an open drainage channel.

The theory behind use of this procedure for canalicular trauma is that a large nasal osteotomy may allow greater lacrimal drainage in the upright position than will a lacrimal sac with an interrupted lacrimal pump. When the sac is opened during DCR, microtubes are forced back laterally towards the nasal-most end of the laceration. The nasal mucoperiosteum is injected with 2 percent lidocaine with epinephrine to aid the dissection after removal of bone. The nares should be packed with 4 percent cocaine solution prior to the initial incision. Methylene blue solution is injected into the nasolacrimal system, if one of the functioning canaliculi can be found, to stain the inside of the lacrimal sac; this helps in identification of the sac at a later stage. A curvilinear incision (Fig. 6-33) is made in the medial canthus 7 to 10 mm from the medial canthal angle, avoiding the angular vessels if possible (Fig. 6-34). The incision is started superiorly at the level of the medial canthal tendon but should not sever the tendon nor extend superior to the tendon. The incision is then extended down to the periosteum, and the periosteum is reflected temporally, revealing the anterior lacrimal crest. The lacrimal sac will then also be reflected temporally along with the periosteum. The underlying anterior lacrimal crest and the fossa of the lacrimal sac can be removed with a Kerrison punch or end-cutting rongeurs if a bony dehiscence is noted in this location. The anterior lacrimal crest is removed with a Hall drill if a dehiscence in bone is not noted. An osteotomy is created in which the anterior lacrimal crest, the wall of the lacrimal groove, and the bone of the posterior lacrimal crest are removed. The nasolacrimal canal is then unroofed the distance of a few millimeters so that the osteotomy is approximately as large as the surgeon's index finger. The lacrimal sac is identified with Bowman probes inserted into the sac through the canaliculi. Anterior and posterior flaps are created by cutting an H shape in the lacrimal sac (Fig. 6-34C); the sac mucosa is easily identified by its blue color from the prior injection of methylene

blue solution. Using absorbable suture material, these anterior and posterior flaps are sutured to adjoining anterior and posterior flaps fashioned out of the nasal mucosa. It is possible to create a continuous lining (respiratory) epithelium between the mucosa of the nose and the lacrimal sac. Silicone tubing should be passed through the punctum, through the lacerated end of the canaliculus, and into the junction of the lacrimal sac and nasal mucosa, exiting through the nares. This causes the intact temporal end of the canaliculus to be stretched towards the osteotomy. The nasolacrimal tubing left in place will allow only minimal tear passage during granulation.

In cases where the canalicular system is totally obliterated, a conjunctivodacryocystorhinostomy is performed. A dacryocystorhinostomy is performed as previously described, and the caruncle in the medial canthus is excised. A 22-gauge needle is inserted through the anatomical location of the caruncle to penetrate through the medial canthus into the region of the osteotomy. The needle should pass between the sutured anterior and posterior flaps (Fig. 6-35). The anterior flaps may be closed after the placement of the "Jones" tube to allow easier visualization. A sharply pointed knife or scissors is used to enlarge the path into the nose that is delineated by the needle. The incision should allow the insertion of a Pyrex glass tube or

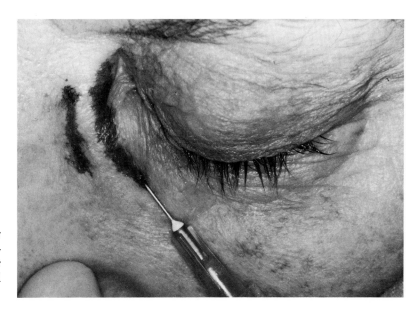

Fig. 6-33. Dacryocystorhinostomy entails exposure through a curvilinear incision that extends superiorly to the level of the medial canthal tendon.

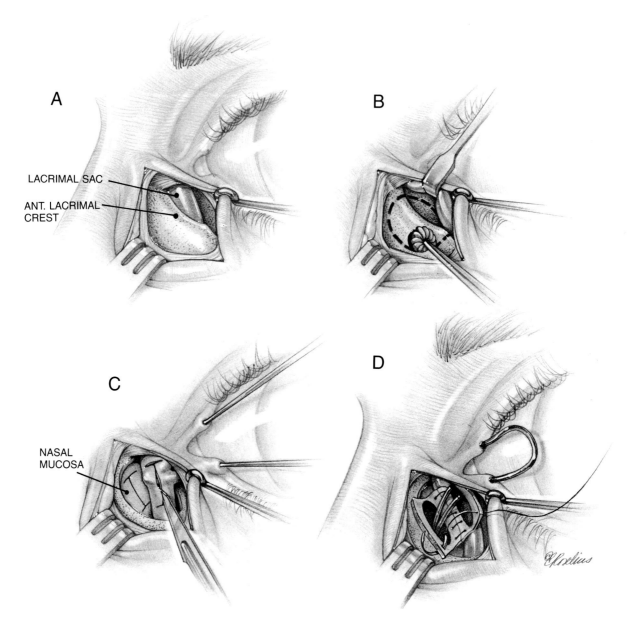

Fig. 6-34. Technique of dacryocystorhinostomy. **(A)** The curvilinear incision is created in the medial canthus, which extends from the medial canthal tendon and curves down around the infraorbital rim. The anterior lacrimal crest is exposed after the periosteum is elevated. **(B)** An osteotomy is created by removing the anterior lacrimal crest. The osteotomy is placed inferonasal to the medial canthal tendon and extends down to the entrance of the nasolacrimal duct. The bony defect should approximate the size of the surgeon's thumb. The osteotomy can be created with a Hall drill and burr or a Kerrison punch. **(C)** The nasal mucosa is tented, and an H incision is made into the nasal mucosa to develop anterior and posterior nasal flaps. The lacrimal sac is tented with Bowman probes to identify the sac and create similar anterior and posterior sac flaps in the form of the letter H. **(D)** The posterior flaps of nasal mucosa and lacrimal sac are sutured with 4-0 chromic microtubes, and silicone microtubes are threaded over the posterior flap prior to closure of the anterior nasal and lacrimal sac flaps. The microtubes are tied together within the nose with 6-0 silk sutures and left to dangle freely.

plastic Jones tube between 6 and 15 mm in length. The tube is threaded over a #1 or #2 Bowman probe and then penetrates through the incision in the medial canthus. A 6-0 silk suture is tied around the head of the tube and anchored through the body of the tube. The head of the Pyrex tube should fit snugly in the medial canthus without occlusion by redundant conjunctiva. The length of Pyrex tubing must be individualized at the time of the procedure so as to extend well into the nose without striking the nasal septum. The anterior portion of the middle turbinate should be resected if Pyrex tubing comes in contact with it. Drainage of irrigation fluid from the conjunctival sac and through the pyrex tube should be tested intraoperatively. The previously placed 6-0 silk suture is used to secure the tube in the medial canthal tissue for the first postoperative week.

This last procedure has an extremely high rate of failure, and postoperative care is extremely important. Patients should be instructed not to blow their nose for at least 4 to 6 weeks postoperatively. They must be taught to clean the tube regularly and clear it when obstructed. This can be accomplished by aspirating saline or water through the tube on a daily basis and intermittently blowing air through the tube to clear minor obstructions. It is sometimes necessary to run a fine wire through the tube or replace it if the patient is unable to clear it on his own. An extruded tube should be replaced within a few hours, since the conjunctivorhinostomy opening can quickly close in a recent surgical site. A patent fistula may be formed after 12 months; however, it is preferable to leave the tubing in place much longer. The tubing should not be removed for long periods of time to test for the development of an epithelialized tract.

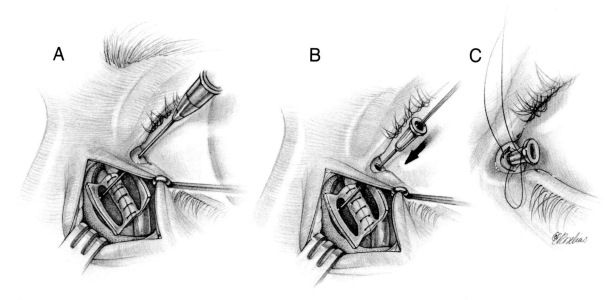

Fig. 6-35. Technique of conjunctivodacryocystorhinostomy (Jones tube). **(A)** Following the creation of nasal and lacrimal sac flaps as in Figure 6-34, the caruncle is removed in the medial canthus. A long 25-gauge needle is used to penetrate the medial canthal tissues to enter in the medial canthus and transfix the prior osteotomy. **(B)** The distance between the medial canthus and the nasal septum is measured, and a Jones Pyrex tube is chosen to bridge this area. The Pyrex tube is threaded over a Bowman probe to lie in the medial canthus and extend over the posterior flaps to enter the nasal cavity. **(C)** A 6-0 silk suture is tied around and through the Jones tube to secure it to the medial canthus and prevent extrusion.

SUGGESTED READING

Anderson RL, Edwards JJ: Indications, complications and results with silicone stents. Ophthalmology 86:1474, 1979

Beyer CK, Smith B: Naso-orbital fractures, complications and treatment. Ophthalmalogica, 163:418, 1971

Beyer CK, Smith B: Naso-orbital fractures: Their complications and treatment. p. 197. In Tessier P, Callahan A, Mustardé JC, Salyer KE, (eds): Symposium on Plastic Surgery in the Orbital Region. C.V. Mosby, St. Louis, 1976

Beyer CK, Fabian R, Smith B: Naso-orbital fractures, complications and treatment. Ophthalmol 89:456, 1982

Browning CW: Alloplast materials in orbital repair. Am J Ophthalmol 63:955, 1970

Butler RM, Morledge D, Holt GP, Kreiger AE: A system of surgical approaches to orbital floor fractures. Trans Am Acad Ophthalmol Otol 75:519, 1971

Cassady JV: Developmental anatomy of the nasolacrimal duct. Arch Ophthalmol 47:141, 1952

Cole HB, Smith B: Eye muscle imbalance complicating orbital floor fracture. Am J Ophthalmol 55(5):930, 1963

Converse JM, Firman F, Woodsmith D, Friedland JA: Conjunctival approach in orbital fractures. Plast Reconstr Surg 52(6):656, 1973

Converse JM, Smith B: Reconstruction of the floor of the orbit by bone graft. Arch Ophthalmol 44:1, 1950

Converse JM, Smith B: Enophthalmos and diplopia in fractures of the orbital floor. Br J Plast Surg 9(4):265, 1957

Converse JM, Smith B: Blow-out fracture of the floor of the orbit. Trans Am Acad Ophthalmol Otol 64:676, 1960

Converse JM, Smith B: Naso-orbital fractures. Trans Am Acad Ophthalmol Otol 67:622, 1963

Converse JM, Smith B: Malunited fractures of the bones of the orbit. p. 645. In Converse JM (ed): Reconstructive Plastic Surgery; Principles and Procedures in Correction, Reconstruction, and Transplantation. Vol. 2. W.B. Saunders, Philadelphia, 1964

Converse JM, Smith B: Naso-orbital fractures and traumatic deformities of the medial canthus. Excerpt Medica Intl Congress Series No. 113; Procedures VIII, Intl. Congress of Otorhinolaryngology, October 1965

Converse JM, Smith B: Naso-orbital fractures and traumatic deformities of the medial canthus. Plast Reconstr Surg 38(2):14, 1966

Converse JM, Smith B: On the treatment of blow-out fractures of the orbit. Plast Reconstr Surg 62:100, 1978

Converse JM, Smith B, Lisman RD: Differential diagnosis and its influence on the treatment of orbital blow-out fractures. p. 96. In 3rd International Symposium of Plastic and Reconstructive Surgery of the Eye and Adnexa. Williams & Wilkins, Baltimore, 1982

Converse JM, Smith B, O'Bear MF, Woodsmith D: Orbital blow-out fractures: a ten year survey. Plast Reconstr Surg 39:20, 1967

Cramer LM, Tooze FM, Lerman S: Blow-out fractures of the orbit. Br J Plast Surg 18:171, 1965

Crawford JD: Intubation of obstructions in the lacrimal system. Can J Ophthalmol 12:289, 1977

Dayal Y, Ghose S, Sood NN: Blow-out fracture of the orbit. I. Observations on the surgical anatomy of the rhesus monkey orbit as compared to man; East Arch Ophthalmol 7:7, 1979

Dayal Y, Ghose S, Sood NN: Blow-out fracture of the orbit. II. A new experimental model. East Arch Ophthalmol 7:19, 1979

Deutschberger O, Kirshner H: Intraorbital fractures. Ann Ophthalmol 3:380, 1971

Dodick JM, Galin MA, Littleton JT, Sod LM: Concomitant medial wall fracture and blow-out fracture of the orbit. Arch Ophthalmol 85:273, 1971

Dortzbach RK, Callahan A: Repair of cicatricial entropion of upper eyelids. Arch Ophthalmol 85:82, 1971

Dortzbach RK, France TD, Kushner FJ, Gonnering RS: Silicone intubation for obstruction of the nasolacrimal duct in children. Am J Ophthalmol 94(5):585, 1982

Duke-Elder S, Cook C: Normal and abnormal development. p. 240. In Duke-Elder S (ed): System of Ophthalmology. Vol. 3, C.V. Mosby, St. Louis, 1963

Emery JM, von Noorden GK, Schlernitzauer DA: Management of orbital fractures. Am J Ophthalmol 74:299, 1972

Emery JM, von Noorden GK, Schlernitzauer DA: Orbital floor fractures; long term follow-up cases with and without surgical repair. Trans Am Acad Ophthalmol Otol 75:802, 1971

Goldman RJ, Hessburg PC: Appraisal of surgical correction in 130 cases of orbital floor fracture. Am J Ophthalmol 76:152, 1973

Greenwald HS, Keeney AH, Shannon GM: A review of 128 patients with orbital fractures. Am J Ophthalmol 78:655, 1974

Grove A, Smith B, Guibor P: Fractures of the orbit. Clin Ophthalmol 2:48, 1976

Guerry D, Kendig EL: Congenital impatency of the nasolacrimal duct. Arch Ophthalmol 39:193, 1948

Harris GJ, DiClementi D: Congenital dacryocystocele. Arch Ophthalmol 100:1763, 1982

Harris GJ: Marsupilization of a lacrimal gland cyst. Ophthalmic Surg (1):75, 1983

Hurwitz JJ: A practical approach to the management of lacrimal gland lesions. Ophthalmic Surg 13(10):829, 1982

Hurwitz JJ: The slit canaliculus. Ophthalmic Surg 13(7):572, 1982

Jackson H, Lambert TD: Congenital mucocele of the lacrimal sac. Br J Ophthalmol 47:690, 1963

Jones LT, Wobig JL: Surgery of the eyelids and lacrimal system. Aesculapius, Birmingham, Alabama, 1976

Katowitz JA: Silicone tubing in canalicular obstructions. Arch Ophthalmol 91:459, 1974

Kaye BL: Orbital floor repair with antral wall bone grafts. Plast Reconstr Surg 37:62, 1966

Keith CG: Intubation of the lacrimal passages. Am J Ophthalmol 65:70, 1968

LeFort R: Fractures de la machoire superieure. XIII Congress International Medica, Paris, 1900. Section de Chirurgie Generale 23:275, 1901

Lerman S: Blow-out fracture of the orbit. Br J Ophthalmol 54:90, 1970

Levy NS: Conservative management of congenital amniotecele of the nasolacrimal sac. J Pediatr Ophthalmol Strabismus 16:254, 1979

Linberg JV, Anderson RL, Bumsted RM, Barreras R: Study of intranasal ostium external dacryocystorhinostomy. Arch Ophthalmol 100:1758, 1982

Milauskas AT, Feuger GF, Schulze RR: Clinical experiences with orbitography in the diagnosis of orbital floor fractures. Trans Am Acad Ophthalmol Otol 70:25, 1966

Miller G: Blindness developing a few days after a mid-face fracture. Plast Reconstr Surg 42(4):384, 1968

Nicholson DH, Guzak SV: Visual loss complicating repair of orbital floor fractures. Arch Ophthalmol 86:369, 1971

Patrick RK: Lacrimal secretion in full-term and premature babies. Trans Ophthalmol Soc UK 94:283, 1974

Peterson RA, Robb RM: The natural course of congenital obstruction of the nasolacrimal duct. J Pediatr Ophthalmol Strabismus 15:246, 1978

Putterman AM, Stevens T, Urist MJ: Nonsurgical management of blow-out fractures of the orbital floor. Am J Ophthalmol 77(2):232, 1974

Quickert MH: Lacrimal drainage surgery. p. 95. In Soll DB (ed): Management of Complication in Ophthalmic Plastic Surgery. Aesculapius, Birmingham, Alabama, 1976

Quickert MH, Dryden RM: Probes for intubation in lacrimal drainage. Trans Am Acad Ophthalmol Otol 74:431, 1970

Rumelt MB, Ernest JT: Isolated blow-out fracture of the medial orbital wall with medial rectus muscle entrapment. Am J Ophthalmol 73:451, 1972

Savar DE: High-dose radiation to the orbit. Arch Ophthalmol 100:1755, 1982

Schaeffer JP: Variations in the anatomy of the nasolacrimal passages. Ann Surg 54:148, 1911

Schwarz M: Congenital atresia of the nasolacrimal canal. Arch Ophthalmol 13:301, 1935

Scott WE, Fabre JA, Ossoinig KC: Congenital mucocele of the lacrimal sac. Arch Ophthalmol 97:1656, 1979

Shingleton BJ, Biengang DC, Albert DM, et al: Ocular toxicity associated with high dose carmustine. Arch Ophthalmol 100:1766, 1982

Smith B: Diplopia in depressed orbital fractures. Plast Reconstr Surg 20(4):318, 1957

Smith B: Naso-orbital fractures in contemporary oculoplastic surgery. p. 89. In Smith B, Buibor P (eds): Symposia, Miami, 1974

Smith B: Reduction of nasal orbital fractures and simultaneous dacryocystorhinostomy. Trans Am Acad Ophthalmol Otol 82:527, 1976

Smith B, Barr DR, Langham EJ: Complications of orbital fractures. NY State J Med 71(20):2407, 1971

Smith B, Beyer, CK: Medial canthoplasty. Arch Ophthalmol 82:344, 1969

Smith B, Converse JM: Early treatment of orbital floor fractures. Trans Am Acad Ophthalmol Otol 61:602, 1957

Smith B, Converse JM: Editorial on the treatment of blow-out fractures of the orbit. Plast Reconstr Surg 62(1):100, 1978

Smith B, Lisman RD: Blow-out fractures in children and young adults. p. 388. In Harley RD (ed): Pediatric Ophthalmology. 2nd Ed., W.B. Saunders, Philadelphia, 1982

Smith B, Lisman RD: Dacryoadenopexy as a factor in upper lid blepharoplasty. Plast Reconst Surg 5:629, 1983

Smith B, Lisman RD: External orbital fractures. p. 237. In Fraunfelder F (ed): Current Ocular Therapy. W.B. Saunders, Philadelphia, 1983

Smith B, Lisman RD: Internal orbital fractures (blow-out fractures). p. 238. In Fraunfelder F (ed): Current Ocular Therapy. W.B. Saunders, Philadelphia, 1983

Smith B, Nesi F: Orbital fractures and medial canthal reconstruction. Clin Plast Surg 5:505, 1978

Smith B, Nightingale J: Fractures of the orbit: blow-out and naso-orbital fractures. In Tenzel R (ed): Internat'l Ophthalmology Clinics, Ocular Plastic Surgery. Vol. 18, No. 3. Little Brown & Co., Boston, 1978

Smith B, O'Bear M, Leone CL Jr: The correction of enophthalmos associated with anophthalmos of glass bead implantation. Am J Ophthalmol 64(6):1088, 1967

Smith B, Petrelli R: Herniation of the lacrimal glands. Trans Am Acad Ophthalmol Otol 84(6):988, 1977

Smith B, Putterman AM: Fixation of orbital floor implants. Arch Ophthalmol 83:598, 1970

Smith B, Regan WF Jr: Blow-out fracture of the orbit. Am J Ophthalmol 44(6):733, 1957

Stasior OG: Blow-out fractures. p. 990. In Sorsby A (ed): Modern Ophthalmology, 2nd Ed. J.B. Lippincott, Philadelphia, 1972

Taiara C, Smith B: Palpebral dacryoadenectomy. Am J Ophthalmol 75(3):462, 1973

Walter WL: The use of the pigtail probe for silicone intubation of the injured canaliculus. Ophthalmic Surg (6):488, 1982

Weinstein GS, Giglan AW, Patterson JH: Congenital lacrimal sac mucoceles. Am J Ophthalmol 94:106, 1982

Wilder LW, Smith B: Repairing blow-out fractures. Kans Med Soc 5:238, 1969

Worst JG: Method for reconstructing torn lacrimal canaliculus. Am J Ophthalmol 53:520, 1962

Zizmor J, Smith B, Fasano C, Converse JM: Roentgen diagnosis of blow-out fractures of the orbit. Am J Roentgenol, Radium Therapy and Nuclear Medicine 82:(6):802, 1962

Zolli CL: Tarso-septal z-plasty combined with skin grafting for the late correction of traumatic upper lid contractures. Ophthalmic Surg 13(7):576, 1982

Fractures of the Zygoma and Zygomatic Arch

7

F. Ronald Feinstein
Thomas J. Krizek

In the early 19th century, Guillaume Dupuytren, an eminent surgeon in Paris, considered surgery to correct fractures of the zygoma far too risky. He believed the deformity was not serious enough to warrant taking such risks.[1] Today, elective aesthetic alteration of the noninjured normal but unattractive zygoma is accepted. The "high cheek-boned" model has confirmed the importance of this anatomic part in our concept of beauty. Current practice dictates that the displaced zygoma should be repositioned for restoration of function and aesthetic balance.

As our society has become more mobile and urbanized, the incidence of zygomatic fractures has increased. Indeed, zygomatic and maxillofacial fractures have become an important part of the trauma surgeon's experience. Matsunaga[2] at the Los Angeles County/University of Southern California Medical Center reported 1,200 malar fractures out of a total of 1,900 maxillofacial trauma-related cases between 1966 and 1973. The frequency and etiology of zygomatic fractures depend primarily on the patient population being studied and on the location of the hospital relative to highways, urban centers, and sporting events. The Los Angeles County Hospital is near major highways, and therefore a high percentage of the zygomatic fractures seen there are from motor vehicle accidents. By comparison, Winstanley,[3] in a series of 137 zygomatic fractures from Manchester, England, found 85 percent to be the result of direct trauma such as assault, sporting injury, or fall, and 8 percent from traffic accidents. Regardless of the etiology of zygomatic fractures, their frequency, more than any other factor, attests to the zygoma's prominent and vulnerable position. Zygomatic fractures are present in nearly two-thirds[2] of *all* facial fractures.

The zygoma's suceptibility to fracture can be explained in part by studies conducted by the Federal Aviation Agency. When subjected to controlled amounts of impact force, the zygoma required a force of only 50 to 80 g to cause fracture, which ranks second to nasal bones in susceptibility.[4,5] It is prominent and it is weak!

SURGICAL ANATOMY

The zygoma articulates with four bones: the maxilla, sphenoid, frontal, and temporal bones[6] (Fig. 7-1). This relationship has often been confused by the misnomer of "tripod" fractures, which is commonly applied to these injuries. Three of these

123

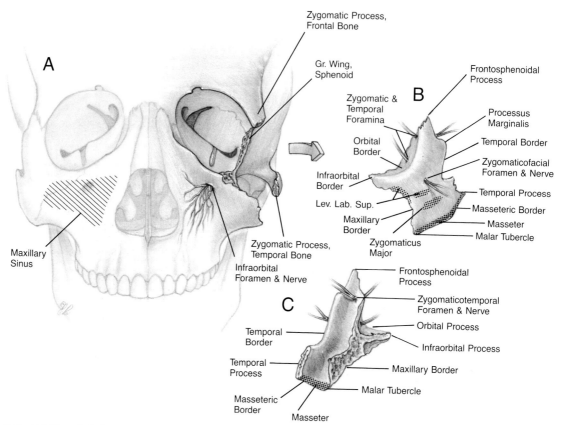

Fig. 7-1. (**A**) Facial skeleton showing areas of articulation of the zygoma with the maxilla, sphenoid, frontal, and temporal bones (see Fig. 7-3A). (**B**) Malar and orbital surfaces of the zygoma. (**C**) Temporal surface of the zygoma.

bones constitute significant buttresses[7] of the face that resist displacement of the zygoma (Fig. 7-1). The zygomatic process of the temporal bone buttresses the zygoma against force that would displace it backward under the cranium. The greater wing of the sphenoid affords resistance to displacement in a vertical direction, as does the zygomatic process of the frontal bone. The usual displacements of zygomatic fractures bear out the infrequency with which fractures actually violate these buttresses.[8,9]

In addition to knowing the zygoma's relationship to the skull, familiarity with surface anatomy is of considerable value in appreciating and evaluating the extent of injury to this structure. Of the three surfaces that comprise the zygoma, the malar surface is best known; it is this that establishes prominence of the cheek. Exiting on the surface through foramina are the zygomaticofacial and zygomaticotemporal nerves, sensory branches of the fifth cranial nerve supplying sensation to the cheek and anterior temporal area, respectively[6] (Fig. 7-1).

Numbness or paresthesias in the distribution of these nerves may be encountered in fractures of the zygoma. Sensory disturbances in the distribution of the infraorbital nerve are also seen because of proximity to the zygoma as it passes through the infraorbital sulcus in the floor of the orbit to exit through the infraorbital foramen (Fig. 7-1A). Muscles originating from the malar surface are the levator labii superior and the zygomaticus major, which are supplied by the seventh cranial nerve and contribute to facial expression.[6] The concave temporal surface transmits the zygomaticotemporal nerve and has an area of masseter muscle attachment.[6] The orbital surface of the zygoma forms part of the floor and lateral wall of the orbit. Disruption of the floor can lead to enophthalamos and diplopia and, on rare occasions, rupture of the globe by the bony spicules of a disrupted orbital floor. The lateral canthal tendons are attached to the lateral portion of the zygoma. Displacement of the canthus inferiorly in a fracture can give an antimongoloid slant to the palpebral aperture.

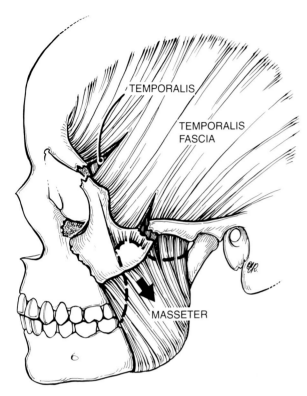

Fig. 7-2. Representation of the downward pull of the masseter, which contributes to displacement of the fractured zygoma.

The temporalis fascia by its attachment to the frontal process of the zygoma and zygomatic arch adds resistance against the downward displacement of a fracture fragment. If the force causing a fracture is severe enough to disrupt the temporalis fascia, significant downward displacement may occur. The downward pull of the masseter will aggravate this (Fig. 7-2). If adequate fixation is not secured after reduction of the fractured bones, loss of the malar prominence may occur.[10]

The zygomatic arch, formed by the temporal process of the zygoma and the zygomatic processes of the temporal bone, may be fractured with the zygoma or may present as an isolated injury (Fig. 7-3).

CLASSIFICATIONS

Since zygomatic fractures may be complex, classification systems have been proposed to aid in understanding the problem and facilitating treatment. A

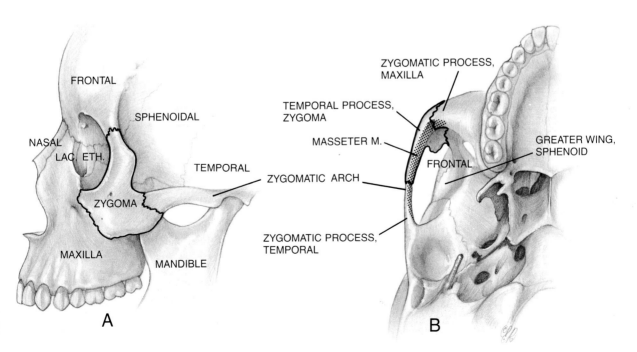

Fig. 7-3. **(A)** Relationship of the zygoma and zygomatic arch to the facial skeleton. **(B)** Basal view.

better understanding of specific fractures may be obtained by systematically grouping them into categories based on anatomic displacement. These groupings can then serve as a guide to management, leading to better and more predictable results. The essential question to be answered is what type of reduction and fixation, if any, is required to achieve a stable zygoma in an acceptable anatomic position.

The most widely accepted classification of zygomatic fractures was proposed by Knight and North in 1962.[8] By analyzing the preoperative anatomic position and eventual treatment outcome of 120 zygomatic fractures, they concluded that the stability of the fracture after reduction could be predicted by the type of displacement noted on the standard Waters radiograph. Once the position of the fracture was ascertained, a protocol for management of the fracture could be outlined.

Although the Knight and North classification has been widely used as a predictor of post-reduction stability, several important deficiencies have been pointed out by Yanagisawa.[9] He evaluated 200 zygomatic fractures and modified the classification of

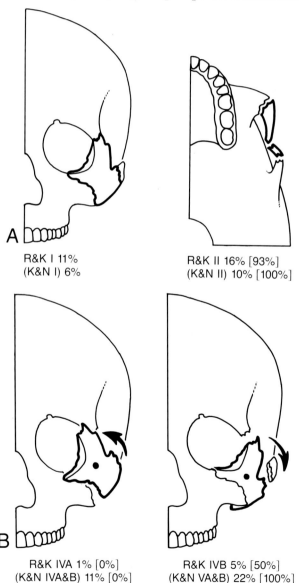

R&K I 11%
(K&N I) 6%

R&K II 16% [93%]
(K&N II) 10% [100%]

R&K IVA 1% [0%]
(K&N IVA&B) 11% [0%]

R&K IVB 5% [50%]
(K&N VA&B) 22% [100%]

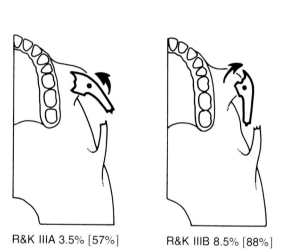

R&K IIIA 3.5% [57%]

R&K IIIB 8.5% [88%]

Fig.7-4. Comparison of modified Rowe and Killey (R&K) classification of zygomatic fractures with that proposed by Knight and North (K&N) (%, incidence of fracture type; [%], post-reduction stability.) (Classifications from refs. 8, 9). **(A)** R&K I and K&N I, Nondisplaced fractures; R&K II and K&N II, Zygomatic arch fractures; R&K III A, Medial rotation around vertical axis; R&K III B, Lateral rotation around vertical axis. **(B)** R&K IV A, Medial rotation around longitudinal axis; K&N IV A, Medial rotation upwards at the infraorbital margin; K&N IV B, Medial rotation inwards at the frontal malar suture; R&K IV B, Lateral rotation around longitudinal axis; K&N V A, Lateral rotation upwards at the infraorbital margin, K&N V B, Lateral rotation outwards at the frontal malar suture. **(C)** R&K V A, Medial displacement without rotation; R&K V B, Lateral displacement without rotation; R&K V C, Posterior displacement without rotation, K&N III, Unrotated fractured bodies; R&K V D, Inferior displacement without rotation. **(D)** R&K VI A&B, Rim fracture; R&K VIII, Complex fractures; K&N VI, Complex fractures.

Rowe and Killey.[11] Yanagisawa's classification dealt with the limitations inherent in the Knight and North classification (Fig. 7-4). The Knight and North classification did not include rotation around a longitudinal (anterior-posterior) as well as vertical axis. The new classification includes this. Fracture types I and II are almost universally accepted. These represent nondisplaced fractures of the zygoma and all fractures of the zygomatic arch, respectively. Type III fractures describe rotation around a vertical axis that is medial and/or lateral. Type IV includes fractures around the longitudinal

axis, again either medial or lateral. In Type V there is displacement but *no* rotation; these have either medial or lateral displacement. Type VI is the rim fracture and Type VII includes all complex fractures. Because the zygoma can rotate around a vertical or longitudinal axis, a complete classification should include this observation. The Waters projection does not allow for adequate evaluation of posterior displacement and rotation because the x-ray beam is in the same direction as the displacement and in the same plane of rotation. In the modified Rowe and Killey classification, posterior dis-

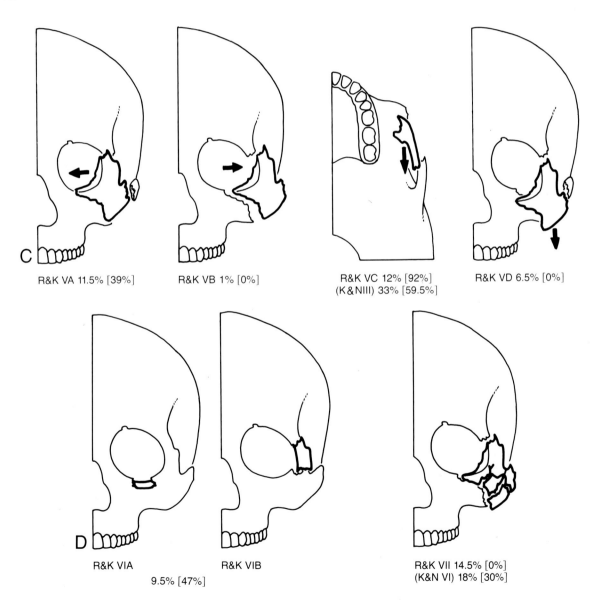

R&K VA 11.5% [39%] R&K VB 1% [0%] R&K VC 12% [92%] (K&NIII) 33% [59.5%] R&K VD 6.5% [0%]

R&K VIA R&K VIB 9.5% [47%]

R&K VII 14.5% [0%] (K&N VI) 18% [30%]

placement was added to Type V because of its uniqueness and apparent frequency (12 percent of zygoma fractures). Blowout fractures were deleted because they are an associated condition, rather than a primary fracture.

These classifications serve as aids in anatomically defining fractures, thereby facilitating their management. Since the surgeon's ultimate concern is stability following treatment, Larsen and Thomson[12] have proposed a simplified classification. They group fractures into two main categories: nondisplaced fractures requiring no treatment, and displaced fractures requiring treatment. They further subdivide displaced fractures into fractures which are either stable or unstable after reduction. Also, they are quick to point out that if there is any doubt at the preoperative evaluation as to the stability of a nondisplaced fracture, reevaluation should occur 1 week after injury and thereafter as required.

These classification systems help visualize anatomic displacement of zygomatic fractures and

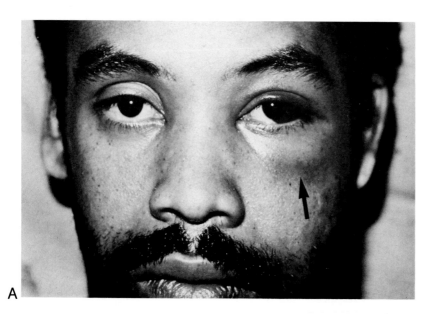

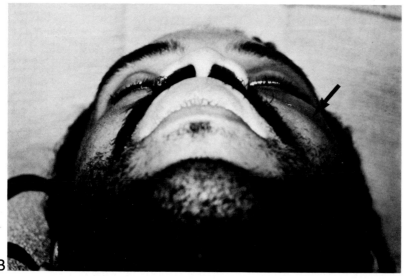

Fig. 7-5. (A & B) Clinical findings of a zygomatic fracture. Note the loss of malar prominence (arrow) and the subconjunctival hematoma in the lower lateral aspect of the sclerum. (Case contributed by Parvaiz-Malik, M.D., Southern California Permanente Medical Group, Los Angeles.)

alert the surgeon to potential problems in their management. They should not, however, be a substitute for a sound clinical approach, which consists of thorough physical examination, appropriate radiographs, computed tomography (CT) scans when necessary, and intraoperative assessment of the fracture.

TREATMENT

History and Clinical Examination

In patients hospitalized with facial trauma, 50 to 70 percent have other injuries.[5] Therefore, the surgeon called to evaluate the facial fracture should be aware of the circumstances of the injury. Any complaints relating to other systems should be evaluated prior to obtaining specifics about the facial fracture. An orderly and systematic evaluation, beginning with the general history and physical examination, should be performed to assure that no other significant injury has occurred.

The specific symptoms of zygomatic fractures are few. There may be localized discomfort. The patient may have pain or difficulty opening or closing the mouth. Visual changes including double vision may be present. The patient may have noted numbness in the lip, side of the nose, or malar area related to injury of the branches of the fifth cranial nerve.

Specific Findings Associated with Zygomatic Fractures

In zygomatic fractures there is often asymmetry caused either by swelling in the area of injury or displacement of the zygoma and zygomatic arch (Fig. 7-5A&B). Displacement of the malar prominence can be noted by both inspection and palpation. In addition to palpating the malar bone relative to the uninjured side, a step-off is often felt

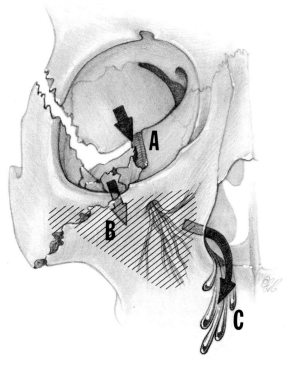

Fig. 7-6. Relationship of the infraorbital nerve to the zygomatic fracture (*A*), maxillary sinus (*B*), and unilateral epistaxis secondary to hemorrhage into the maxillary antrum (*C*). (Redrawn from Converse JM: Surgical Treatment of Facial Injuries. Vol. 1. Williams & Wilkins, Baltimore, 1975. © 1975 the Williams & Wilkins Co., Baltimore.)

along the orbital rim at the zygomaticomaxillary suture and occasionally at the frontozygomatic suture. Bleeding may lead to unilateral epistaxis secondary to hemorrhage into the maxillary antrum (Fig. 7-6) or to periorbital and subconjunctival hematoma (Fig. 7-5C). Intraoral hematoma may also be noted in the upper buccal sulcus. Fractures of the orbital process of the zygoma can result in disruption of the orbital floor and the suspensory ligament of Lockwood, and signs of entrapment may be noted. Examination of extraocular motion may demonstrate incomplete upward, lateral, or medial movement accompanied by diplopia. Confirmatory evidence of entrapment, especially of the inferior rectus muscle, can be obtained by a forced duction test. This is performed by topically

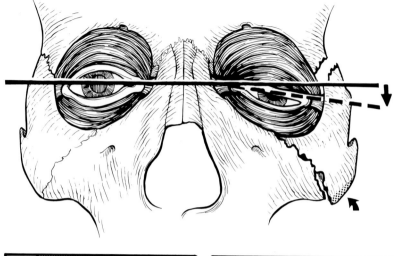

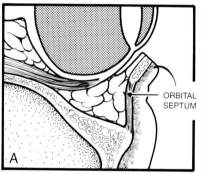

ORBITAL
SEPTUM

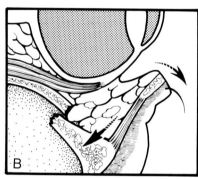

Fig. 7-7. An antimongloid slant to the palpebral fissure can be caused by the inferior displacement of the lateral canthus (dotted line) in a zygomatic fracture. Note the stippled area, which shows the inferior portion of the zygoma corresponding to the masseter muscle insertion. (Redrawn from Dingman RO, Natvig P: Surgery of Facial Fractures. W.B. Saunders, Philadelphia, 1964, with permission from W. B. Saunders Co.)

Fig. 7-8. (**A & B**) Downward displacement of the zygoma causes retraction of the lower eyelid because of attachments between the orbital septum and orbital rim. (Redrawn from Converse JM: Surgical Treatment of Facial Injuries. Vol. 1. Williams & Wilkins, Baltimore, 1975. © 1975 the Williams & Wilkins Co., Baltimore.)

anesthetizing the area and putting forceps traction on the muscle. If there has been significant inferior displacement of the lateral canthus, antimongoloid obliquity to the palpebral fissure may be noted (Fig. 7-7). Retraction of the lower eyelid may also result from downward displacement of the zygoma because of attachments of the orbital septum to the orbital rim (Fig. 7-8).

The infraorbital nerve may be affected, and numbness or paresthesias in the distribution of this nerve can be elicted from the patient. Trismus is not always present, but can occur if there has been impingement of the zygoma or the zygomatic arch on the coronoid process of the mandible (Fig. 7-9). When fractures of the zygomatic arch are present, either in combination with the zygoma or by themselves, a noticeable depression in that area may be seen and confirmed by palpation. Almost all fractures of the zygoma can be detected by obtaining a thorough history and conducting a complete physical examination. These studies should be per-

formed and well documented initially, as signs and symptoms may evolve over a period of days or weeks.

Radiographic evaluation is essential for confirmation of clinical findings and supplying a detailed picture of the extent of injury. Radiographic views most useful for initial assessment of zygomatic fractures are the Waters view (Fig. 7-10) submento-vertex view (Fig. 7-11) and Caldwell view (Fig. 7-12). The Waters view is the best single projection and is the basis for the Knight and North classification. Yanagisawa[9] has shown that posterior displacement of the zygoma as well as rotation around the longitudinal and vertical axes may not be adequately assessed by the Waters view alone. He suggests that longitudinal axis displacement be evaluated by the Caldwell view and posterior axis displacement by the submento-vertex view. Fractures of the zygomatic arch are best seen by the submento-vertex view. In cases where more detailed views of an associated orbital fracture are

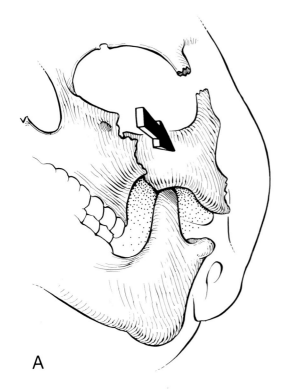

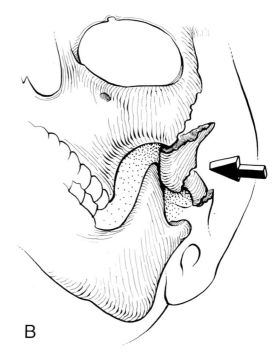

Fig. 7-9. Trismus caused by impingement of the fractured (**A**) zygoma or (**B**) zygomatic arch on the coronoid process of the mandible. (Redrawn from Converse JM: Surgical Treatment of Facial Injuries. Vol. 1. Williams & Wilkins, Baltimore, 1975. © 1975 the Williams & Wilkins Co., Baltimore.)

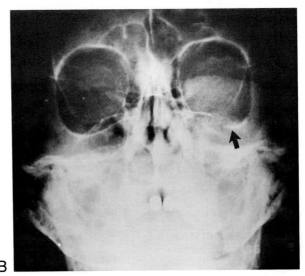

Fig. 7-10. (**A**) Waters view. (**B**) Waters view radiograph of a left zygomatic fracture. Note the disruption of the orbital floor (arrow).

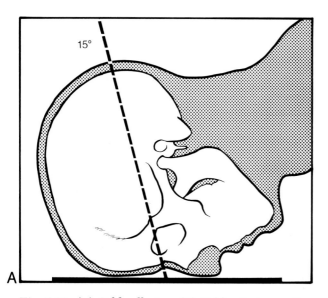

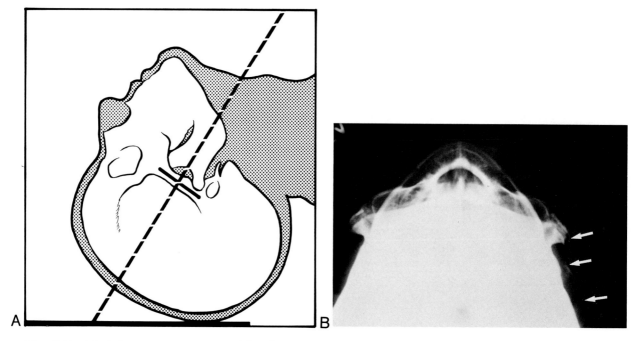

Fig. 7-11. (**A**) Submento-vertex view. (**B**) Submento-vertex view radiograph of a left zygomatic arch fracture showing the typical three-point fracture (arrow).

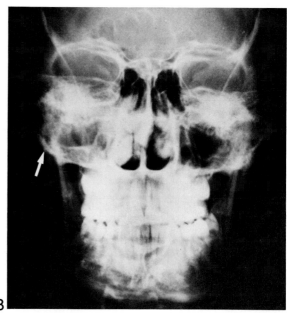

Fig. 7-12. (**A**) Caldwell view. (**B**) Caldwell view radiograph of a right zygomatic fracture. Note the clouded right maxillary antrum (arrow).

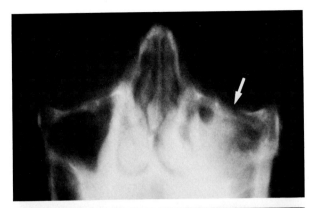

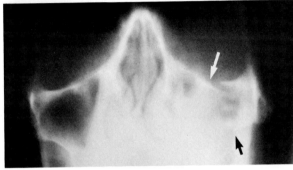

Fig. 7-13. Facial tomograms of a patient with a left zygomatic fracture. Note the disruption of the orbital floor (arrow), and the clouding of the left maxillary antrum.

Fig. 7-14. Computed tomography (CT) scan of a left zygomatic fracture. (A) Disruption of the medial and lateral walls of the maxillary sinus is evident (arrows). (B) The malar eminence is posteriorly displaced (arrows), and the maxillary sinus shows clouding secondary to hemorrhage. *(Figure continues.)*

needed, tomograms can be particularly helpful in assessing displacement of the bony orbit (Fig. 7-13). Use of CT scans in the evaluation of facial trauma has become a common practice as the equipment has become more available. In the acutely injured patient being scanned for head trauma, axial CT scans of the facial skeleton can (and should) be obtained, since they are useful for evaluating injuries to the zygomaticomaxillary complex (Fig. 7-14). Although coronal views may be helpful, especially for orbital floor fractures, this view is often precluded in the multiple trauma patient who cannot be readily positioned for this study. The value of CT scans has been amply demonstrated in evaluating complex injuries involving the orbital area. These fractures are not often seen in sufficient detail with standard radiographic studies. In the patient with altered vision, a CT scan may be helpful in determining the need for optic nerve decompression. Soft tissues around the orbit can be displayed in detail as finely as bone structures, and a significant amount of information regarding the orbital contents and the optic nerve can be obtained.[13-17] By altering the density and thickness of CT cuts, small bone fragments can be seen that are often missed by routine radiogaphs. CT scans are replacing tomograms in many hospitals and may be the only studies needed for evaluation of facial fractures.

In addition to the systematic approach just outlined, ophthalmologic consultation must be obtained in all patients with periorbital trauma.

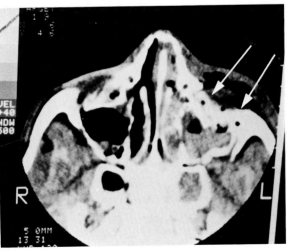

A
B

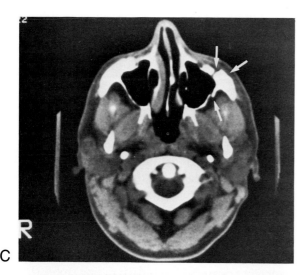

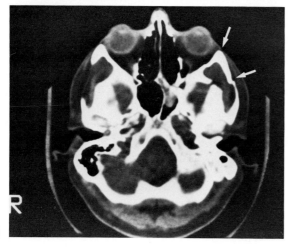

Fig. 7-14 *(Continued).* **(C)** CT scan of a patient with a zygomatic fracture. Note the fracture line (arrow). **(D)** CT scan showing the depression and fracture of the zygomatic arch (arrows).

Classifying the fracture aids initial decision making. It is also helpful to anatomically classify fractures into two therapeutic groups: those fractures requiring "observation only," and those requiring some form of operative treatment.

Nonoperative Therapy

Nondisplaced malar fractures without signs of orbital floor disruption require no surgical treatment. However, these patients should be reevaluated once a week for 2 weeks, and again at 4 to 6 weeks to check for any signs of fracture displacement. If at any time during the observation period, changes in the status of the fracture are noted, appropriate therapy should be instituted. For example, patients with nondisplaced fractures who show signs of entrapment or diplopia suggestive of orbital floor disruption are managed according to the protocol for blowout fractures described in Chapter 6. In patients with minimally displaced fractures of the zygoma and no functional problems, the presence of a slight contour deformity becomes the only complaint. Some of these patients may wish to forego corrective surgery, but this therapeutic compromise must be a mutual agreement between patient and surgeon. It is appropriate in all cases, but in this instance, critical, that careful photographic documentation of the injury and deformity be obtained and kept in the record. Displaced zygomatic arch fractures not impinging on the coronoid process may be managed in a similar fashion. Nondisplaced zygomatic arch fractures require no therapy.

THERAPY FOR FRACTURES OF THE ZYGOMA AND ZYGOMATIC ARCH

Treatment of individuals with facial trauma begins with the initial systemic evaluation and care of any life-threatening problems. If no other injuries demand immediate attention, treatment of the fractured zygoma may proceed in an orderly fashion.

Operative Treatment

Zygomatic fractures exhibiting contour deformities or signs of displacement of the globe, with or without signs of nerve and muscle entrapment, should be reduced and adequate fixation established. A surgical protocol, both in regards to timing and extent of the procedures, assures a thorough approach to treatment. Fractures requiring surgery should be operated on within 7 to 10 days following injury, since surrounding fibrous fixation may make later reduction difficult. This is particularly true for children in whom reduction within a week should be the goal.

In selecting the best approach for reducing a zygomatic fracture, the type of fixation required to maintain the bone in a stable position is the determining factor. Knight and North[8] as well as Larsen and Thomsen[12] have pointed out that 60 to 64 percent of zygomatic fractures will be stable after reduction without fixation. Dingman and Natvig,[10] however, observed that adequate reduction and continued stability usually require direct visualization and wiring because palpation alone is not always sufficient for determining adequacy of reduction, and initially stable fractures may become displaced later owing to masseter muscle pull or other factors. This latter observation would imply that all displaced fractures requiring surgery should have some form of fixation. We suggest that once the decision for reduction has been made, adequate fixation is indicated. In this way, fewer incidences of late displacement and contour loss may be achieved.

Methods of Reduction

Methods of reduction commonly employed utilize either direct or indirect approaches to the displaced zygomatic bone. The two most popular indirect approaches are intraorally through the buccal sulcus (Keen approach) or through the temporal region (Gillies approach). Direct approaches employ periorbital incisions and provide direct visualization of the fracture sites and orbital floor, facilitating wire fixation after reduction.

Indirect Methods of Reduction. The intraoral approach was first described by Keen in 1909. (Fig. 7-15) An elevating instrument is inserted through an incision in the upper buccal sulcus and placed behind the zygoma. The fracture is reduced with an upward and outward motion while palpating the orbital rim and malar eminence to determine adequacy of reduction.

The second and more commonly employed method of indirect reduction was described by Gillies in 1927[18,19] (Fig. 7-16) and employs an approach through the temporalis fascia. A small verti-

cal area posterior to the hairline overlying the temporalis muscle is shaved and infiltrated with lidocaine with epinephrine. Local anesthesia with epinephrine is used alone or as an adjunct to general anesthesia, which provides hemostasis and aids dissection. The incision is made vertically, with care taken to avoid the superficial temporal vessels. It is carried through both the temporoparietal and temporalis fascia over the muscle. A sturdy elevator is passed beneath the zygoma, and using the other hand as a guide, the bone is elevated into position. Through this same approach, any accompanying fracture of the zygomatic arch (Fig. 7-16A) can be readily reduced as well.

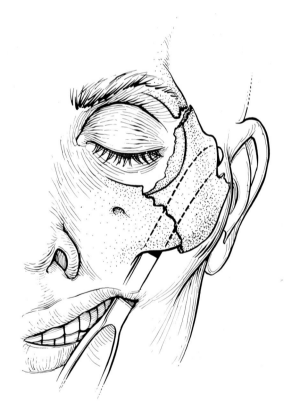

Fig. 7-15. Intraoral (Keen) approach for the reduction of zygomatic fractures. An elevating instrument is placed through an incision in the upper buccal sulcus and passed behind the zygoma; the fracture is reduced with an upward and outward motion while palpating the orbital rim and malar eminence. (Redrawn from Converse JM: Surgical Treatment of Facial Injuries. Vol. 1., Williams & Wilkins, Baltimore, 1975. © 1975 the Williams & Wilkins Co., Baltimore.)

If there was minimal disruption of the frontozygomatic suture preoperatively and if the zygoma feels firm and stable after indirect approach for reduction, further stabilization may not be required. While this is considered adequate treatment in some centers,[12,20] it is our feeling that some form of fixation should also be achieved. The method of internal pin fixation first described by Brown[21,22] in 1942 and later refined by Matsunaga[2] provides sufficient stability without direct wiring and seems ideally suited when closed reduction techniques are used. Matsunaga, using leverage models, demonstrated that the temporal approach provided the best leverage for reduction and the

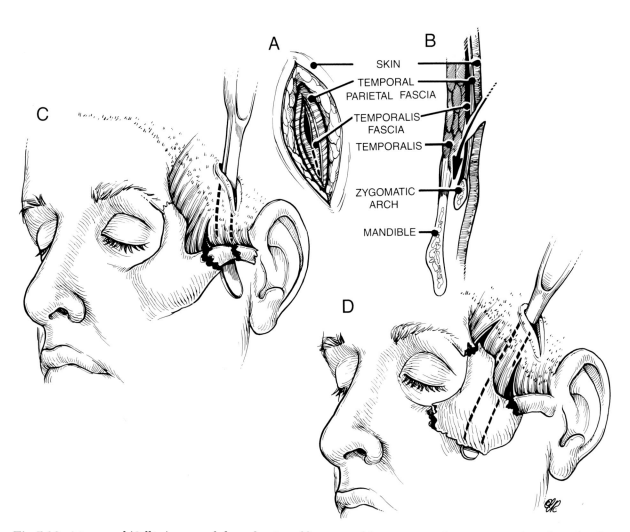

Fig. 7-16. A temporal (Gillies) approach for reduction of fractures of the zygoma and zygomatic arch, as described by Killey. (**A**) A small area posterior to the hairline and overlying the temporalis muscle is shaved and infiltrated with lidocaine and epinephrine. The vertical incision is carried through both the temporal parietal and temporalis fascia. (**B**) The elevator (as indicated by the arrow) is inserted behind the zygoma or the zygomatic arch. (**C**) The elevator is shown in position for elevation of the zygomatic arch. (**D**) The elevator is shown in position for reduction of the zygomatic fracture.

pin technique provided sufficient fixation in more than 75 percent of a large series of malar fractures treated at the Los Angeles County/University of Southern California Medical Center. Once reduction is accomplished, a 1/8th inch to 3/16th inch unthreaded Steinman pin or K-wire is driven obliquely through the zygoma and antrum into the hard palate approximately 2 cm posterior to the nasal spine. This angle of pin fixation is eccentric to the usual axis of rotation through the zygomatico-maxillary and frontozygomatic suture lines and resists displacement around that axis (see Fig. 7-17H for pin placement).

Direct Approach for Reduction and Fixation. Whenever there is orbital floor involvement or comminution, indirect reduction with or without fixation will not suffice. If pin fixation is established and instability persists, more direct means of stabilization are required. The approach described by Dingman and Natvig[10] for open reduction and internal fixation appears to be the most versatile and secure, and can be combined with pin fixation when necessary. The frontozygomatic suture disruption is approached first. We prefer an incision just medial to the orbital rim (Fig. 7-17A). The incision heals quite well in this location, especially

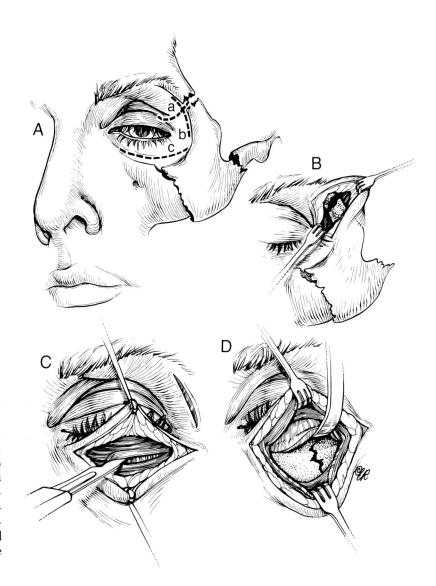

Fig. 7-17. (**A**) Dotted lines mark the preferred placement of incisions for exposure of the (*a* & *b*) frontozygomatic and the (*c*) zygomaticomaxillary suture lines. (**B**) The frontozygomatic fracture site is exposed. (**C**) A subtarsal incision exposes the zygomaticomaxillary suture line. (**D**) The orbital rim is exposed and the periosteum incised and elevated for inspection of the orbital floor. (*Figure continues.*)

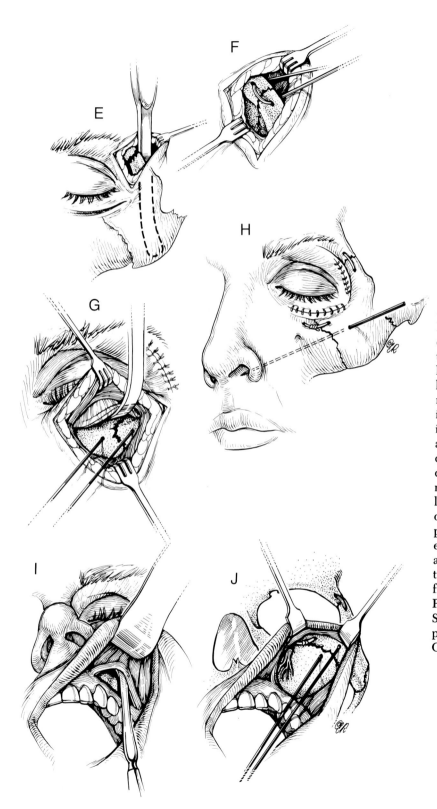

Figure 7-17 *(Continued)*. **(E)** The elevator is placed for reduction of the zygomatic fracture under direct vision. Wires secure the fracture at the **(F)** frontozygomatic and **(G)** zygomaticomaxillary sutures. **(H)** A Steinman pin is placed either as a third point of fixation, as shown here, or alone in selected cases, as described by Matsunaga (Ref. 2). Note that the angle of pin fixation is eccentric to the usual axis of rotation through the zygomaticomaxillary and frontozygomatic suture lines, thereby resisting displacement around that axis. **(I)** The maxillary buttress is exposed through an incision in the buccal sulcus. The area is first infiltrated with lidocaine and epinephrine, and the incision is made through the buccal mucosa and carried down to the level of the maxilla, where the periosteum is incised. Then, in a subperiosteal plane, the fracture line is exposed. **(J)** A fixation wire is placed at the maxillary buttress to secure a third point of fixation. (Redrawn from Converse JM: Reconstructive Plastic Surgery. Vol. 2. W.B. Saunders, Philadelphia, 1977, with permission from W. B. Saunders Co.)

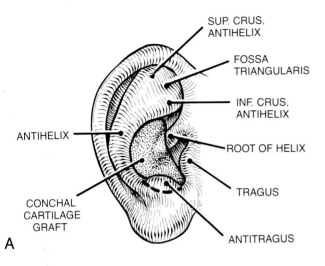

if the eyebrow is avoided. Local anesthesia with epinephrine for hemostasis is used in combination with general anesthesia. Dissection is performed to expose the fracture site (Fig. 7-17B) while a malleable retractor holds orbital contents medially. An incision is then made through the lower eyelid skin in the subtarsal fold (Fig. 7-17C). The skin is undermined 2 mm, and the obicularis muscle fibers are split horizontally, thereby avoiding scar inversion that may occur when muscle and skin incisions are placed at the same level.[7,23] Access may also be accomplished through a subcillary or transconjunctival incision. It has been pointed out by Converse[23] that the subciliary incision requires dissec-

Fig. 7-18. (A) A Conchal cartilage graft donor site is delineated by the stippled area. The cartilage can be harvested from either an anterior or posterior (preferred) approach. The area is infiltrated with lidocaine and epinephrine. An incision is made posteriorly through the subcutaneous tissue, which is then dissected to expose the conchal cartilage. The incision is then carried through the cartilage, taking care to stay below the antihelix. An eliptical donor site is then outlined, and the full-thickness cartilage is incised and removed anteriorly in the subperichondrial plane. Landmarks, such as the antihelix, antetragus, and tragus, should be observed. In dressing the wound, it is important to pack the conchal cavity, preferably with Vaseline-impregnated gauze, to prevent wrinkling of the skin. Large, bulky dressing is placed over the concha and ear. (B) An approximately 5-cm² conchal cartilage graft has been scored to facilitate its adaptation to the orbital floor. (C) The conchal cartilage is placed over the orbital floor defect and secured with 5-0 nonabsorbable Mersilene sutures.

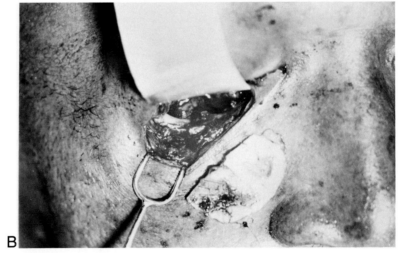

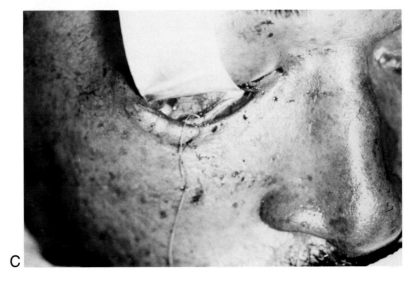

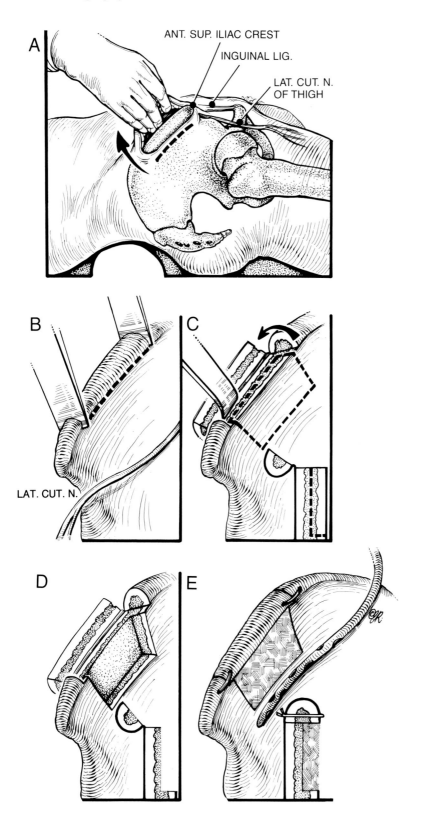

ANT. SUP. ILIAC CREST

INGUINAL LIG.

LAT. CUT. N.
OF THIGH

A

B

LAT. CUT. N.

C

D

E

Fig. 7-19. Iliac bone graft. (**A**) The incision is made approximately 2 cm lateral to the iliac crest and about 2 cm posterior to the anterior iliac spine. It is then carried through the subcutaneous tissue; the skin is then retracted medially to expose the iliac crest. The periosteum of the iliac crest is incised, and the inner table of the ilium exposed subperiosteally. Placement of the incision and exposure in this manner preserve the anterior-superior iliac crest, avoid potential damage to the lateral femoral cutaneous nerve of the thigh, and reduce postoperative morbidity found with incisions placed directly over the crest. (**B**) Osteotomes are used to cut through the iliac crest approximately 2 to 3 cm deep. (**C**) A curved osteotome (or an oscillating saw) is used to cut through the inner table of the ilium just below the iliac crest, as marked, which leaves the iliac crest attached to the periosteum laterally. A graft from the inner cortical plate of the ilium is removed. (**D**) A view of the donor site shows the extent of the harvested graft. (**E**) The donor site is packed with bone wax. The iliac crest is then realigned and wired or sutured in place; a drain is placed as shown.

tion over the pretarsal fibers and may result in vertical shortening of the lid. The transconjunctival approach is performed by making an incision through the conjunctiva and periosteum, exposing the orbital rim. This is a rapid technique, affords ready access to small blowout fractures of the orbit,[23] and has the advantage of a hidden scar. If more exposure is needed, a lateral canthotomy extension is required, thereby eliminating the advantage of a hidden scar.[24] For these reasons, the subtarsal approach is favored over the subciliary and transconjunctival approaches by most maxillofacial

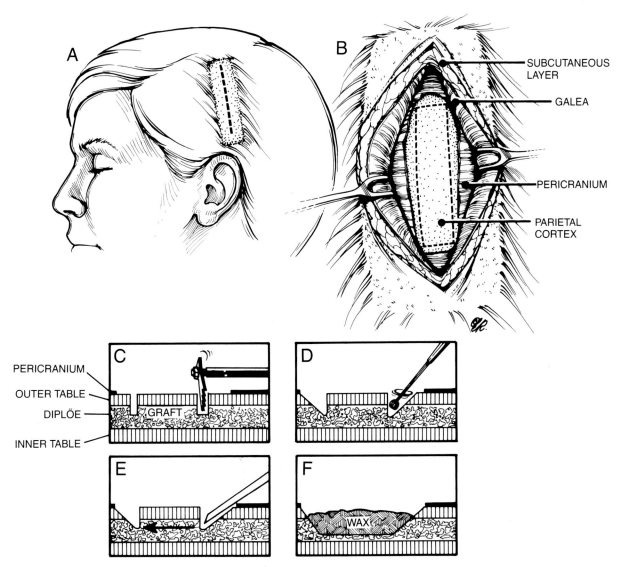

Fig. 7-20. Calvarial bone graft. **(A)** A vertical area over the pericranial region is shaved and infiltrated with lidocaine and epinephrine. **(B)** The incision is carried through all layers, and the size of graft required is marked as needed. **(C)** An oscillating saw is used to cut through the outer table to the level of Diplöe. **(D)** Using a round burr, the outer edge of the trough created by the saw is beveled. **(E)** Using a chisel positioned as shown, the calvarial bone graft is then harvested. The donor site is packed with bone wax and the incision closed in layers. If more extensive amounts of bone are neded, exposure through a coronal incision would be preferred.

surgeons. Once the orbital rim is exposed, the periosteum is incised and elevated to expose the orbital floor for inspection (Fig. 7-17D). After the fracture site has been identified, the superior orbital incision is retracted laterally. A sturdy elevator is placed behind and under the zygoma and the bone reduced under direct observation of the fracture site (Fig. 7-17E). The fracture lines are inspected directly, and an anatomic reduction is accomplished. Care is required, however, because while the fracture line may look reduced, it is possible for the malar prominence to have been depressed when the bone was rotated. In some cases, direct intraoral inspection of the maxillary buttress, as suggested by Karlan[25] for obtaining three-point alignment, may be necessary for accurate reduction prior to fixation. Once normal anatomic position has been obtained, drill holes are placed on either side of the fracture lines and secured with 26- or 28-gauge wires (Fig. 7-17F&G). If the fracture still feels unstable, a third point fixation can be established intraorally at the maxillary buttress or by passing a Steinman pin percutaneously as previously described. (Fig. 7-17H,I&J). These additional procedures should alleviate most delayed loss of malar prominence after two-point fixation. If the orbital floor needs reconstruction, conchal cartilage grafts may be used with defects up to 5 cm² (Fig. 7-18). With larger defects iliac bone grafts (Fig. 7-19) or preferably calvarial bone grafts (Fig. 7-20) can be used quite effectively. Our preference for calvarial bone grafts relates to the ease of harvesting this bone as well as to reduced postoperative morbidity compared to the iliac bone graft site.[26] Prosthetic materials such as thin Silastic sheets are effective, but foreign body implants with their associated problems are best avoided whenever possible.

Zygomatic arch fractures can also be reduced through the orbital rim or temporal approaches and rarely require fixation. If some form of stabilization is necessary, packing the temporal fossa with a Penrose drain or an inflated Foley catheter is effective. This can be removed within 7 to 10 days, once organization and early fibrosis around the fracture site has occurred. External support techniques have also been utilized by either K-wire fixation or transcutaneous suspension from a halo or biphase appliance.

OPEN FRACTURES

Open fractures of the zygomaticomaxillary complex are the result of severe trauma, such as that experienced in an automobile accident. (Fig. 7-21). Because of the possibility of foreign bodies in the open wound, thorough irrigation under pressure and debridement of devitalized tissue must be accomplished. Once the wound has been cleansed and bony fragments located, direct reduction and fixation of the fracture can be accomplished, often through the wound. Access may be facilitated by extending the laceration with conservative incisions along expression lines. Packing the maxillary antrum for support of the orbital floor has been discouraged by some in elective procedures where "blind" packing through a Caldwell-Luc approach has been used. It may however be of particular benefit in open fractures. If an open fracture of the zygomaticomaxillary complex affords ready access to the maxillary antrum and there is comminution and disruption of the orbital floor, the sinus can be packed under direct vision with Vaseline or antibacterial-impregnated gauze brought through a Penrose drain. The Penrose drain is then brought through a nasal antrostomy beneath the inferior turbinate and out the nares. Packing brought out of the wound or through the Caldwell-Luc incision increases the risk of infection and fistulization.[27] The Caldwell-Luc approach facilitates reduction of the orbital floor and is relatively safe when performed under direct vision. The volume of the maxillary antrum in an adult is about 17 ml. Overpacking or overinflation of a Foley balloon used to support the orbital floor should be avoided.

Once reduction and fixation have been established and wound margins conservatively debrided, the wounds can be closed in layers. If packing was placed in the maxillary antrum, it should be removed in stages 7 to 10 days postoperatively, when sufficient organization and early fibrosis around the fractures afford adequate stability. In open fractures involving the maxillary sinus and fractures into the oral cavity, prophylactic antibiotics are recommended. They should be given at the time of injury, prescribed specifically for oral organisms most likely to cause infection, and discontinued at 24 to 36 hours after injury. When antibiotics are used in this way, the incidence of infection can be reduced, and the emergence of resistent organisms is less likely to occur.

COMMINUTED FRACTURES

In cases where severe comminution and multiple fractures affect the zygomaticomaxillary complex and periorbital area, a bicoronal approach may afford the best access for anatomic reduction and fixation (Fig. 7-22). This procedure is described in detail in Chapter 2 and should be part of the armamentarium of anyone treating maxillofacial trauma. After adequate exposure has been obtained, direct wiring technique is performed, beginning at the most stable point and reassembling bone fragments into monobloc fixation. If bony destruction or loss is substantial, direct wiring alone may be inadequate to establish skeletal integrity. In these instances, primary bone grafting as described by Pollack and Gruss in Chapter 12 may be required to achieve stability and restore bony contour.

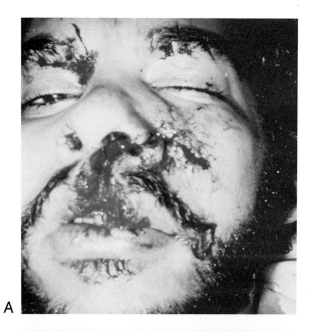

A

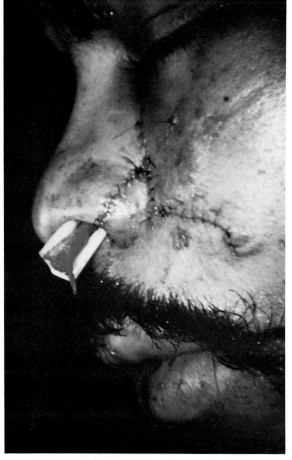

B

Fig. 7-21. (A) Open fracture of zygomaticomaxillary complex resulting from severe trauma in an auto accident. **(B)** Early postoperative photo following thorough cleansing of wound and debridement of devitalized tissue. Fractures of the orbital rim and anterior wall of the maxillary sinus were reduced and wired. Under direct vision, the maxillary antrum was packed for support of the orbital floor. The packing was brought through a Penrose drain beneath the inferior turbinate through a nasal antrostomy and out the nares.

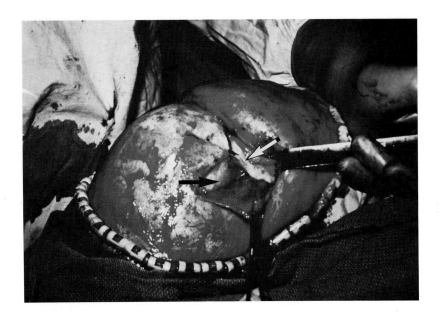

Fig. 7-22. Bicoronal approach for exposure of frontozygomatic and periorbital area. White arrow points to frontozygomatic suture, and black arrow to the temporal fossa, with temporalis muscle and fascia retracted laterally.

DELAYED RECONSTRUCTION

Zygomatic fractures are rarely a surgical emergency, and repair may be delayed until more serious injuries are managed. In cases where treatment has been delayed, attention should be directed toward the specific problem that persists and the least difficult approach utilized to correct it. If malunion has resulted in the loss of malar prominence only, augmentation of the area with onlay bone grafts or prosthetic materials may suffice. When malunion results in a more complex problem of enophthalmos with diplopia, as well as the loss of cheek prominence, correction becomes more difficult. Kawamoto[28] has shown that grafting the orbital floor to correct the enophthalmos that results from malunion is often not sufficient. He recommends that the zygoma be refractured through a combined coronal and orbital rim approach. After the zygoma is repositioned, the orbital floor and walls can be reconstructed with cranial bone grafting as needed. This can be a formidable undertaking and should be reserved for surgeons with craniofacial experience. Surgery may also be required for intrinsic eye muscles if diplopia persists.

ZYGOMATIC FRACTURES IN CHILDREN

In most large series of patients with facial fractures, approximately 4 to 6 percent occur in the pediatric (younger than 15 years old) age group.[29-31] Of these, fewer than 10 percent involve the zygoma.[29] The relatively smaller facial size and more flexible bony skeleton in children may explain this low incidence.[29] The lack of complete formation of the maxillary sinus in early childhood accounts for the scarcity of orbital blowout fractures.

Owing to the low incidence of zygomatic fractures in children, it is difficult to compile a large enough series in one institution to compare management methods. Over a period of years, the combined experience of several centers has established some basic principles of management. Once initial evaluation eliminates any major, critical problem, specific signs and symptoms related to possible zygomatic fracture should be elicited. Since young children are often uncooperative, sedation may be helpful, if not contraindicated by other injuries. Specific signs such as facial asymmetry, infraorbital paresthesias, and enophthalmos should be sought.

Radiologic examination is essential and should include the series of Waters, Caldwell, and submento-vertex views. In the severely injured child who may be receiving a CT scan for intracranial assessment, axial projection views of the facial skeleton should be obtained. Coronal views require positioning of the head in a manner that may be contraindicated in the severely traumatized patient. Once the diagnosis of zygomatic fracture is made and the extent outlined, displaced fractures should be openly reduced and fixation established. The extent of fracture is usually limited to displacement at the frontozygomatic suture line and a "greenstick" type fracture at the zygomaticomaxillary suture. The displaced frontozygomatic suture can be approached through a lateral upper eyelid incision and wired directly. The majority of zygomatic fractures in children require only fixation at this suture point. If other conditions permit, these fractures should be treated earlier than in an adult, since fibrous union is more rapid in children and reduction may be extremely difficult beyond 7 to 10 days. Delay in treatment may result in significantly more difficult problems. When the diagnosis is in doubt, frequent reassessment and reexamination are essential to ensure adequate treatment.

COMPLICATIONS

It is helpful to divide complications into those that occur early and are related to the initial trauma or surgery, and those that occur late and are most often associated with malunion.

Because of its proximity to the fracture, the eye is often involved in the initial injury. A thorough eye exam should be performed by the surgeon, an ophthalmologic consultation obtained, and findings recorded in detail. Complications such as corneal abrasion, hyphema, glaucoma, subluxation of the lens, vitreous hemorrhage and ruptured globe should be recognized and appropriate consultation sought. In cases of decreased visual acuity, a CT scan is indicated to rule out involvement of the optic nerve, either by direct injury or compression in the optic canal. The importance of a good eye exam preoperatively cannot be overemphasized, since at the time of reduction of the zygoma, there is always potential for damage to the globe and optic nerve. Two cases were reported by Converse[18] in which there was loss of vision after reduction of a zygomatic fracture, presumably due to bony spicules impinging on the optic nerve. Retrobulbar hemorrhage leading to compression of the optic nerve can also cause loss of vision after reduction of zygomatic fractures.[32] Bleeding in the retrobulbar area can be treated by decompression as well as by medical means of reducing fluid and tissue edema. It is essential that the patient's postoperative visual acuity be monitored frequently.

Whenever an open fracture is present, there is potential for development of osteomyelitis. Tetanus as a result of osteomyelitis in an open zygomatic fracture has been reported,[33] and tetanus prophylaxis in open fractures is recommended. With fracture into the maxillary sinus, acute or chronic sinusitis may be a troublesome complication. Proper management of the wound and appropriate use of antibiotics will significantly reduce the potential for these problems.

Most late-occuring complications are related to malunion or, in rare cases, nonunion of zygomatic fractures. In malunion with a contour defect or abnormal position of the eye, procedures for restoring contour and position of the zygoma have already been discussed. Since persistent enophthalmos and diplopia may be extremely difficult to correct, proper initial assessment and management should prevent most ophthalmic complications. Fibro-osseous ankylosis of the coronoid process has developed from impingement by the zygomatic arch; it has been recommended that the coronoid process be excised via an intraoral approach.[10]

Symptoms associated with trauma to the infraorbital nerve are not uncommon with zygomatic fractures and are present initially in 40 to 50 percent of cases.[25] If symptoms persist beyond 12 to 18 months, exploration and possible decompression of the infraorbital nerve may be considered. The nerve is best approached through a lower eyelid subtarsal incision exposing the orbital rim and floor, as described previously. The patient should be alerted to this problem at the time of initial injury and informed that although return of sensation is expected, this may not be the case, even after decompression.

CONCLUSIONS

"High," "prominent," "beautiful" cheekbones represent our society's attitude toward the normal or aesthetically pleasing zygomatic prominence. If only for aesthetic significance, careful repositioning and fixation or augmentation is worthwhile. Its keystone position relative to the orbit and orbital floor and its important neighbors such as the mandible and maxillary antrum make careful identification of fractures and meticulous repositioning and maintenance of fractured parts functionally significant as well.

REFERENCES

1. Goldwyn RM: Discussion of tetanus resulting from osteomyelitis of the zygoma. Plast Reconstr Surg 65:682, 1980
2. Matsunaga RS, Simpson W: Simplified protocol for the treatment of malar fractures. Arch Otolaryngol 103:535, 1977
3. Winstanley RD: The management of fractures of zygoma. Int J Oral Surg 10(s):235, 1981
4. Edgerton MT Jr: Emergency care of maxillo-facial injury. p. 286. In Zuidema GD (ed): The Management of Trauma. W.B. Saunders, Philadelphia, London, Toronto, 1979
5. Luce EA, Tubb TD, Moore AM: Review of 1000 major facial fractures and associated injuries. Plast and Reconstr Surg 63(1):26, 1979
6. Goss CM (ed): Gray's Anatomy. 28th Ed. Lea & Febiger, Philadelphia, 1966
7. Grant JC: Grant's Atlas of Anatomy. 5th Ed. Williams & Wilkens, Baltimore, 1962
8. Knight JS, North JK: The classification of malar fractures: An analysis of displacement as a guide to treatment. Br J Plast Surg 13:325, 1961
9. Yanagisawa E: Symposium on maxillo-facial trauma. III. Pitfalls in the management of zygomatic fractures. Laryngoscope 83:527, 1973
10. Dingman RO, Natvig P: Surgery of facial fractures. W.B. Saunders, 64:211 and 311, 1964
11. Rowe NL, Killey HC: Fractures of the facial skeleton. 2nd Ed. E. & S. Livingstone, Edinburgh, London, 1968
12. Larsen OD, Thomsen M: Zygomatic fractures. I. A simplified classification for practical use. Scand J Plast Reconstr Surg 12:55, 1978
13. Finkle D: Correspondence on CAT scan for facial trauma. Plastic Reconstr Surg 72(1):112, 1983
14. Mantredi SJ, Mohammad R, Sprinkle P: Computerized tomographic scan findings in facial fractures associated with blindness. Plast Reconstr Surg 68(4):479, 1981
15. Noyek AM, Kassell EE, Gruss J, et al: Sophisticated CT in complex maxillo-facial trauma. Laryngoscope, 92(27):1, 1982
16. Noyek AM, Kassell EE, Wortzman G, et al: Contemporary radiologic evaluation maxillo-facial trauma. Otolaryngol Clin North Am 16(3):473, 1983
17. Zilkha A: Computed tomography in facial trauma. Radiology 144(3):515, 1982
18. Converse JM: Reconstructive plastic surgery. W.B. Saunders, Philadelphia, London, Toronto 2:708, 1977
19. Huffman WC, Lievle DM: Zygomatic fractures-dislocations. Trans Am Acad Ophthalmol & Otol 56:543, 1952
20. Larsen OD, Thomsen M: Zygomatic fractures. II. A follow-up of 137 points. Scand J Plast Reconstr Surg 12:59, 1978
21. Brown JB, Fryer MP: Internal wire pin stabilization for middle third facial fractures. Surg Gynecol Obstet 93:676, 1951
22. Fryer MP, Brown BJ, Davis G: Internal wire-pin fixation for fracture dislocation of the zygoma. Plast Reconstr Surg 44(6):576, 1969
23. Converse JM: Discussion of a randomized comparison of four incisions for orbital fractures. Plast Reconstr Surg 67(6):731, 1981
24. Holtzman B, Wray C, Little AG: A randomized comparison of four incisions for orbital fractures. Plast Reconstr Surg 67(6):731, 1981
25. Mathog RH: Maxillo-facial trauma. Williams & Wilkens, Baltimore, London, 1985
26. Tessier R: Autogenous bone grafts taken from the

calvarium for facial and cranial applications. Clin Plast Surg 9:531, 1982

27. Wavak P, Zook EG: Immobilization of fractures of zygomatic bone with an antral pack. Surg Gynecol Obstet 149:587, October 1979

28. Kawamoto HK: Late post-traumatic enopthalmos, a correctable deformity. Plast Reconstr Surg 69(3):423, 1982

29. Bales CR, Randall P, Lehr HB: Fractures of the facial bones in children. J Trauma 12(1):56, 1972

30. McCoy FJ, Chandler RA, Crow ML: Facial fractures in children. Plast Reconstr Surg 37(3):209, 1966

31. Mulliken JB, Kaban LE, Murray JE: Management of facial fractures in children. Clin Plastic Surg 4:491, 1977

32. Lederman IR: Loss of vision associated with surgical treatment of zygomatic orbital floor fracture. Plast Reconstr Surg 68(1):94, 1981

33. Robson MC, Frank D, Heggers JP: Tetanus resulting from Osteomyeliti of the zygoma. Plast Reconstr Surg 6(5):679, 1980

SUGGESTED READINGS

Adams WM, Adams LH: Internal wire fixation of facial fractures, a 15 year follow-up report. Am J Surg 92:12, 1956

Constantian MB: Use of auricular cartilage in orbital floor reconstruction. Plast Reconstr Surg 69(6):951, 1982

Converse JM: Kazangian's and Converse's surgical treatment of facial injuries. Williams & Wilkens, Baltimore 1:287, 367–396, 1975

Finkle DR, Ringler SL, Luttenton CR, et al: Comparison of the diagnostic methods used in maxillo-facial trauma. Plast Reconstr Surg 75:32, 1985

Fortunato MA, et al: Facial bone fractures in children. Oral Surg 53:225, 1982

Freeman BS: The direct approach to acute fractures of the zygomatic maxillary complex and immediate replacement of the orbital floor. Plast Reconstr Surg 29(5):587, 1962

Georgiade N, Georgiade G, Serafin D: Twenty-five year evaluation of halo fixation for severe maxillo-facial injuries. Plast Reconstr Surg 68(3):444, 1981

Gruss JS, Mackinnon SE, Kassei EE: The role of primary bone grafting in complex maxillo-facial trauma. Plast Reconstr Surg 75:17, 1985

Jabaney M, Lehrman M, Shaders HJ: Ocular injuries in orbital fractures, a review of 119 cases. Plast Reconstr Surg 56(4):410, 1975

Johnson DH: CT of maxillo-facial trauma. Radiol Clin N Am 22(1):131, 1984

Kaplan LJ: Unilateral disk edema following tripod fracture repair necessitating optic nerve decompression. Plast Reconstr Surg 70(3):375, 1982

Manstein GH, Manstein G, Seitchik MW: Technique for reducing fractured zygomas using local anesthesia. Ann Plast Surg 6(3):213, 1981

Marsh JL, Gado M, Vannier MW: Discussion of comparison of the diagnostic methods used in maxillo-facial trauma. Plast Reconstr Surg 75:39, 1985

Nahum N: The biomechanic of maxillo-facial trauma. Clin Plast Surg 2:59–64, No 1, January 1975

Neumann P, Zilkha A: Use of the CAT scan for diagnosis in the complicated facial fracture patient. Plast Reconstr Surg 70(6):683, 1982

Ord FA, LeMay M, Duncan JG, et al: Computerized tomography and B-scan ultra sonography in diagnosis of fractures of medial orbital wall. Plast Reconstr Surg 67(3):281, 1981

Press B, Boies L, Shons A: Facial fractures on trauma victims: The influence of treatment delay on ultimate outcome. Ann Plast Surg 11(2):121, 1983

Reil B, Kranz S: Traumatology of the maxillo-facial region in children. J Maxillo-facial Surg 4:197, 1976

Reynolds John R: Late complications vs. method of treatment in a large series of mid-facial fractures. Plast Reconstr Surg 61:871–875, No 6, June 1978

Romm S, Goldstein S, Gottlieb S, et al: Computed tomography; new horizons for plastic surgeon. Plast Reconstr Surg 73:476–491, No 3, March 1984

Roncevic R, Malinger B: Experience with various procedures in the treatment of orbital floor fractures. J Maxillofac Surg 9:81, 1981

Schulta RC, Carbonell AM: Medfacial fractures from vehicular accidents. Clin Plast Surg 2(1):173, 1975

Shaw RC, Parsons RW: Exposure through a coronal incision for initial treatment of facial fractures. Plast Reconstr Surg 56:254, 1975

Tegmeier RE: A protector for the zygoma after fracture reduction. Plast Reconstr Surg 64(3):421, 1980

Tenzel RR, Miller GR: Orbital blowout fracture repair, Conjunctival approach. Am J Ophthal 71:1141, 1971

Wray RC, Holtman B, Ribaudo JM: A comparison of conjunctival and subciliary incisions for orbital fractures. Br J Plast Surg 30:142, 1977

Yamashita DDR, Arnet GF: A procedure for stabilization of intra-orbital rim in comminuted malar complex fractures. Plast Reconstr Surg 67(3):357, 1981

Zawarski RE: A simple support for unstable fractures of the zygomatic arch. Plast Reconstr Surg 65(5):673, 1980

Maxillary Fractures

8

Walter G. Sullivan

The most frequent causes of facial fractures are interpersonal trauma and vehicular accidents, and their reported incidences are 37 percent and 35 percent respectively.[1] The incidence of maxillary fracture varies greatly depending on the series, from 12 percent to over 50 percent.[2-7] The maxilla is relatively sensitive to transversely directed shear forces and can be fractured by a single blow.[8] Maxillary fractures reported by major trauma centers as resulting from high-speed automobile accidents are usually comminuted, associated with other severe injuries, and are a mixture of different classic types.[9]

ANATOMY

What is usually referred to as the *maxilla* is composed of four bones: two paired maxillae joined in the midline and the palatine bones. The body of the maxilla contains the maxillary sinuses. In the child the sinus is small, with the maxilla occupying a proportionally smaller surface area of the face, thereby making it a smaller target to trauma. The growth of the sinus allows the maxilla to increase in size without a proportional increase in mass. The anterior wall becomes quite thin and is more easily fractured. There are four processes: alveolar, frontal, zygomatic, and palatine. The alveolar process contains the teeth. With the loss of teeth there is a gradual resorption of the alveolar process. In the edentulous patient, resorption may be complete up to the nasal spine with little bone between the sinus and the oral cavity. The frontal process supports the nasal bones laterally. The palatine process joins the horizontal plate of the palatine bone posteriorly.

The maxilla forms a major part of the orbit and the nasal and oral cavities. It is related functionally and structurally to the mandible and cranium. The lower maxilla acts as an antagonist and stopping place for the mandible. The contact occurs at the occlusal surface of the teeth. Although a normal class I occlusion is usually present, the incidence of class II and class III malocclusions is such that either may be the patient's pre-traumatic occlusion (see Chapter 9). Loss of the maxillary teeth secondary to trauma or due to age may allow the over-rotation of the mandible, resulting in a pseudo-prognathic appearance.

The attachment of the maxilla to the cranium

149

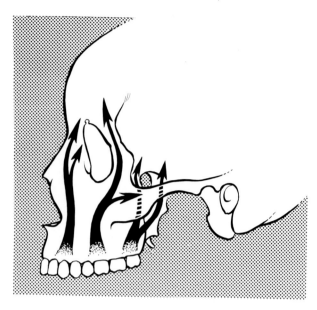

Fig. 8-1. Structural pillars showing the relationship of the maxilla to the cranium.

allows severe stress to be dissipated by fracture of the midface, which thus acts to protect the cranium and spine. Critical to this relationship and to the pathophysiology of maxillary fractures is the system of buttresses or structural pillars relating the maxilla to the cranium[9] (Fig. 8-1). There are three paired pillars: anterior, middle, and posterior. The anterior or nasomaxillary buttress extends from the region of the alveolar process of the cuspid, forms the lateral boundary of the pyriform aperature, and runs to the frontal bone via the nasal process and anterior medial orbital wall. The zygomatic buttress begins in the alveolar bone of the anterior molar teeth and extends to the zygomatic process of the frontal bone via the frontal process of the zygoma. Related to this buttress is a temporal extension through the zygomatic arch to the cranial base. The pterygomaxillary buttress has two components. The pterygoid component extends from the posterior maxillary alveolus to the cranial base through the pyramidal process of the palatine bone. The maxillary component relates the maxilla to the cranial base via the sphenoid. The structural pillars encircle the maxillary sinus, orbit, nasal cavity, and dental arch. As vertically oriented cushions, they protect the maxilla principally from vertically directed forces. Consequently, the maxilla is

most at risk for transversely oriented fractures. This was first extensively studied by LeFort, whose experimental studies led to the classification of maxillary fractures that bears his name.

Unlike the mandible, which has multiple muscles acting to displace the fragments after fracture, the maxilla has no strong muscle group attachments. Only the lateral pterygoid acting directly through its origin on the sphenoid bone has any appreciable effect on the maxilla. Consequently, the major displacement of the maxilla occurs through the mechanism of injury rather than through the pull of attached muscles.

The maxillary nerve, the second branch of the fifth cranial nerve, exits through the foramen rotundum into the pterygopalatine fossa. It passes through the inferior orbital fissure to become the infraorbital nerve. Traversing the infraorbital canal and exiting through the infraorbital foramen, it supplies the upper lip and lateral aspect of the nose. Among the branches are the anterior-superior alveolar nerve, which arises from the infraorbital nerve and traverses the roof of the maxillary sinus to the anterior wall where it gives off branches to the incisor, canine, pre-molar and first molar teeth; the adjacent gingiva; the maxillary sinus; and the floor, lateral wall, and septum of the nasal cavity anteriorly. The posterior alveolar nerve arises from the maxillary nerve in the pterygomaxillary fissure where it lies along the posterior maxilla and then enters the bone to supply the molar teeth and join the anterior-superior alveolar nerve in a plexus.

CLASSIFICATION

Alveolar Fractures

The dentoalveolar process may be fractured alone or in combination with other maxillary fractures (Fig. 8-2). The mechanism is one of direct force applied anteriorly or laterally. The mandible may

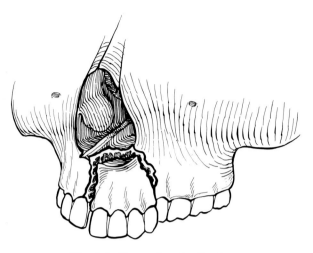

Fig. 8-2. Dentoalveolar fracture.

serve as an intermediary that directs the force of a blow upward and outward against the teeth of the maxilla. The fractured segment generally contains several teeth. Blood supply is usually secure, being pedicled on the soft tissue of the labial-buccal sulcus or the palatal mucosa.

LeFort Fractures

In 1901, Rene LeFort published the results of his experiments in which he inflicted blows to the head of cadavers by striking them with a wooden club

and throwing them at the edge of a table.[10,11] This monumental work formed the foundation of the classification of the major fractures of the maxilla used to this day.

LeFort I Fractures

First described by Guérin in 1866, the LeFort I fracture is occasionally called the transverse fracture of the maxilla (Fig. 8-3). The line of the fracture extends transversely above the apices of the teeth, through the maxillary sinus and the nasal septum. It runs posteriorly across the pyramidal process of the palatine bone and the pterygoid process of the sphenoid bone.

LeFort II Fractures

Also known as the pyramidal fracture, the LeFort II fracture follows the same path as the LeFort I fracture posteriorly (Fig. 8-4). It continues anteriorly and then curves upward near the zygomaticomaxillary suture and infraorbital foramen, through the inferior orbital rim onto the orbital floor, up through the medial orbital wall, and across the frontal process, nasal bones or nasofrontal suture, and nasal septum.

LeFort III Fractures

The LeFort III fracture represents a craniofacial dysjunction (Fig. 8-5). The fracture line extends from the nasofrontal suture through the frontal

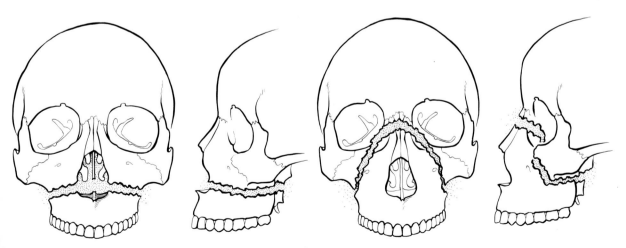

Fig. 8-3. LeFort I fracture.   **Fig. 8-4.** LeFort II fracture.

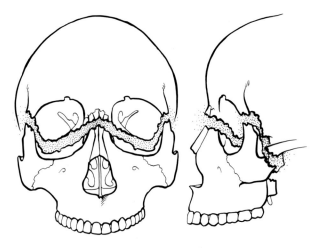

Fig. 8-5. LeFort III fracture.

orly. The fracture may, in addition, follow the transverse course of the LeFort I type or cross the infraorbital rim into the orbit and down through the zygomaticomaxillary suture area. Many types are possible. It is less common than the LeFort fractures and rarely occurs in pure form. It is thought to be caused by a force directed from the side.[12]

In the clinical situation, comminution and combinations of the different types of maxillary fractures are the rule. Associated nasal, orbital, zygomatic, and nasoethmoid fractures are common. This classification scheme, however, allows a more systematic approach to these frequently complex fractures.

process, down the medial orbital wall, across the frontozygomatic suture. It runs through the arch and continues through the pterygoid process of the sphenoid.

Sagittal Fractures

The sagittal fracture runs in a sagittal plane through the maxilla (Fig. 8-6). It typically passes to one side of the vomer and exits through the midline posteri-

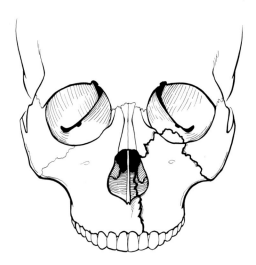

Fig. 8-6. Sagittal fracture into the orbit.

EVALUATION

Clinical Examination

Usually there is concomitant significant soft tissue trauma as evidenced by facial and intraoral lacerations and edema. (Fig. 8-7). Periorbital edema, ecchymoses with conjunctival edema as well as enophthalmos and entrapment may be present and suggest an associated orbital floor fracture. Nasal bleeding, though nonspecific, may be present and may initially obscure the presence of cerebrospinal fluid (CSF) rhinorrhea. Decreased sensation in the distribution of the infraorbital nerve may be due to simple soft tissue trauma, but anesthesia of the gum and teeth is suggestive of an intraosseous nerve injury.

Displacement of the maxilla is usually in a downward and backward direction. This gives the classic "dishface" appearance of the retruded maxilla, in addition to the "horse-like" elongation of the midface (Fig. 8-8). With displacement a malocclusion will be apparent on inspection (Fig. 8-9). However, with LeFort III fractures, occlusal changes may be slight. In fractures with only slight displacement, the patient may report, when questioned, that his or her teeth feel "different." It should be kept in

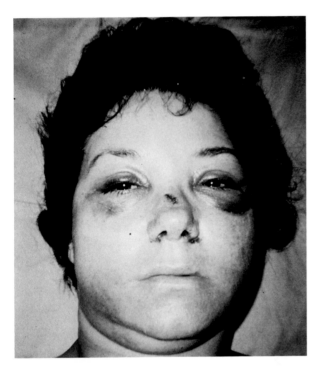

Fig. 8-7. Significant facial swelling and periorbital ecchymoses are present in a LeFort II and bilateral zygomatic fracture.

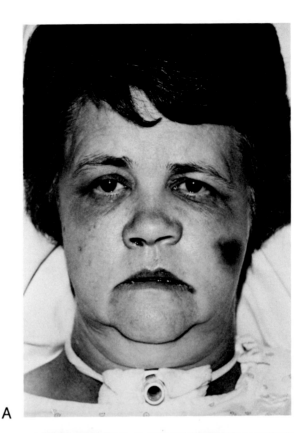

Fig. 8-8. (A) Preoperative view of a patient with a LeFort II fracture, 4 weeks following injury. (B) Lateral view of the same patient showing midface elongation and retrusion. *(Figure continues.)*

A

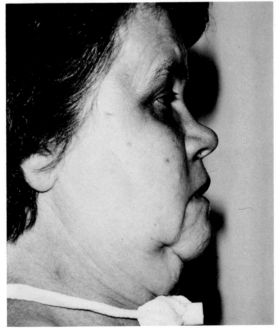

B

mind that mandibular fractures may also give a malocclusion.

By palpation, a step-off may be noted at the inferior and lateral orbital rims, zygomatic arches, and nasofrontal region. These may be obscured by edema. By grasping the anterior maxillary teeth, independent movement of an alveolar segment will be detectable. This should be repeated laterally. All types of impacted fractures, however, may show little movement.

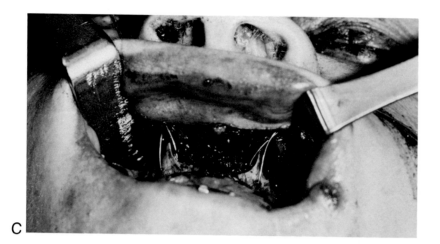

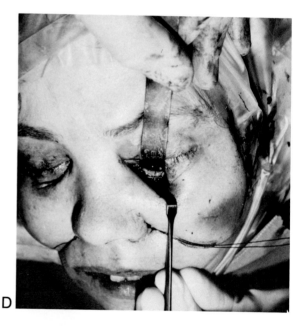

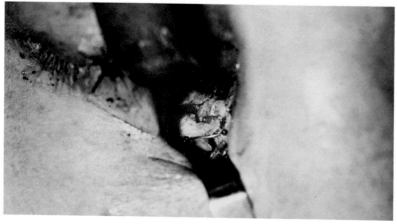

Fig. 8-8 *(Continued).* **(C)** Exposure of pyriform apertures with placement of suspension wires. **(D)** Exposure and wiring of left orbital rim fracture. **(E)** Direct reduction and wiring of right orbital rim fracture. *(Figure continues.)*

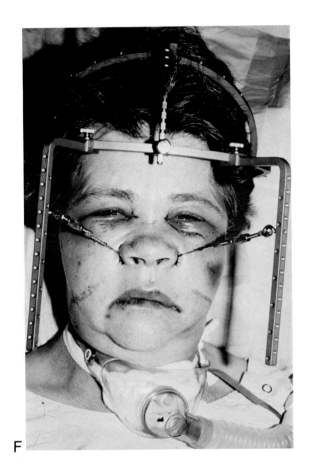

F

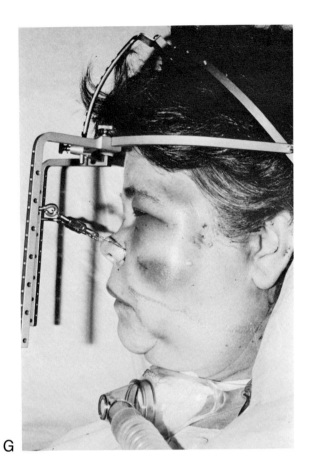

G

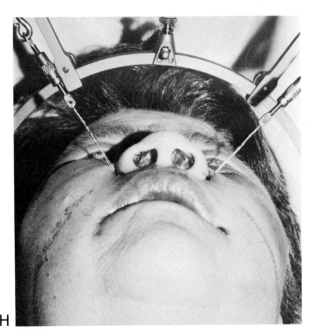

H

Fig. 8-8 *(Continued).* **(F)** Early postoperative view with halo suspension of retruded midface. **(G)** Early postoperative lateral view. **(H)** Early postoperative basal view. *(Figure continues.)*

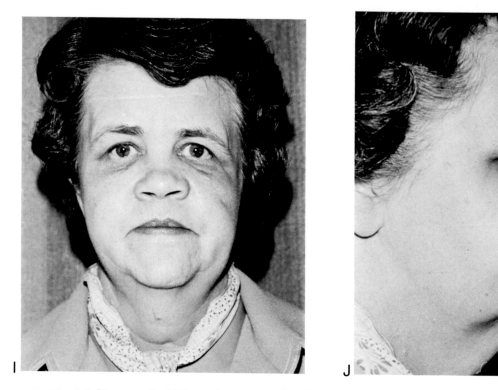

Fig. 8-8 *(Continued).* **(I)** Frontal view 8 weeks after surgery. **(J)** Lateral view 8 weeks after surgery.

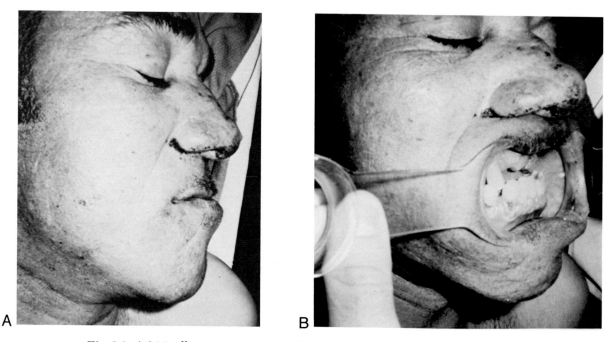

Fig. 8-9. (A) Maxillary retrusion in a LeFort I fracture. **(B)** Class III malocclusion.

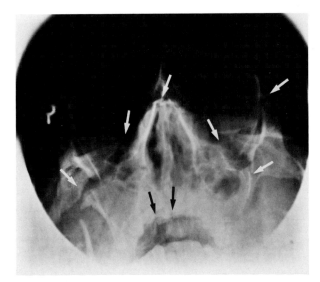

Fig. 8-10. Waters view of a LeFort II fracture with a palatal split. White arrows indicate the plane of fracture. Note the palatal split (black arrows).

Radiographic Evaluation

The most useful roentgenogram is the Waters view[13,14] (Fig. 8-10). The oblique view of the upper facial bones (Fig. 8-11A&B) allows a relatively unobstructed view of the orbital rims, zygoma, and maxillary sinus. Occlusal views, although not generally part of the facial series, are useful for sagittal and alveolar fractures. The panorex film is useful not only for the mandible but for the lower maxilla as well. The use of tomograms (Fig. 8-11C), though occasionally helpful, has given way to the use of computed tomograms (CT), which more clearly show the extent of the fractures, including intracranial and posterior orbital extensions.[15,16] A CT scan of the facial bones can be performed emergently at the same time intracranial injuries are investigated (Fig. 8-12). The axial view is standard, but coronal views may be helpful, particularly in looking at the orbital floor. However, the coronal cuts require extension of the neck and are contraindicated in the presence of a suspected neck injury. Sagittal cuts can be reconstituted from axial views. Computed tomography is the state of the art in radiography of facial fractures. When available, it should be utilized in all patients with severe maxillary fractures, prior to exploration, in preference to any other radiographic technique.[17]

TREATMENT

Severe midface fractures and associated injuries can be life threatening, with compromise of the airway being the principal immediate concern. Although infrequently necessary, tracheostomy should always be considered. The need for a more adequate airway may become apparent only after immobilization in intermaxillary fixation. Hence, a tracheostomy, although not emergently needed, may become necessary as treatment progresses (see Chapter 1). Patients with head injuries may go from adequate ventilation before treatment to inadequate exchange in the presence of intermaxillary fixation and nasal obstruction from blood clots.

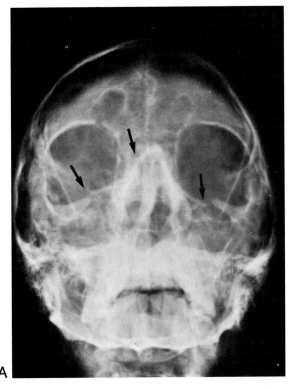

Fig. 8-11. (A) Waters view of a LeFort II fracture. Arrows indicate line of fracture. *(Figure continues.)*

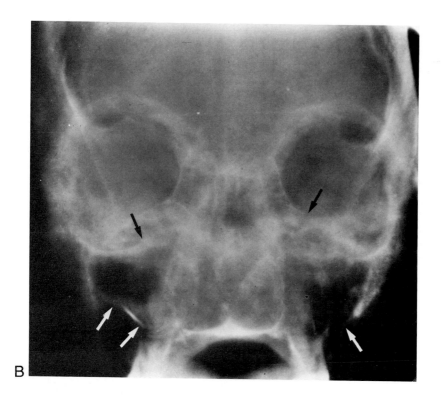

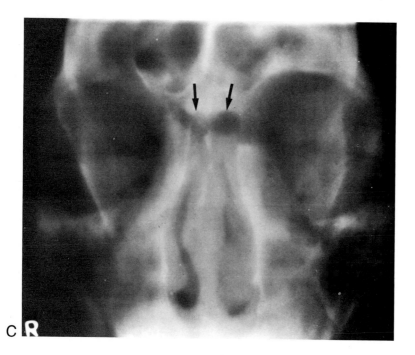

Fig. 8-11 *(Continued).* (B) Caldwell view of a LeFort II fracture (arrows). (C) Tomogram showing midfacial disjunction (arrows) at the level of the cribriform plate in a LeFort II fracture.

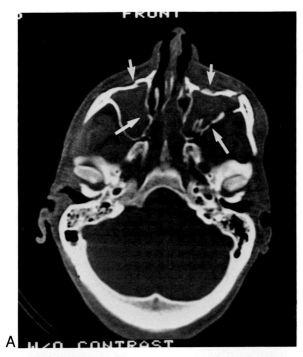

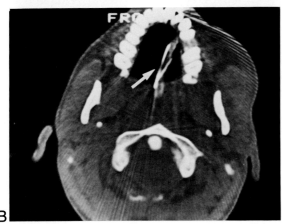

A

B

Fig. 8-12. Computed tomography (CT) scans of a LeFort II/III fracture with a floating palate. (**A**) Arrows indicate disruption of the maxilla. (**B**) Arrow indicates disjunction of septum and palate.

Alveolar Fractures

When there is an intact maxilla on either side, the displaced dentoalveolar segment is reduced and ligated to the adjacent teeth. This is most easily accomplished by utilizing an arch bar to fix the seg-

ment relative to the intact maxilla (Fig. 8-13). Associated soft tissue injury is repaired. When there are other fractures of the maxilla that make secure immobilization of the segment impossible, intermaxillary fixation should be performed. When the alveolar segment is large, added stability may be gained by the fabrication of an acrylic splint.[18] Making such a splint is relatively easy. Impressions are made of the upper and lower jaws. A plaster cast is then made. This is split, duplicating the fracture. The fractured plaster segment is then reduced. Wax is used to secure the reduction and more plaster is applied to make handling the now reduced fragments safer. The plaster models are mounted on an articulator and the proper pre-traumatic occlusion is established. An acrylic splint is then made on the lingual surface of the upper model. This is fitted onto the maxilla after reduction. If reduction is difficult, the fracture site is explored directly through a labial-buccal vestibule incision. An alternative approach obviating the need for an open reduction is the use of rubber band intermaxillary fixation.[19] The mandible will gradually force the segment into place over a period of hours. Failure to achieve reduction by this technique will require open reduction. Treatment of a fracture of the dentoalveolar segment requires immobilization for 3 to 4 weeks.

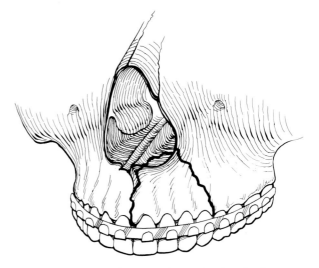

Fig. 8-13. Arch bar fixation of a simple alveolar fracture.

LeFort Fractures

The concept of treatment of LeFort fractures is evolving from one based on reduction, intermaxillary fixation, and craniomaxillary suspension to one based on open reduction, interfragment wiring, intermaxillary fixation, and less use of craniomaxillary suspension wires. Midfacial fractures are commonly comminuted. The impaction associated with suspension wires may lead to excessive shortening of the maxilla and premature contact of the molar teeth, which causes an anterior open bite. Shortening of the maxilla (loss of vertical height), a very difficult condition to correct later, is more common than lengthening of the midface following treatment.[9] Recently, interest has been generated in use of miniplate fixation that eliminates the necessity of intermaxillary fixation[20] (see Chapter 10). The reestablishment of the patient's pre-traumatic occlusion and intermaxillary fixation remain however the foundation of LeFort fracture treatment.

LeFort I Fractures

The mandible is the key to reduction of the maxilla. Any mandibular fractures are reduced and fixed relative to the cranial base. The maxilla is then reduced and placed in proper occlusion with the mandible. The incidence of pre-traumatic malocclusion is significant and should be considered if any difficulty is encountered in placing the maxilla in class I occlusion. The wear pattern of the teeth can be a reliable guide to proper occlusion. Although it is reported that the maxillary fracture will heal without malunion or facial elongation with intermaxillary fixation (IMF) alone,[21] some additional means of stabilization is commonly added. A suspension wire may be passed percutaneously around the zygomatic arch and attached to the upper or lower arch bar. This route offers the disadvantages of a posteriorly directed force that may tend to retrude the maxilla. Alternatively, a hole may be drilled through the inferior orbital rim and used to anchor the suspension wires. Obviously, this requires an open approach. Another approach is to explore the fracture through the labial-buccal sulcus with direct fragment wiring in the region of

the zygomatic buttress and the pyriform aperture. Additionally, from the same holes suspension wires can be passed from the strong triangle of bone where the pyriform aperture meets the maxillary sinus (Fig. 8-14). This approach however may still lead to excessive shortening of the maxilla in cases of severe comminution. If this occurs, simple internal fixation is appropriate. Regardless of the method used for suspension, it is suggested that this loop be twisted closed just inside the labial-buccal sulcus with an auxillary loop dropped from here to the upper or lower arch bar. Tightening of the stretched wire may be necessary for several weeks postoperatively. As this wire may break, it is easily replaced without jeopardizing the suspension wire. This suspension loop, visible in the upper sulcus, is easily removed after the period of intermaxillary fixation is over. Union is usually uneventful and nonunion rare. Intermaxillary fixation is maintained for 4 to 6 weeks.

LeFort I fractures in edentulous patients often require no therapy. On occasion, reduction and

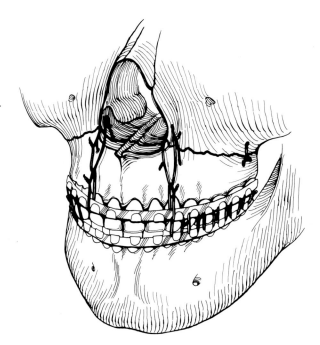

Fig. 8-14. Open reduction internal fixation and intermaxillary fixation of a LeFort I fracture with suspension wires running from the pyriform aperture.

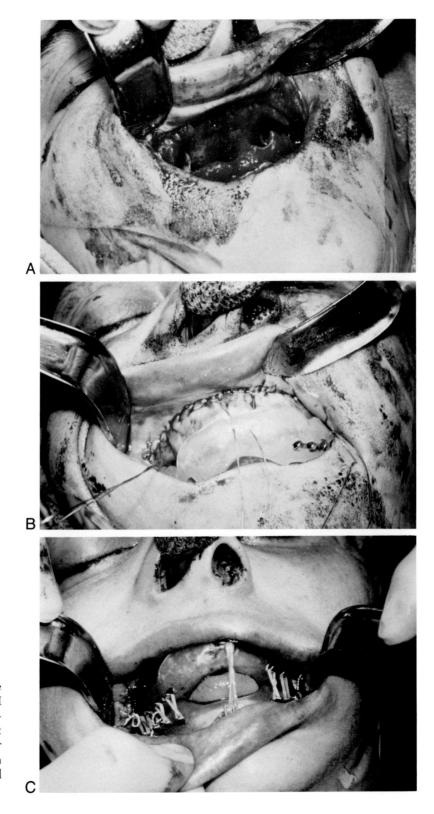

Fig. 8-15. (A) Intraoperative photo showing a LeFort I fracture in an edentulous patient. (B) The maxillary stent is wired in place. (C) A rubber band intermaxillary fixation connects the maxillary and mandibular stents.

fixation of these fractures are necessary to reestablish and maintain normal maxillomandibular relationships. The patient's dentures are ideal for use in this reduction. If dentures are unavailable, Gunning's splints may be constructed to maintain fixation (Fig. 8-15).

LeFort II Fractures

The maxilla is usually retruded, and reduction is frequently facilitated with the use of Rowe or Hayton-Williams disimpaction forceps. Pre-traumatic occlusion is reestablished and the maxillae are placed in intermaxillary fixation. Commonly, craniomaxillary suspension wires are then dropped from the zygomatic arch or inferior orbital rim to complete treatment. However, open reduction of the upper maxilla is preferred to simple suspension wires for reasons already mentioned. Internal fixation is done at the nasofrontal suture, infraorbital rim, and zygomatic buttress. Superiorly, exposure is gained through any existing laceration, a local incision, or preferably through a biocoronal approach. This exposure also allows treatment of any naso-orbital fracture or traumatic telecanthus, if

either is present. Wires are placed between the stable frontal bone and nasal bones of the maxillary segment. Any frontal bone fractures are first stabilized by anchoring them to intact cranium. The inferior orbital rim is reduced and stabilized through a lower eyelid incision or laceration, if there is one. Additional stability is gained through an upper labial-buccal sulcus incision to wire the maxilla at the zygomatic buttress (Fig. 8-16). Routine drainage of the maxillary sinus is controversial, as no clear advantage has been shown. Intermaxillary fixation is maintained for approximately 6 weeks.

Occasionally, direct exposure and wiring of fracture fragments may not be desirable. Significant delays in treatment necessitated by other injuries may make mobilization and fixation of the midface difficult. In these instances, external fixation and suspension of the midface with a halo is a treatment alternative (Fig. 8-8).

LeFort III Fractures

Reduction and immobilization is approached as in the LeFort II fracture. The maxilla is reduced and placed into intermaxillary fixation. Craniomaxillary suspension wires can be dropped from the superior lateral orbital rim after reduction and interosseous wire fixation of the frontozygomatic suture region of the fracture (Fig. 8-17). However, direct wiring of the major fracture is preferred (Fig. 8-18). A bicoronal flap is raised. The nasofrontal region is wired. The lateral orbital rim is easily exposed and wired through the bicoronal incision. In addition, this incision affords a direct approach to the zygomatic arch, which is difficult to achieve through local incisions because of the danger of injury to the temporal branch of the facial nerve. A lower eyelid incision can allow inspection of the orbital floor and treatment of an associated orbital floor fracture. In extensive orbital floor fracture or nasoethmoid fracture, primary bone grafting may be indicated (see Chapter 5). Outer table of skull is preferred and is easily accessible through the bicoronal incision. The utility of bone grafts in the pterygomaxillary area is unproven.[22] Intermaxillary fixation is continued for approximately 6 weeks.

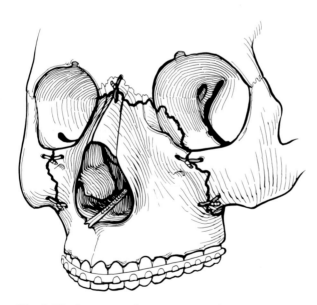

Fig. 8-16. An open reduction internal fixation and intermaxillary fixation of a LeFort II fracture.

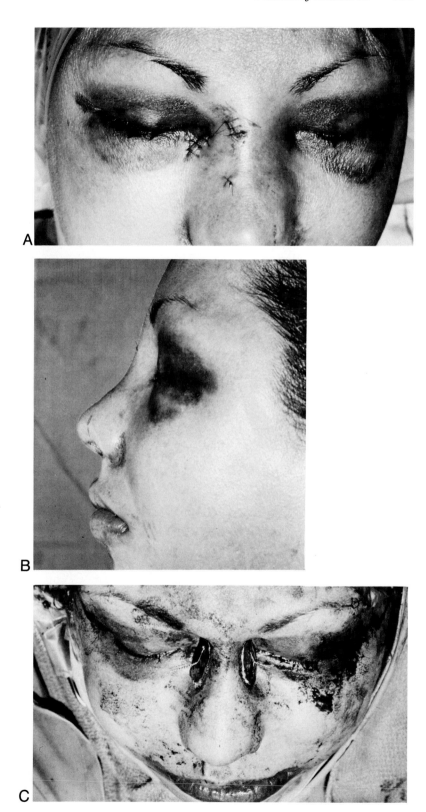

Fig. 8-17. (A) Preoperative photo of a patient with a Le-Fort III fracture. **(B)** Lateral view of the same patient. **(C)** Intraoperative photo showing a lead plate reduction of the nasal fracture. *(Figure continues.)*

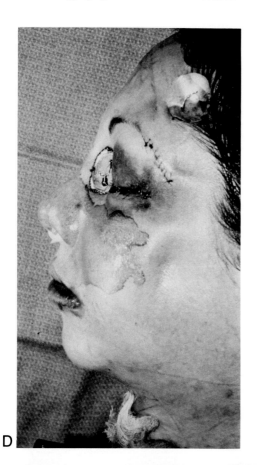

D

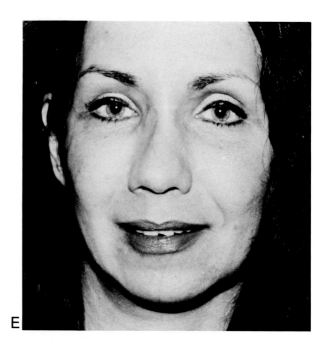

E

Fig. 8-17 *(Continued).* **(D)** Intraoperative lateral view showing a suspension wire pullout button, lead plates, and lateral brow incision. **(E)** Postoperative view. **(F)** Postoperative lateral view. **(G)** Postoperative basal view.

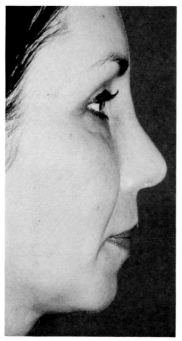

F

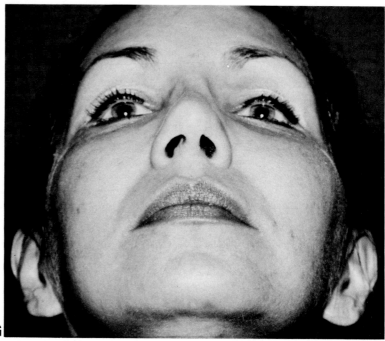

G

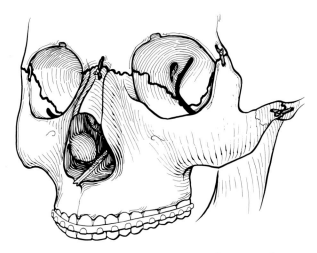

Fig. 8-18. An open reduction internal fixation and intermaxillary fixation of a LeFort III fracture.

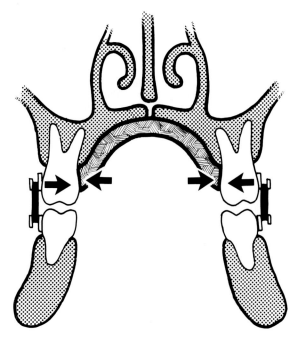

Fig. 8-19. A palatal splint in place to prevent palatal rotation of the lateral maxillary segments.

Sagittal Fractures

Simply placing the maxilla into intermaxillary fixation allows palatal rotation of the lateral maxillary segments toward the midline. To prevent this, a palatal splint is fabricated to hold the lateral segments in proper occlusion (Fig. 8-19). In addition, it is suggested that an interosseous wire is necessary at the pyriform aperature, which is approached through a superior labial sulcus incision. Fractures that also extend laterally in the manner of a LeFort I fracture are additionally wired in the zygomatic buttress area. Sagittal fractures that extend into the orbit and across the lateral orbital rim are similarly wired (Fig. 8-20). Occasionally, displacement posteriorly in the palate is treated by raising a mucoperiosteal flap and securing the posterior palate with an interosseous wire. Intermaxillary fixation is maintained for 6 to 8 weeks.

The Edentulous Patient

The patient's dentures are utilized to bring the maxillae into their normal relationship (see Chapter 9). The dentures are secured by circummandibular wires and either by wires around the pyriform aperature or by suspension wires from the pyri-

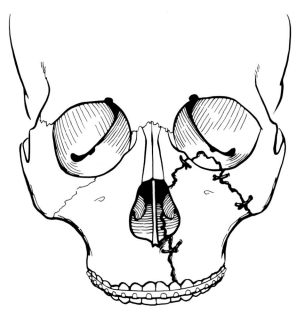

Fig. 8-20. An open reduction internal fixation and intermaxillary fixation of a sagittal fracture involving the orbit.

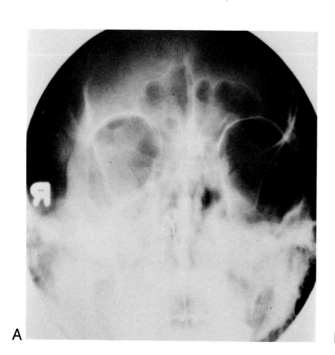

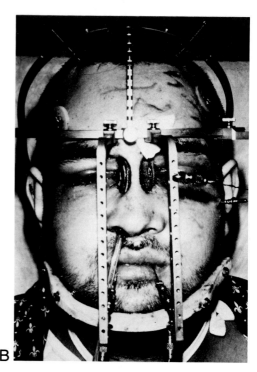

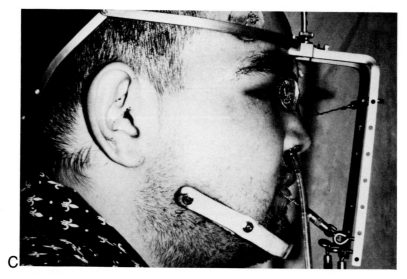

Fig. 8-21. **(A)** Waters view showing a panfacial fracture. **(B & C)** Postoperative photographs illustrating the use of a Joe Hall Morris external fixation with a Georgiade's halo.

form area, the inferior orbital rim, or the zygomatic arch. In the patient without dentures, a Gunning splint is prepared (Fig. 8-15). In minimally displaced fractures in the elderly patient, fixation may be avoided and the patient's dentures merely adjusted to fit the slightly different maxillary relationship.

Children

The maxilla is small and not fully pneumatized in children and therefore is relatively infrequently fractured. Treatment is similar to that of adults, with a few exceptions.[23] Healing is very rapid and reduction should be accomplished as soon as possible, probably within 7 days. In addition, the zygomatic arch is quite delicate and should not be used for suspension wires if these are used. The pyriform area is significantly stronger.

External Skeletal Fixation

Intermaxillary fixation and interosseous wiring may not be sufficient to prevent collapse of severely comminuted fractures. Lateral and anterior traction may be necessary to prevent collapse. In this exceptional situation, external skeletal traction, such as provided by Georgiade's halo apparatus, the "crown of thorns," may be necessary[24] (Fig. 8-8). Usually, when external skeletal fixation is needed, it is applied to the mandible in the form of a Joe Hall Morris appliance. The mandible can then be used for proper reduction of the maxilla (Fig. 8-21).

Timing

When facilities are available, patients even with severe injuries may be taken to the operating room within hours of trauma, before swelling becomes great. An emergency CT scan will not only demonstrate the facial fractures clearly but also will eliminate the guesswork about whether the patient has a significant intracranial injury. At this stage fractures are easily reduced and treatment can be undertaken concomitantly with other procedures (e.g., exploratory laparotomy, tracheotomy). However it is frequently not possible to operate immediately. In this case, swelling has usually subsided substantially by the fifth post-traumatic day, and surgery may be performed more easily between this time and approximately the tenth post-injury day. If possible, the patient is placed in intermaxillary fixation as soon as possible. This not only increases patient comfort but makes eventual reduction and fixation easier.

COMPLICATIONS

The early complications of bleeding, airway problems, and infection are common to facial fractures in general. Specific to the maxilla is a low incidence of maxillary sinusitis. Airfluid levels in the sinus associated with unidentified fever should be followed by drainage through a labial sulcus incision.

CSF Rhinorrhea

CSF Rhinorrhea is reported in 25 to 35 percent of LeFort II and LeFort III fractures.[17,5,25] Without operative treatment, most CSF leaks close in a few days, and 95 percent will close spontaneously within 3 weeks. The value of antibiotics to prevent meningitis has not been demonstrated, although they are commonly used. Easily treated dural tears (e.g., frontal sinus fracture) can be repaired at the time of exploration. CSF leaks persisting after 3 weeks are treated, usually with a dural patch.

Blindness

Blindness is usually a complication of the initial injury.[26,27] The mechanism is thought to be an optic nerve laceration caused by displaced bone fragments.

LATE COMPLICATIONS

Nonunion

Nonunion is quite rare and is usually seen in untreated fractures or those in which comminution was severe and fixation was not adequate for the extent of the injury. Treatment consists of exposure of the fracture site, bone grafting, and fixation. Slight mobility of the maxilla, now commonly seen in elective LeFort I procedures, may be present for months. Eventual firm union can be expected.

Malunion

Untreated fractures or those with inadequate reduction may demonstrate malunion or malocclusion. In one study, occlusal disharmony was seen in approximately 20 percent of patients with approximately 90 percent of these corrected by simple means not requiring surgery.[28]

Severe late deformities, such as an elongated face or retruded maxilla, may be corrected with LeFort osteotomies. Where occlusion is satisfactory, onlay bone grafts may correct a nasal or zygomatic deformity. Where the upper maxilla is satisfactory, a LeFort I may be performed to correct malocclusion. A short face resulting from suspension wires used in the presence of severe comminution is very difficult to correct electively, and recurrence is common.

Nerve Injury

Anesthesia of the teeth is expected after transverse maxillary fracture. Recovery is usual, and patients should be instructed to inform their dentists, as unnecessary root canal therapy may be instituted in the months before pulp testing returns to normal. Injury to the infraorbital nerve is common, being reported in 40 percent of LeFort fractures. Persistent infraorbital nerve symptoms are reported in half of these patients. Decreased sensation may be permanent and less annoying to the patient over time. Pain may be a significant problem and should be approached through decompression of the infraorbital canal if no relief occurs within 6 to 12 months.[28]

Osteomyelitis

Osteomyelitis is rarely reported after treatment of maxillary fractures; treatment should include debridement, bone grafting, and fixation.

Lacrimal System

The nasolacrimal duct may be interrupted in the LeFort II fracture. LeFort II and LeFort III fractures may be associated with injuries of the lacrimal sac. Persistent epiphora is reported in 4 percent of patients.[28] Reconstructive procedures, (e.g., dacryocystorhinostomy, Jones tube insertion), may be indicated (see Chapter 6).

Others

Anosmia is reported in 2 to 3 percent of patients.[28] It is slightly higher in patients undergoing craniotomy for associated cranial injuries. Diplopia is found in approximately one-third of patients with LeFort II and LeFort III fractures. This resolves in 70 percent of patients, with the remainder having persistent diplopia, usually due to the entrapment of the lateral oblique muscle. Extraoccular muscle surgery is successful in the majority of patients. Chronic maxillary sinusitis is rarely seen.

ACKNOWLEDGEMENT

Special thanks to Martin C. Robson, M.D., Eti Gursel, M.D., and June Unger, M.D. for the use of their clinical photographs and radiographs; and to Henry K. Kawamoto, Jr., M.D., D.D.S. for his assistance.

REFERENCES

1. Gwyn PP, Cardway JH, Horton CE, et al: Facial fractures: Associated injuries and complications. Plast Reconstr Surg 47:225, 1971
2. Afzelius LE, Rosen C: Facial fractures: A review of 368 cases. Int J Oral Surg 9:25, 1980
3. Kelly DE, Harrigan WF: A survey of facial fractures: Bellevue Hospital, 1948–1974. J Oral Surg 33:146, 1975
4. McCoy FJ, Chandler RA, Magnan CG, et al: Analysis of facial fractures and their complications. Plast Reconstr Surg 29:381, 1962
5. Morgan BDG, Madan DK, Bergerot JPC: Fractures of the middle third of the face: A review of 300 cases. Br J Plast Surg 25:147, 1972
6. Schultz RC, Carbonell AM: Midfacial fractures from vehicular accidents. Clin Plast Surg 2:173, 1975
7. Turvey TA: Midfacial fractures: A retrospective analysis of 593 cases. J Oral Surg 35:887, 1977
8. Nahum AM: The biomechanics of maxillofacial trauma. Clin Plast Surg 2:59, 1975
9. Manson PN, Hoopes JE, Su CT: Structural pillars of the facial skeleton: An approach to the management of LeFort fractures. Plast Reconstr Surg 66:54, 1980
10. LeFort R: Experimental study of fractures of the upper jaw. I, II. Rev Chir de Paris 23:208, 360, 1901. Transl by P. Tessier in Plast Reconstr Surg 50:497, 1972
11. LeFort R: Experimental study of fractures of the upper jaw. III. Rev Chir de Paris 23:479, 1901. Transl by P. Tessier in Plast Reconstr Surg 50:600, 1972
12. Manson PN, Shack RB, Leonard LG et al: Sagittal fractures of the maxilla and palate. Plast Reconstr Surg 72:484, 1983
13. Dingman RO, Converse JM: The clinical management of facial injuries and fractures of the facial bones. p. 599. In Converse JM (ed): Reconstructive Plastic Surgery. W.B. Saunders, Philadelphia, 1977
14. Noyek AM, Kassel EE, Wortzman G, et al: Contemporary radiologic evaluation in maxillofacial trauma. Otolaryngol Clin North Am 16:473, 1983
15. Johnson DH Jr: CT of maxillofacial trauma. Radiol Clin North Am 22(1):131, 1984
16. Rowe LD, Miller E, Brandt-Zawadzki M: Computerized Tomography in Maxillofacial Trauma. Laryngoscope 91:745, 1981
17. Manson PN: Complex facial injuries. Presented at the Northwestern University Board Review Course, 1983
18. Holmes SM, Kline SN: The use of intraoral splints in the treatment of maxillofacial injuries. Otolaryngol Clin North Am 16(3):525, 1983
19. Dingman RO, Natvig P: Surgery of Facial Fractures. W.B. Saunders, Philadelphia, 1964
20. Munro IR, Kay P, Beals S: Cranio-maxillo-facial surgery and mini-plates: Elimination of intermaxillary fixation. Plast Surg Forum 8:64, 1985
21. Sofferman RA, Danielson PA, Quatela V, Reed RR: Retrospective analysis of surgically treated LeFort fractures. Arch Otolaryngol 109:446, 1983
22. Bonanno PC, Converse JM: Primary bone grafting in management of facial fractures. NY State J Med 75:710, 1975
23. Mullikan JB, Kaban LB, Murray JE: Management of facial fractures in children. Clin Plast Surg 4:491, 1977
24. Georgiade N, Nash T: An external cranial fixation apparatus for severe maxillofacial injuries. Plast Reconstr Surg 38:142, 1966
25. Rowe NL, Killey JC: Fractures of the Facial Skeleton. Williams & Wilkins, Baltimore, 1955
26. Ketchum LD, Ferris B, Masters FW: Blindness without direct injury to the globe: A complication of facial fractures. Plast Reconstr Surg 58:187, 1976
27. Miller GR, Tenzel RR: Ocular complications of midfacial fractures. Plast Reconstr Surg 39:37, 1967

28. Steidler NE, Cook RM, Reade PC: Residual complications in patients with major middle third facial fractures. Int J Oral Surg 9:259, 1980

29. Tessier P: Total osteotomy of the face for faciostenosis or for sequelae of LeFort III fractures. Plast Reconstr Surg 48:533, 1971

SUGGESTED READINGS

Adams WM: Basic principles of internal wire fixation and internal suspension of facial fractures. Surgery 12:523, 1942

Kawamoto HK Jr: Surgery of the Jaws. p. 125. In Lesavoy MA (ed): Reconstruction of the Head and Neck. Williams & Wilkins, Baltimore, 1981

Kazanjian VH, Converse JM: The Surgical Treatment of Facial Injuries. Williams & Wilkins, Baltimore, 1974

Kreutziser KL: Complex maxillofacial fractures: Management and surgical procedures. South Med J 75(7):783, 1982

Sicher H: Oral Anatomy. C.V. Mosby, St. Louis, MO, 1960

Steidler NE, Cook RM, Reade PC: Incidence and management of major middle third facial fractures at the royal melbourne hospital: A retrospective study. Int J Oral Surg 9:92, 1980

Mandibular Fractures

9

Douglas P. Sinn
Stephen C. Hill
Stephen W. Watson

The mandible is one of the most unusual bones of the body. No other has such distinctive shape or a more important function. It is positioned at the base of the face and its aesthetic form is always evident. Injuries to the mandible must be managed with careful attention to the restoration of form, function, and aesthetics.

While midfacial fractures are decreasing in number, primarily due to lowered highway speed limits, the incidence of mandibular fractures has remained fairly constant. The most common etiology of mandibular fractures is aggravated assault, followed by auto accidents, gunshot wounds, and sports injuries. A review of 137 mandible fractures from 1983 to 1984 at Parkland Memorial Hospital in Dallas, Texas, demonstrated that 68 percent of the cases resulted from aggravated assault, 23 percent from motor vehicle accidents, 4 percent from gunshot wounds, and 5 percent from other causes (falls, sports accidents, etc.) The prominent position of the mandible predisposes it to trauma from blows directed at the lower third of the face. The thick cortical bone of the inferior border of the mandible is substantial enough to absorb the en-

ergy from most impacts, but when the compressive strength of the mandible is exceeded, a variety of fractures may occur.

SURGICAL ANATOMY

The mandible is a very efficient stress-absorbing structure. It is a strong horseshoe-shaped bone with an anterior horizontal portion and two vertically oriented posterior struts. The horizontal segment is made up of a thick compact cortical inferior border that is the base for the alveolar bone, which is the supporting matrix for the teeth. The two vertical segments serve as attachments for the major muscles of mastication and terminate superiorly as the condyles, which constitute the mandibular component of the temporomandibular joints.

The mandible is divided into several anatomic

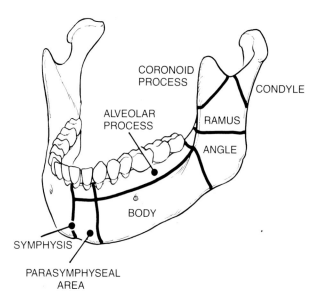

Fig. 9-1. Schematic representation of the anatomic regions of the mandible.

parts whose nomenclature must be thoroughly understood by those who manage mandibular fractures (Fig. 9-1). The mandibular symphysis makes up the anterior curve of the mandible and extends between the mandibular canine teeth. It is thick and has ridges and depressions which are related to associated anatomic structures and muscle attachments. The body of the mandible is a curvilinear strut of bone that houses the teeth, from canine to molar. Medially, the strut has a depression for the sublingual gland and a ridge that traverses posteri-

orly and superiorly to form the internal oblique ridge and serves as the attachment of the mylohyoid muscle. Laterally, the bone of the mandibular body is slightly expanded to accommodate the tooth roots and sweeps posteriorly and superiorly into the external oblique ridge. The internal and external oblique ridges come together at the retromolar trigone and form the thin cortical extension towards the coronoid process. Posterior and inferior to the coronoid process, the cortical plates are closely situated and form the vertical ramus of the mandible. The vertical ramus extends superiorly, and its terminal structure is the condyle, which serves as the articulating element with the cranium.

The blood supply to the mandible arises from the muscle attachments and the inferior alveolar artery. The inferior alveolar artery traverses from a medial entrance into the vertical ramus at the mandibular foramen to exit through the mental foramen, which is laterally located on the mandibular body. During its passage through the bone, the inferior alveolar artery branches to both teeth and bone. However, the attachments of the muscle groups, which have many perforating periosteal arterioles, provide the bulk of the blood supply to the mandible in the region of their insertions.

The nerve supply to the mandible and its teeth originates in the inferior alveolar nerve, which has the same course as its arterial counterpart.

Normal mandibular growth and form are dependent upon good function and a normal enveloping

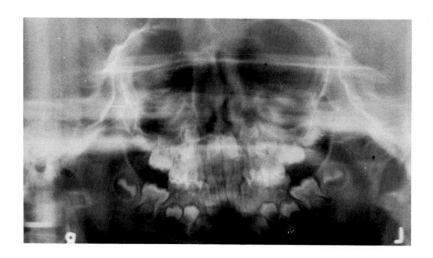

Fig. 9-2. Panoramic radiograph of the mixed dentition of a 7-year-old, which reveals the presence of multiple unerupted and developing permanent teeth.

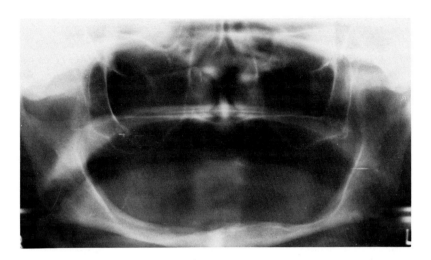

Fig. 9-3. Panoramic radiograph of an edentulous mandible. Note the bilaterally atrophied body regions, which increase the susceptability to fracture.

soft tissue matrix. Overall mandibular shape is also affected by the presence or absence of teeth. Early in development, the mandible is weakened by the presence of many unerupted and developing permanent teeth (Fig. 9-2). These erupting or impacted teeth decrease the amount of bone available for structural support and create regions that are susceptible to fracturing. The absence of teeth results in atrophy of alveolar bone and a decrease in the vertical height of the tooth-bearing portion of the mandible (Fig. 9-3). This occurs owing to resorption of alveolar bone when there is no func-

tional stimulus from teeth. Interestingly, alveolar bone will not develop if tooth eruption does not take place.

The Temporomandibular Joint

The temporomandibular joint (TMJ) is the unit of the mandible that articulates with the cranial base. An absolute requirement for proper management of mandibular fractures is a thorough understand-

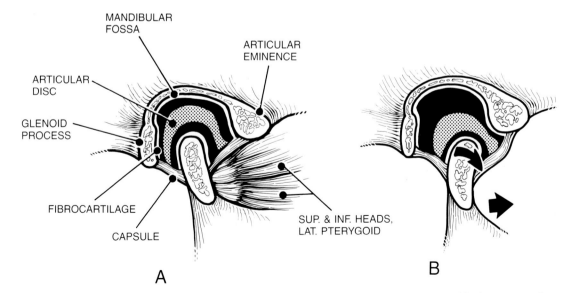

Fig. 9-4. Schematic representations showing (**A**) structures of the temporomandibular joint and (**B**) the rotational and translational movements of the mandibular condyle.

ing of this complex unit comprising a compressed fibrous disc interposed between the mandibular condyle and the articular fossa of the cranial base. The temporomandibular joint functions with both hinge movement and translation and is the only such joint in the body (Fig. 9-4). The rotational movement about the center of the condyle occurs early in jaw opening, and the sliding translational motion takes place when opening wide. This sliding motion brings the floor of mouth structures forward so as not to impede the airway. The joint is surrounded by a fibrous capsule, which is thickened laterally by the lateral temporomandibular ligament; it is a synovial joint. Some of the lateral pterygoid muscle fibers insert into the capsule, disc, and condyle and are intimately involved in their complex movements. When the normal condyle-disc relationship is disrupted, an internal derangement of the temporomandibular joint occurs with resultant dysfunction, such as TMJ pain, clicking, or locking.

FUNCTIONAL ANATOMY

Mandibular functional anatomy refers to those structures that provide and allow for movement of the mandible. Since loss of mandibular function results in a severe disability, reestablishment of satisfactory jaw function following injury is the main objective of treatment. Therefore, an understanding of functional anatomy is essential to proper management of mandibular injuries.

Muscles and Their Relationship to the Mandible

Four major muscle groups, the temporalis, masseter, pterygoid, and suprahyoid groups, comprise the muscles of mastication; they are primarily responsible for elevation of the mandible as well as lateral and protrusive movements (Fig. 9-5). The temporalis and masseter muscles are primarily re-

sponsible for elevation. Considering the length and size of these two muscles, their strength is enormous. They are capable of producing 50 pounds per square inch of crushing pressure at the occlusal surface of the teeth during mastication. They are short, stout, and their attachment to the mandible is extensive, which allows an enormous amount of force to be delivered when they are in the contractile state. Without good temporalis and masseter function, the crushing strength of the jaw is drastically reduced. The temporalis has its origin along the side of the skull and extends inferiorly beneath the zygomatic arch to the coronoid process and the anterior surface of the mandibular ramus. The masseter muscle takes its origin along the inferior portion of the zygomatic arch and zygomatic body and extends inferiorly to the mandibular angle where it has a large insertion into the lateral ramus and the heavy inferior cortical border. The masseter muscle insertion extends anteriorly to just below the tooth root of the second and third molars and posteriorly to the angle of the mandible. During mastication, the temporalis and masseter muscles work together to create an upward and retrusive force on the mandible that seats the temporomandibular joint in the glenoid fossa.

The lateral pterygoid muscle actually consists of two muscles. The inferior lateral pterygoid muscle takes its origin along the lateral surface of the lateral pterygoid plate and inserts into the scaphoid fossa at the anterior aspect of the condyle. The superior lateral pterygoid muscle originates from the infratemporal crest of the sphenoid bone and inserts into the fibrous capsule and meniscus of the temporomandibular joint. The main function of the inferior lateral pterygoid muscle is protrusion of the mandible, while that of the superior lateral pterygoid muscle is thought to be stabilization of the meniscus during the power stroke of chewing. Inhibited protrusion of the mandible, which can occur following any injury that interfers with lateral pterygoid muscle function, causes deviation, during opening, towards the side of the injury. Dysfunction of the lateral pterygoid muscle is quite evident to the examiner and is observed as a lack of anterior movement of the ipsilateral condyle. Such inhibited movement is frequently noted following condylar fractures or hemarthrosis of the temporomandibular joint.

The medial pterygoid muscle extends from the

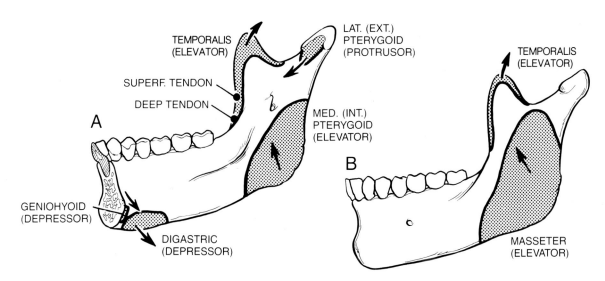

Fig. 9-5. Schematic representation of the mandible for (**A**) medial and (**B**) lateral surfaces showing attachments of muscles and their direction of function.

medial pterygoid plate inferiorly to a large insertion on the medial aspect of the mandibular ramus. Its anterior-posterior width is approximately the same as the masseter muscle, and together these muscles form an encasing sling around the mandible. This protective sling helps shield the ramus from injury and protects the neurovascular bundle as it traverses the pterygomandibular space and enters the medial surface of the mandible. When fracture occurs within the muscle mass, displacement is frequently minimal, unless there is extensive tearing of the muscle. However, when fractures occur outside the muscle mass, displacement easily takes place (Fig. 9-6).

The remaining muscles of interest are those which attach to the medial aspect of the mandible anteriorly. Frequently referred to as the suprahyoid muscle groups, they are the muscles responsible for opening the jaw (along with the lateral pterygoid muscle) and stabilizing the mandible during retraction.

The mylohyoid muscle, which takes its origin along the mylohyoid ridge of the mandible and inserts on the hyoid bone, is a fan-shaped muscle that serves as a support structure for the floor of the mouth as well as stabilizes the mandible during opening.

The geniohyoid muscle is positioned closely to the mylohyoid muscle and extends from the genial tubercles on the medial aspect of the mandibular symphysis to the hyoid bone. The geniohyoid mus-

cle functions during opening of the jaw, upon swallowing, and during other movements of the tongue.

The genioglossus muscle also takes its origin on the genial tubercles superior to the geniohyoid muscle and extends into the body of the tongue. It is primarily responsible for protrusion of the tongue mass. Its role in mandibular fractures is minimal.

The other muscles of the suprahyoid group that are significant in their relationship to mandibular fractures are the digastric muscles. They act pri-

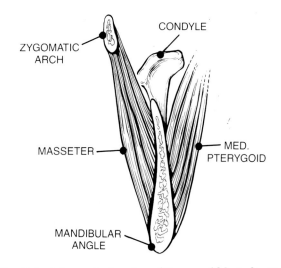

Fig. 9-6. Schematic drawing of the mandible indicating the encasing sling formed by the masseter and medial pterygoid muscles.

marily as depressors of the mandible and can contribute to mandibular fracture displacement.

Teeth

When all teeth are present and erupted, the human adult has a total of 32 teeth. This includes the four wisdom teeth, which are usually impacted to some degree and frequently are not visible in the oral cavity. An understanding of the way teeth normally interdigitate and the variations that occur are essential to proper management of mandibular fractures. Occlusion is classified based on the relationships of the first molar, cuspid, and incisor teeth (Fig. 9-7). Angle's class I occlusion occurs when the mesiobuccal cusp of the maxillary first molar is closely related to the embrasure between the buccal cusps of the mandibular first molar, the maxillary cuspid articulates with the embrasure between the mandibular first bicuspid and cuspid, and the maxillary incisors slightly overlap the mandibular incisors (Fig. 9-7A). Angle's class II occlusion occurs when the mandibular dentition is shifted to some degree in a posterior direction, which results in the lower teeth shifting behind the maxillary teeth. This occlusion causes a typical overbite appearance (Fig. 9-7B). Angle's class III occlusion occurs when the lower jaw and its teeth are anteriorly positioned, which usually causes a prognathic appearance (Fig. 9-7C).

Each of these occlusal relationships can be the result of skeletal deformities of either the upper or lower jaw. Such malocclusions may be variants of normal and be present in an individual without a mandible fracture; therefore, it is important to question the patient or family concerning the pre-injury occlusion. This allows the surgery to attain a jaw position as close to the pre-injury situation as possible. When teeth are absent or malaligned, there is more difficulty in identifying the pre-injury occlusion. Occasionally, it is necessary to take dental models and articulate these dental units with one another to absolutely identify the occlusal relationship. Unfortunately, many patients who sustain mandible fractures do not have ideal occlusions, nor do they have all their teeth. In this situation, a thorough understanding of occlusion is required to identify the correct position.

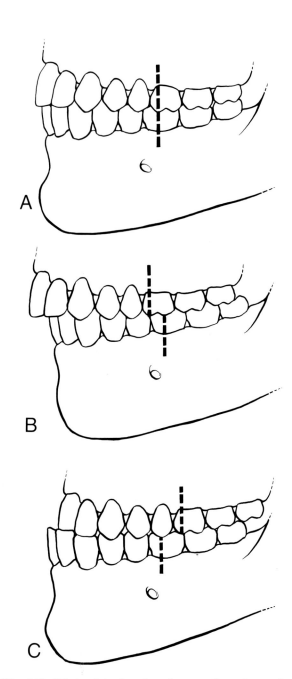

Fig. 9-7. **(A)** Angle's class I occlusion. The relationship of the mesiobuccal cusp of the maxillary first molar and the embrasure of the mandibular first molar is indicated by a dotted line. This is the "key" by which to distinguish occlusions. **(B)** Angle's class II occlusion. Note the mesiobuccal cusp of the maxillary first molar is anterior to the embrasure (mesiobuccal groove) of the mandibular first molar. **(C)** Angle's class III occlusion. Note the mesiobuccal cusp of the maxillary first molar is posterior to the mesiobuccal cusp of the mandibular first molar.

CLASSIFICATION OF FRACTURES

Mandibular fractures, from a descriptive standpoint, should be classified by location and by whether they are open or closed, displaced or nondisplaced, complete or incomplete, and linear or comminuted (Fig. 9-8).

An open fracture includes any fracture of the mandible that is exposed to the external elements by a tear in the mucosa or skin. Additionally, all fractures that are near the root of a tooth and extend into a tooth socket are considered open, as these fractures communicate with the oral cavity through the tooth socket.

Fractures of the mandibular ramus, angle, coronoid process, and condyle are usually closed fractures. However, if the angle fracture is associated with an impacted tooth that pierces the oral mucosa, it should be considered an open fracture. All other fractures of the mandible that do not involve communication with the intraoral or extraoral environment are considered to be closed fractures.

The distinction between displaced and nondisplaced fractures is self explanatory. Those fractures which are displaced by either the amount of trauma sustained or by muscle contraction are often evident upon clinical and radiographic examination. The fractured segments will frequently be displaced as muscles distract the parts following injury. The correlation of displacement with angulation of fracture lines (in the past referred to as favorable and unfavorable) is not of major significance. Since the fracture line does not offer a favorable or unfavorable attitude in all circumstances, displacement is more related to muscle relationships and conditions along the fracture line itself.

Nondisplaced fractures are frequently seen in the area of the mandibular condyle, coronoid, and ramus, as these regions all have large muscle masses that serve to splint and stabilize fractures. Displacement of fractures in the mandibular body, symphysis, and angle are more common owing to their lack of support by major muscle groups and the displacing action of muscle forces on these regions.

Incomplete fractures are those fractures that do not extend all the way through the mandible and in which continuity of the mandible across the fracture site is maintained.

Greenstick fractures are a special type of incomplete fracture that usually occurs in the mandibles of young patients. Young bones seem to be more elastic and have a tendency to bend rather than cleanly fracture. Frequently, in young patients one will see mandible fractures that have a minimal amount of displacement and multiple connections across the fracture line.

Linear fractures are the most common mandibular fracture and are represented in radiographs by a single line.

Comminuted fractures are those fractures which have multiple fragments. These fractures frequently are difficult to manage because of the lack of stability that can be achieved from their reduction. Comminuted fractures present multiple segments with compromised vascularity, and this must be considered in their management. The surgeon should make every attempt to maintain the marginal vascularity that is present in these situations.

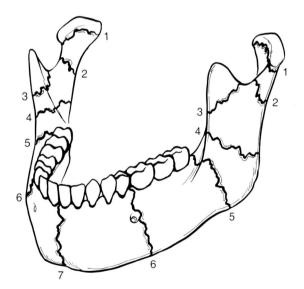

Fig. 9-8. Locations of mandibular fractures: (1) condylar (intracapsular), (2) subcondylar, (3) coronoid, (4) ramus, (5) angle (open through third molar socket), (6) body (open through tooth socket), and (7) symphysis fractures.

In describing mandibular fractures one must also note the anatomic area that the fracture traverses. It is essential that correct nomenclature be utilized in describing the different regions of the mandible that are involved by fractures. In a review of 137 cases at Parkland Memorial Hospital, the most commonly fractured area of the mandible was the mandibular angle, which was involved in 35 percent of the injuries. The mandibular symphysis (24 percent), body (18 percent), and condyle (17 percent) were other commonly fractured areas (Fig. 9-9).

The mandibular condyle is frequently fractured owing to the small cross-sectional area of the condylar neck that extends spirally upwards. The anatomic configuration of the mandible transmits the kinetic energy from a blow along the mandible to the condylar neck, where the compressive strength of the bone is exceeded and fracturing occurs. The mandibular angle is predisposed to fracturing, since it is frequently both the site of impacted third molar teeth and the point of application of a blow. The impacted or partially submerged tooth decreases the amount of osseous support and weakens the mandible so that fractures commonly occur along the socket of the impacted tooth and extend inferiorly through the mandibular angle (see Fig. 9-6).

The cuspid area is another region of the mandible that frequently fractures owing to the presence of teeth, in this case the cuspids, which are the longest teeth in the mandible. The mental foramen is close to this area and further serves to decrease the resistance to fracture.

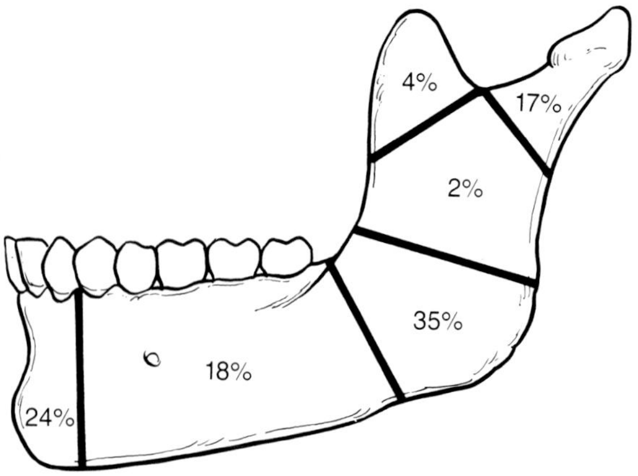

Fig. 9-9. Frequency of fractures in various anatomic regions of the mandible.

of the injury, and whether it occurred by one or multiple blows. One should always be alert to the possibility of associated trauma, such as intracranial insult or visceral injuries, that could be life threatening. Motor vehicle accidents with their high velocity have the greatest frequency of associated traumatic injuries and, therefore, require thorough evaluation.

Contrecoup injuries are very common in mandibular fractures. When a patient sustains trauma to the left side of the jaw, it is not uncommon to find fractures on the right side of the mandible. This relates to the transmission of kinetic energy through the mandible to the opposite side, creating stress buildup and fracture. Consequently, the examiner should not overlook a subtle fracture by concentrating on the more apparent injury. A thorough and systematic history and clinical examination are the most efficient means for reaching an accurate diagnosis.

CLINICAL HISTORY

In developing an understanding of a mandibular fracture, it is important to have a detailed history of how the injury took place. This can be helpful in identifying areas that may be fractured as well as the likelihood of associated injuries. It is important to know the velocity of the trauma, the magnitude

CLINICAL SYMPTOMS

The most common complaints of patients with mandibular fractures are pain, malocclusion, trismus, swelling, anesthesia, paresthesia, hemorrhage, and ecchymosis. Other than pain at the site of injury and an altered bite, the most common clinical finding is that of trismus. Trismus refers to an inability to open the mouth due to muscle pain. Mandibular fracture patients who have trismus are most commonly fractured somewhere near the posterior aspect of the mandible, and the resulting pain upon attempting function causes a limitation in motion. Pain can also result from the involvement of nerves as well as elevation of mucoperiosteum that exposes the underlying bone. The pain from the blow that causes the acute injury is transient, but with subsequent movement of the fractured segments, nerve endings of blood vessels and periosteum are stimulated, and pain is elicited.

Swelling and ecchymosis are also commonly associated with mandibular fractures and, when present, can facilitate location of the injury. If the injury is acute, ecchymosis and swelling are significant findings and closely related to the site of fracture. However, in the older injury, pain and swelling may be more closely associated with an inflammatory process. Ecchymosis is hemorrhage that has seeped into the soft tissues near the fracture site. However, secondary to hemorrhagic dissection, ecchymotic areas may migrate along fascial planes, with the direction of movement dictated by gravity and connective tissue anatomy.

CLINICAL EXAMINATION

Clinical examination of the patient with a suspected mandibular fracture should be orderly and systematic. Initially, the examiner should evaluate the patient for any surface injuries, contusion, excoriation, or lacerations that may require therapy or signify the region of a fracture. The examiner should then evaluate the intraoral condition of the patient, checking for similar contusions, ecchymosis, or lacerations. The dental status should be assessed for avulsed, loose, or fractured teeth, which may be evidence of a mandibular fracture, dentoalveolar fracture, or dental injury. Sudden

variations in the level of the occlusal surfaces of the teeth or hemorrhage around the teeth may also indicate a fracture site. The patient's occlusion should be examined to determine the type and degree of any malocclusion that may be present. Multiply crowded and rotated teeth or many missing teeth should alert the examiner to the difficulty of reducing and stabilizing the fractures.

After visual inspection, the examiner should palpate the mandible in an attempt to detect areas of tenderness or the edges of fractures. The temporomandibular joint region should also be palpated via the external auditory canal and the preauricular area. Tenderness experienced during this maneuver may be evidence of intracapsular damage, including hemarthrosis, internal derangement (i.e., a displaced meniscus), or condylar fracture. The examiner should next digitally manipulate the mandible, attempting to detect the presence and amount of fracture site mobility. A functional evaluation should be performed that includes millimeter measurements of the incisal opening as well as right and left lateral excursion movements. Deviation upon opening signifies limitation of translatory movement of the condyle on the side where the deviation occurs. Deviation may also be seen upon protrusion of the mandible. This may be indicative of condyle fracture, hemarthrosis, or internal derangement of the temporomandibular joint. Neurological assessment of the presence and degree of nerve injury should also be performed. Examination of sensibility should include documentation of anesthesia or paresthesia of the inferior alveolar, lingual, and mental nerves. In some cases, a detailed evaluation, including light directional discrimination, two-point discrimination, and other tests of sensation, may be warranted.

RADIOGRAPHIC EXAMINATION

The most commonly used radiographic survey for evaluation of mandible fractures is the mandibular series. This refers to a four-view plain film analysis

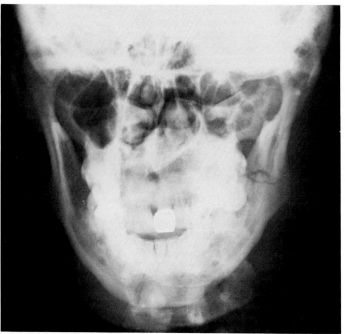

A

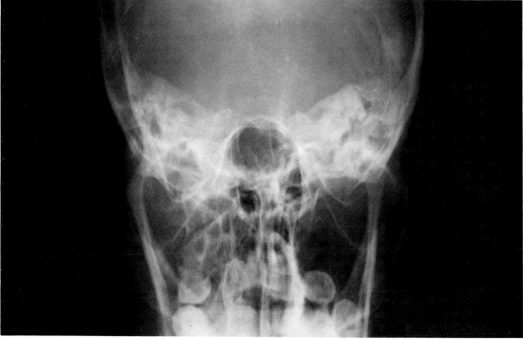

B

Fig. 9-10. (A) Posterior-anterior view of the mandible revealing an open, complete, nondisplaced symphysis fracture on the right; and an open, complete, nondisplaced mandibular angle fracture on the left. (B) Towne's view radiograph revealing a fracture on the left of the mandibular subcondylar region *(Figure continues.)*

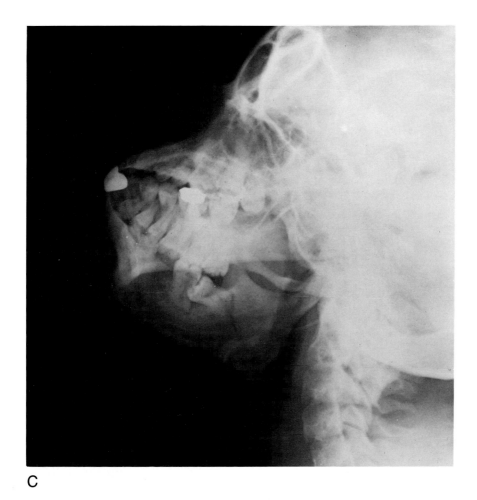

C

Fig. 9-10 *(Continued).* (C) Lateral oblique view showing an open, complete, nondisplaced mandibular angle fracture extending through the unerupted third molar.

of the mandible. It includes a posterior-anterior view of the mandible, a Towne's view (for evaluation of the mandibular condyles), and right and left lateral oblique views of the mandible for visualization of the mandibular angle, body, and symphysis (Fig. 9-10). The Towne's view is the most difficult to read, as frequently the area about the condyle is clouded by superimposition. A correctly made film will allow the examiner to evaluate the condyle and subcondylar area for fractures.

The panoramic radiograph has become very popular as an adjunct in diagnostic evaluation of patients who may have sustained mandibular fractures. This radiographic technique allows the observer to see the total mandible in one complete view. It is a plain film and does not allow three-dimensional appreciation; however, it easily visualizes fractures of the condyle and condylar neck as well as fractures through the remainder of the mandible. The panoramic radiograph also identifies the relationship of fractures to the mandibular and maxillary teeth, which is important in formulating an overall plan of treatment (Fig. 9-11).

Displacement as it appears on the panogram must be taken under close scrutiny, as it may not be totally accurate. The panogram should be supported by views in other dimensions and clinical evaluation of fracture mobility.

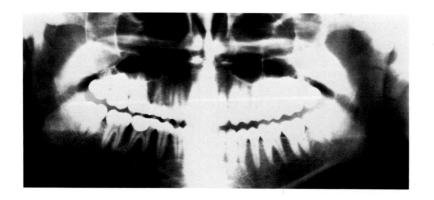

Fig. 9-11. Panoramic radiograph of the mandible. An open, complete, nondisplaced angle fracture is noted on the right while a closed, complete, nondisplaced subcondylar fracture is seen on the left.

THERAPY

Nonoperative

Nonoperative management of mandibular fractures is indicated when there is a minimal amount of displacement noted in the fractured areas and the patient can bite to normal occlusion without excessive discomfort. However, the surgeon must always consider temporarily immobilizing any mandibular fracture with intermaxillary (maxillomandibular) wire fixation. Circumstances peculiar to the case will usually suggest the appropriate technique. If the patient is unable to undergo application of arch bars and intermaxillary wire fixation for reasons related to associated injuries or other specific problems, the surgeon can consider treatment alternatives that do not include an operative approach. This primarily consists of close follow-up and observation for any tendency toward fracture displacement. Most mandibular fractures will require some type of reduction and immobilization.

Operative Treatment

Immobilization techniques for mandibular fractures are indicated in all cases where stability is required for fracture healing to take place. It is necessary to immobilize the jaw so that healing will occur with the mandibular teeth in the correct relationship to the maxillary teeth. This will provide a normal comfortable occlusion after healing has been completed. The length of immobilization required varies according to type of fracture, degree of injury, patient age, and associated injuries or illness. Intermaxillary fixation normally ranges from a few days to 6 weeks; however, in rare situations this may be extended.

Timing

These fractures should be reduced as soon after injury as possible, providing the patient is stable and can undergo the operative procedure. Early management decreases pain and also the incidence of infection. Although not desirable in terms of patient comfort and healing, the surgeon can delay definitive care of mandibular fractures for a few days without catastrophic results. Should a delay in management be necessary, temporary stabilization of the fracture should be accomplished. According to the location of the fracture, this may require a Barton bandage, arch bars, or a bridle wire (around teeth adjacent to the fracture). In any case, delayed management should be combined with diligent efforts to maintain good oral hygiene, including toothbrushing and oral irrigation.

Closed Versus Open Reduction

The choice of reduction technique (closed or open) is frequently dictated by the location and condition of the fracture. For example, almost all condylar

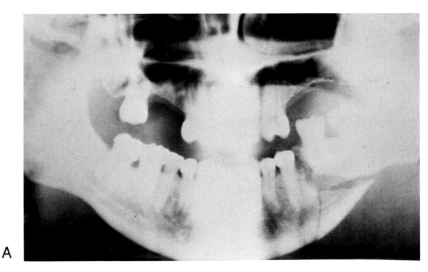

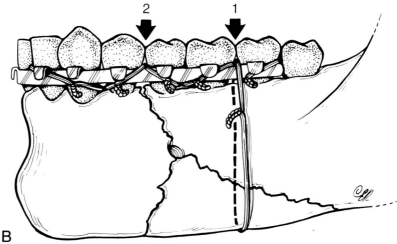

Fig. 9-12. (A) Panoramic radiograph revealing an open, complete, grossly displaced left mandibular body fracture with a triangular-shaped comminuted fragment along the inferior border. (B) Schematic drawing showing the placement of a circummandibular wire to help reduce the comminuted fracture segment. Note that the circummandibular wire passes above the arch bar (1). Also note that the circumdental wires on either side of the fracture pass over the arch bars (2).

and subcondylar fractures should be treated by closed techniques; it is only the rare situation where an open reduction may be indicated. Mandibular symphysis and angle fractures are more frequently treated with an open reduction and internal fixation than other mandible fractures due to their tendency to displace postoperatively when treated with closed techniques. If the patient has good dentition, most mandibular body fractures can be managed in a closed fashion. However, in those cases where most or all of the dentition is missing, an open reduction with internal fixation may be required. In some cases (frequently owing to excessive swelling or hematoma) the operator may be unable to determine at surgery if the fracture is adequately reduced. In this situation the surgeon should consider making a limited intraoral vestibular incision and performing an open reduction under direct vision. It is unnecessary to wire every fracture that is visualized. The placement of interosseous wire fixation should be considered only when stable reduction of the fracture cannot be obtained or if early postoperative mobilization of the mandible is required. Comminuted fractures, unless already exposed through a laceration, usually fare better when treated by closed reduction. Frequently, a circummandibular wire around the arch bar and the largest inferior fragment helps to reduce these fractures (Fig. 9-12).

Placement of maxillary and mandibular arch bars for a closed or open reduction involves cutting the malleable metal arch bars (Erich-type arch bar) to

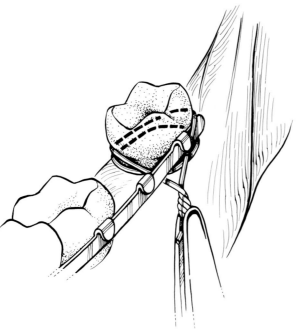

Fig. 9-13. Schematic drawing of a double (Dingman) wire loop that is passed around a solitary tooth. The arch bar is secured as indicated by the arrow.

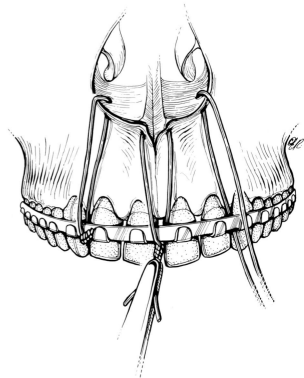

Fig. 9-14. Schematic drawing of skeletal suspension wires passing from the bony pyriform rim and the anterior nasal spine.

extend from the first molar on one side of the arch to the first molar on the opposite side. Occasionally it may be necessary to extend the arch bar back to the second or even third molar tooth in order to bridge a fracture site. These bars are contoured to fit their respective dental arches and are wired into position at the cervical region of the teeth by passing circumdental wires and twisting them tightly in place. If a solitary tooth is present a double loop wire will usually serve to satisfactorily stabilize the arch bar (Fig. 9-13). Occasionally, because of periodontally involved or loose teeth, a circummandibular wire is required to stabilize the mandibular arch bar. In the maxillary arch, a pyriform rim or anterior nasal spine wire performs a similar function (Fig. 9-14).

In fractures involving the dentition, arch bars are usually placed on the largest mandibular fragment and then loosely applied to the lesser fragments. With the fracture reduced and teeth held in maximum interdigitation, the circumdental wires on lesser segments are tightened, thereby reducing

the fracture. Bridle wires placed around a tooth on either side of a fracture are a very helpful means of temporary reduction and can also aid in final reduction of the fracture when used in conjunction with arch bars (Fig. 9-15).

TREATMENT OF FRACTURES

Condylar and Subcondylar Fractures

Management of mandibular condylar and subcondylar fractures has been controversial throughout the years. However, multiple reviews of condylar

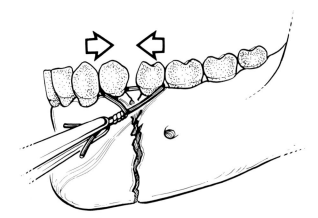

Fig. 9-15. Schematic drawing showing the placement of a bridle wire around premolar teeth for a temporary reduction of a mandibular body fracture.

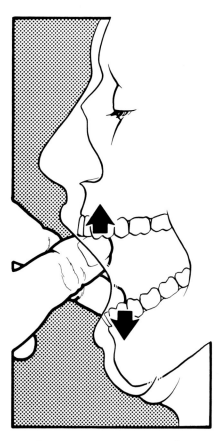

Fig. 9-16. Schematic representation of active physiotherapy. The thumb is placed on the maxillary incisors, and the index finger is placed on the mandibular incisors. The jaws are then pried apart with the fingers working in a scissor-like fashion, as indicated by the arrows.

fractures, animal experiments, and significant clinical experience support the use of closed reduction of these fractures. In a review of 137 mandible fractures at Parkland Memorial Hospital, 43 fractures involved the mandibular condyle, and all were successfully treated with closed reduction. An open reduction of a condylar or subcondylar fracture should only be performed if (1) the displaced condyle fragment is a physical impediment to function, (2) no other means of stabilizing the posterior vertical height of the mandible is applicable, or (3) the condylar fragment is displaced into the middle cranial fossa. It is frequently difficult to determine preoperatively if a displaced condylar fragment will interfere with function; therefore, the surgeon should generally not decide to open a condylar fracture until after a closed reduction has been performed and physical limitation of function is detected in the early postoperative period.

The regimen employed for managing condylar fractures that involve the intracapsular portion of the mandible is of paramount importance. Initially arch bars and intermaxillary fixation should be placed if malocclusion is present, or if the patient is uncomfortable upon functioning. Intermaxillary fixation should be released in 10 to 14 days and a regimen instituted of nighttime intraoral elastics (to control the occlusion) and daytime increased function of the jaw. This function should include

physiotherapy with stretching exercises consisting of initially active incisal opening and lateral excursions, then active and digitally assisted levering of the jaw (Fig. 9-16). In some cases a side-action mouth prop may help the patient attain a normal range of function. Throughout physiotherapy the patient should be followed closely and progress in jaw function monitored by the measuring of incisal opening and lateral excursions. Physiotherapy proceeds for 2 to 3 months following release of intermaxillary fixation until the incisal opening is greater than 40 mm and lateral excursions are greater than 7 mm. Mandibular fractures that are low on the condylar neck should be treated like ramus fractures and do not require special consideration.

Pediatric mandibular condylar fractures rarely require open reduction and are managed much like adult fractures except for a reduced length of immobilization time of 5 to 8 days. With the enormous potential for healing noted in children, bridging mandibular body and symphysis fractures with bridle wires and arch bars will provide enough union within 7 to 10 days to allow mobilization of any associated mandibular condylar fractures. Pediatric condylar fractures generally heal very well without noticeable interference with growth or movement when adequate function is restored through diligent postoperative physiotherapy. Interestingly, adults tend to have more problems with dysfunction and asymmetry than children following condylar fractures.

Ramus and Coronoid Fractures

Fractures of the mandibular ramus are not common and are frequently splinted by the surrounding muscle masses. Comminution occasionally occurs with severe direct blows, but is supported and usually held in satisfactory position. Seldom do these fractures require any type of operative treatment other than immobilization of the jaw by placement of maxillary and mandibular arch bars. Occasionally a low mandibular condylar neck fracture will be associated with loss of posterior vertical facial height. In this case the fracture is usually low enough on the ramus to allow access via a Risdon approach, which entails an incision made below and behind the angle of the mandible. Interosseous wiring can be used to complete stabilization of this low condylar neck or ramus fracture. A small bone plate may also be ultilized to stabilize this segment, although wires are usually satisfactory. The objective of this treatment is to maintain the patient's posterior vertical facial height and prevent collapse of the interarch distance. Fractures of the mandibular coronoid process seldom require operative treatment and are managed conservatively with short-term immobilization.

Mandibular Angle Fractures

Mandibular angle fractures are very common and frequently occur in association with impacted third molar teeth. Management of this fracture often requires use of an open reduction with internal fixation. This decision is based, as in all fractures, upon stability of the initial reduction and need for early postoperative mobilization. Presence of the third molar tooth in the line of fracture can complicate this situation.

If the mandibular third molar tooth is completely impacted and the fracture does not communicate with the oral cavity, a closed reduction is usually satisfactory. Occasionally, the impacted tooth will physically interfere with the reduction and necessitate its removal. When this occurs, internal fixation is usually performed to ensure postoperative stability of the reduction. If the mandibular third molar tooth is partially erupted, the fracture automatically communicates with the oral cavity and is considered contaminated. The tooth should then be removed if it interferes with the reduction or if the tissue surrounding it is inflamed. An intraoral open reduction, with or without internal fixation, can be completed at the external oblique ridge. In such cases a small mucoperiosteal flap is elevated and the tooth is completely removed. After removal of the tooth, a 25-gauge stainless steel wire can be placed through drill holes made in the external oblique ridge. It is important to place the drill holes in such a manner that the wire will cross the reduced fracture in a perpendicular fashion. This intraoral technique has many advantages over the extraoral approach, including no external scar, decreased operative time, and less possibility of facial nerve injury.

When the third molar tooth is completely erupted and retained in the proximal segment, it will usually occlude with its opponent tooth in the maxillary arch and prevent proximal segment rotation. The third molar should then be kept in position and utilized in a closed reduction of the fracture. When the erupted third molar tooth lies in the distal segment, removal of the tooth may be considered. If an open reduction with internal fixation is required, removal of the third molar tooth is necessary only when there is inadequate space to place a drill hole on the distal fragment.

Mandibular Body Fractures

Fractures of the mandibular body commonly involve the dentition and are frequently contaminated either by tearing of the oral mucosa or by contamination along a tooth root. It is necessary to stabilize the fracture by bridging it with a bridle wire as well as mandibular arch bar. Maxillary and mandibular arch bars with intermaxillary fixation usually allow stabilization of the occlusion and reduction of the mandibular body fracture. If displacement continues to be noted, it may be necessary to do an open reduction with internal fixation, either by an intraoral or extraoral approach. The intraoral route allows access to the fracture without leaving an external scar but is more difficult and can result in damage to the inferior alveolar nerve. An extraoral approach provides excellent access to the fracture site but involves an external scar and possible injury to the marginal mandibular branch of the facial nerve. Regardless of the approach, a simple interosseous bicortical wire provides adequate stabilization, and figure-of-eight wires in this area are seldom indicated.

Mandibular Symphysis Fractures

Fractures involving the mandibular symphysis can usually be treated in a closed fashion if no other fractures are present and the patient has good dentition. However, the muscle forces on the mandibular symphysis are considerable and may not be counteracted by a simple arch bar. If early postoperative mobilization is required (e.g., owing to a concomitant condylar fracture), open reduction with internal fixation should be considered. Also, multiple mandible fractures in conjunction with a mandibular symphysis fracture usually necessitate open reduction and internal fixation to prevent displacement of the fractured mandible.

This is best accomplished by placement of heavy

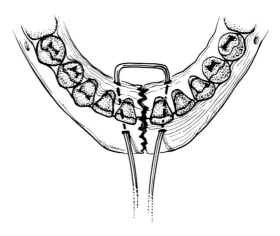

Fig. 9-17. Schematic drawing showing the passage of a double 25-gauge wire in a rhomboidal fashion for reduction of a mandibular symphysis fracture.

stabilization using a double 25-gauge bicortical stainless steel wire that is inserted across the mandibular symphysis fracture in a trapezoidal fashion. The trapezoidal configuration of the wire results from drilling holes that diverge away from the facial surface of the fracture. The larger base of the trapezoid lies on the lingual surface of the mandible and when tightened tends to draw the lingual cortices together and prevents splaying. While this wire can be placed either intraorally or extraorally, the extraoral approach is easier, more effective, and does not leave a noticeable scar (Fig. 9-17).

Complex Mandibular Fractures

Management of a fractured mandible becomes considerably more complex when fractures occur in multiple areas of the jaw. Therapy will frequently require open reduction with internal fixation of at least one fracture site to gain enough stability for control of the segments. Usually open reduction of the most displaced fracture is indicated.

A complex problem that requires special consideration is bilateral condylar and symphysis fractures. When this occurs open reduction with internal fixation of the symphysis is indicated along with intermaxillary fixation. The patient's airway must

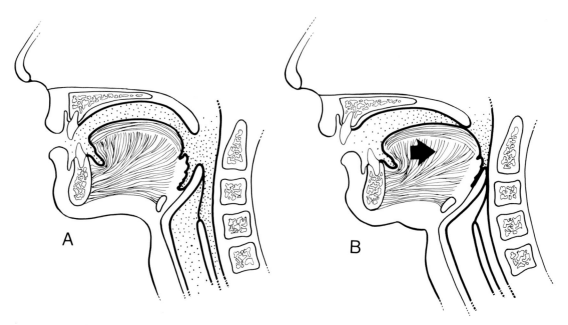

Fig. 9-18. Schematic drawing showing how the collapse of the tongue can occlude the hypopharynx.

be evaluated prior to treatment, as the mandible has lost both anterior and posterior support. This condition has been referred to as a "flail mandible" and may allow soft tissues to collapse and occlude the hypopharynx. Splaying of the body and ramus segments must be controlled by reduction at the symphysis, otherwise the pull of intermaxillary fixation will aggravate the splaying of the mandible (Fig. 9-18).

Another injury that presents problems is a bilateral body fracture of the edentulous mandible. This fracture may also collapse and cause airway problems. A stable reduction of this fracture usually requires bilateral open reduction with interosseous wiring, bilateral bone plates, or external skeletal fixation. Attempts at reduction utilizing splints or dentures are frequently unsatisfactory (Fig. 9-19).

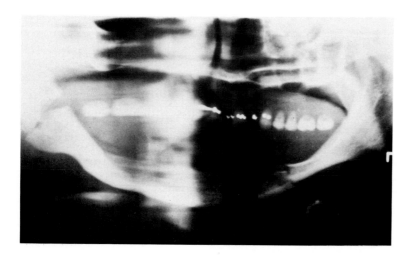

Fig. 9-19. Panoramic radiography showing bilateral fractures of the edentulous mandible.

Use of Splints

The use of lingual splints for management of mandible fractures has been quite popular for many years; however, the technique is time consuming and requires specialized expertise (and occasionally general anesthesia) to get an impression of the maxillary and mandibular teeth. The plaster model is then sectioned and positioned into satisfactory occlusion with the maxillary dental cast and the segments stabilized with wax. A methyl methacrylate splint is then custom made to fit along the lingual surfaces of the mandibular teeth. Interdental wires are used to fix the splint to the dental arch and stabilize the fracture during healing. This allows the patient to have minimally displaced mandibular fractures treated without interosseous wiring and without intermaxillary fixation.

Pediatric Fractures

Fractures in the child offer few differences from those fractures already addressed. Due to the lack of thick cortical surfaces, pediatric fractures are frequently incomplete or greenstick fractures that are best managed by closed reduction. The anatomy of the pediatric dentition is such that a stable occlusion cannot always be easily attained; however, stable arch bars can be applied in most instances. The period of mixed dentition from 9 to 12 years of age frequently results in multiple missing or mobile teeth which may require circummandibular wires, pyriform rim wires, or acrylic splints for fixation. Usually arch bars and intermaxillary fixation can be achieved without an excessive amount of difficulty. Immobilization of pediatric mandibular fractures is usually reduced to 7 to 14 days. Mandibular condylar fractures have a higher incidence of ankylosis in children and should be mobilized as early as possible, or not immobilized at all. Most pediatric fractures can be managed by application of arch bars and utilization of postoperative interarch elastics to control the occlusion. This allows the child to mobilize the mandible and continue to maintain a good occlusion. The use of open reductions in children is rare and difficult

because the position of the developing tooth buds do not allow good access for placement of interosseous wires.

Edentulous Fractures

From a practical standpoint, fractures in the edentulous mandible are the most difficult to manage. There are no teeth present to effect intermaxillary fixation, the mandibular cross section is small due to atrophy, the mandible is primarily cortical bone with little capacity for repair, and the muscle pull easily displaces the fragments. Utilization of skeletal wiring to fixate the maxillary and mandibular dentures alone does not satisfactorily stabilize many edentulous mandibular fractures. This is due to the presence of mobile tissue on most edentulous ridges and an inability to tighten the denture enough to stabilize the underlying bony fracture without causing tissue necrosis. If there is very little displacement and minimal mobility, then careful observation may be the only therapy necessary. Fractures of large edentulous mandibles that have not atrophied can be treated by open reduction and wire fixation or bone plates if they are solitary fractures. The multiply fractured edentulous mandible is a more difficult problem and usually requires stabilization by multiple techniques and/or external skeletal fixation. The severely atrophic mandible usually deserves an attempt at closed reduction and stabilization using external skeletal fixation. Should satisfactory union not occur with this treatment, continued stabilization and bone grafting may be required.

CARE OF TRAUMATIZED TEETH

In the past, management of teeth in the line of fracture entailed extraction, regardless of the situation. This is no longer an acceptable form of treatment. Aside from third molars, which have been previously discussed, teeth that are involved with a fracture are retained if at all possible. Exceptions are nonvital, nonrestorable or severely fractured teeth. Occasionally, even these teeth may be retained for stabilization purposes and extracted following release of intermaxillary fixation. If a fracture transects and fractures the root of a tooth, then this tooth should also be scheduled for extraction. Fractures that enter the periodontal ligament space and run along the surface of a tooth root frequently result in devitalization of the tooth and a secondary infection. When this occurs, the infection is usually noted some weeks after initial injury and requires extraction of the offending tooth and debridement of the fracture site. This must be differentiated from a fracture that becomes infected from avascular necrosis, develops a sequestrum, and requires thorough debridement of the fracture site.

Teeth

Fractures of teeth range from fractures only of the enamel surface to those involving the dental pulp. If the fracture involves only a portion of the crown of the tooth and the root is intact and the tooth stable, the tooth can be retained and treated by restorative dentistry. When the fracture avulses the crown of the tooth, restoration is extremely complex and usually not feasible; therefore, the surgeon should remove the remaining root and reconstruction can later be performed with a fixed prosthesis. Teeth that are completely avulsed should be replanted as quickly as possible. The success rate of tooth replantation is inversely proportional to the amount of time the tooth remains out of the alveolus. All teeth that have been avulsed will require root canal therapy. The highest rate of success results when teeth are stored in saline, replanted within 30 minutes, and treated with root canal therapy within 2 to 3 weeks. When a mandibular alveolar fracture involves multiple avulsed teeth, the teeth should be carefully repositioned and stabilized with interdental wiring techniques or an arch bar. Root canal therapy may be required to save the teeth and prevent external bone resorption.

POSTOPERATIVE CARE

Postoperative care of patients with mandibular fractures requires careful management of the airway and secretions as well as good nutritive, supportive care. Initially, the greatest concern for any patient with intermaxillary fixation is to ensure an adequate airway (see Chapter 1). Patients involved in accidents are presumed to have full stomachs for 6 hours following injury. These patients should have nasogastric suction tubes inserted prior to surgery and maintained following surgery to help prevent aspiration. Endotracheal tubes should remain in place until patients are alert enough to control their own airway, since reinsertion of tubes can be extremely difficult in a patient with intermaxillary fixation. Cutting fixation wires should not be the first step in airway control because wiring is frequently complex and difficult to remove, even by those most knowledgeable. The steps to ensure an adequate airway should progress from positioning, suction, nasopharyngeal airway, nasoendotracheal tube to cricothyroidotomy. A cricothyroidotomy is the procedure of choice rather than an emergency tracheostomy. The cricothyroidotomy is simple to perform, requires less equipment, is more expedient, and has fewer complications than an emergency tracheostomy (see Chapter 1).

All patients should have oral suction equipment at their bedside to help control their secretions. Patients frequently have some oral hemorrhage following surgery which when swallowed contributes to development of nausea and vomiting. Mandibular fracture patients frequently have some difficulty swallowing owing to edema or hematoma formation. Should any vomiting occur, oral suction can help remove any gastric contents that may collect in the oral cavity and decrease the chance of aspiration.

Postoperative nutrition should progress from an initial clear liquid diet, to a high-protein full-liquid diet, to a blended diet such as that recommended for fractured jaw patients. All patients should have a consultation with the dietary service to provide instruction to patients and their families concerning nutrition during intermaxillary fixation. The average weight loss of patients in fixation is five to ten pounds.

Oral hygiene can be a difficult problem for some patients in intermaxillary fixation. A regimen of oral rinses and diligent toothbrushing can serve to maintain adequate oral hygiene during this period. Rinsing with a mixture of equal parts hydrogen peroxide, mouthwash, and saline or water will help to reduce the accumulation of debris in those areas that cannot be reached by toothbrushing.

Antibiotics are indicated in the therapy of open mandible fractures and should be instituted as soon as possible in the emergency room. They should be maintained for a 4- to 5-day period following surgery and then discontinued unless reasons for their continued use are apparent. Antimicrobial therapy should be effective against most oral organisms including anaerobes. The antibiotic of choice is penicillin G, with cephalosporin or erythromycin as alternatives.

COMPLICATIONS

Infection is the most common complication in management of mandibular fractures. These infections develop from a variety of causes including contamination from oral fluids, avascular necrosis of bone or soft tissue, and spread from a nonvital tooth involved in the fracture. Any delay in the delivery of care for a fractured mandible increases the risk of development of wound infection. Administration of antibiotics when a patient presents at the emergency room or office setting and prompt definitive therapy for mandible fracture are the most effective means of preventing wound infection. Should any delay in the definitive care be anticipated, one should provide aseptic local wound care with irrigation and gentle debridement, temporary reduction of the mandible fracture, and diligent oral hygiene. At the time of surgery, any obviously nonvital tissue should be debrided; however, because of the excellent vascularity of the head and neck, this step requires removal of only a minimal amount of material. Should a late infection occur after definitive therapy has been administered, it should be managed as any oral infection with culture of the purulence, incision and drainage of any abscess, and debridement of necrotic soft tissue or bone.

Radiographs should be taken of the fracture site to examine this region for any evidence of free bony particles, which may represent an avascular sequestrum. If evidence of a sequestrum is noted, along with clinical evidence of an infected fracture, the sequestrum should be surgically removed and a thorough debridement of the fracture site performed. If active production of purulence or other evidence of an acute infective process is seen, drainage of the operative site is indicated. Resolution of acute and chronic osteomyelitis is enhanced by inserting an irrigating catheter (such as a red rubber catheter or pediatric feeding tube) through a percutaneous incision into the debrided fracture site. Frequent irrigations can thus be performed with assurance that irrigant fluid is reaching the site of the infection. A separate Penrose drain allows the irrigation to flow freely from the wound. This regimen usually results in a quick resolution of the infective process. However, the amount of debridement required in these cases usually results in a significant continuity defect of the mandible. While many of these defects (if less than 1 cm in length) will heal with good stabilization of the segments, many will require an autogenous bone graft to establish firm union. Frequently the inferior alveolar nerve is severely damaged during the sequence of mandibular fracture, osteomyelitis, and subsequent debridement. This type of significant nerve injury can be conveniently addressed simultaneous with repair of the continuity defect by a combination nerve-bone graft procedure. These defects can also be grafted at the time of initial debridement, but more predictable results can be achieved by allowing the infection to resolve, then performing a bone graft at a later date if required.

Wound infection secondary to a nonvital tooth in the line of fracture commonly occurs weeks to months after initial therapy. When this situation occurs, it can be difficult to decide if the tooth adjacent to a fracture should be removed. This is a clinical judgment; tooth mobility, loss of supportive alveolar bone, or lack of gingival attachment should alert the clinician to the possibility that extraction of the tooth may be required. Extraction may be necessary because loss of viability of the tooth, secondary to the fracture, has allowed bacterial contamination of the fracture to occur. Usually after extraction and curettage, healing will take place rapidly.

Injury to the inferior alveolar nerve following a mandibular fracture is commonly seen owing to the shearing force of the fracture segments as they are displaced. Most mandibular fractures that traverse the inferior alveolar canal will result in a variable disturbance of sensation. When initial examination reveals evidence of inferior alveolar nerve injury, primary nerve repair is not indicated, unless an open wound allows direct visualization of the nerve and it is obvious that the nerve has been transsected. If indicated, a primary nerve repair may be performed with appropriate decortication and mobilization of the inferior alveolar nerve to allow tension-free repair. Otherwise, a normal reduction of the fracture is carried out, and most nerve injuries resolve without additional therapy. Occasionally, a severe nerve injury will occur that for various reasons does not resolve and the patient will complain of persistent paresthesias, anesthesia, or painful dysesthesias of the inferior alveolar nerve distribution. If there is no improvement of these conditions or in nerve sensibility over a 6-month period following the initial injury, a secondary exploration of the nerve with a neurolysis or nerve graft repair is indicated.

Mandibular Hypomobility

A decrease in function immediately following a mandibular fracture is a common finding; however, late hypomobility of the jaw after fracture healing is abnormal and indicative of poor rehabilitation. Mandibular fracture immobilization may range from 2 to 6 weeks and seldom extends beyond a 6-week period. Length of fixation is based on the extent of injury and location of fracture. After fixation is released, the patient is initially placed on a soft diet, with nighttime elastics to maintain occlusion and daytime exercise of the mandible. After 1 or 2 weeks of this regimen, the patient's diet is advanced gradually to a regular diet and nighttime elastics are maintained. The patient is encouraged to perform physiotherapy as described for condylar fractures. This regimen is maintained for as long as the patient continues to progress towards reaching an incisal opening of at least 40 mm. If the patient ceases to make progress, mechanical assistance with a side-action mouth prop may be required to allow the patient to reach a minimally acceptable opening of 40 mm. This physiotherapy is as important to the overall result as the initial fracture reduction and stabilization.

Post-fracture hypomobility can result from muscle scarring or TMJ dysfunction and postoperative physiotherapy is required to resolve both of these problems. In some cases TMJ dysfunction may be related to an internal derangement (or displaced meniscus) that may eventually require secondary TMJ surgery. In rare situations TMJ fibrous or bony ankylosis can occur, usually following a comminuted intracapsular condylar fracture and inadequate physiotherapy. This condition results in a severe limitation of function with almost total lack of TMJ motion and extremely limited incisal opening. When ankylosis occurs, a TMJ arthroplasty or a gap arthroplasty of the mandibular ramus is indicated to restore function.

Malunion

Malunion of the mandible may occur following wound infection or when fractured segments are improperly positioned, or inadequately stabilized. When these situations occur, a malunion of the mandible often results in malalignment of the healed fracture segments and malocclusion. This may require osteotomies of the mandible and repositioning of the segments to achieve a satisfactory occlusion. Prolonged elastic traction in the initial weeks following release of intermaxillary fixation can frequently correct a minor malalignment of a fracture and provide satisfactory occlusion. Nonunion of mandibular fractures is a rare occurrence and should usually be labeled a fibrous union rather than nonunion. Nonunions are noted only when large segments of bone are lost secondary to extensive trauma, as in a severe gunshot wound. Fibrous unions can usually be managed by debridement of the fibrous tissue from the fracture area, stabilization of the fracture, and secondary bone grafting to eliminate any significant continuity defect.

CONCLUSIONS

Mandibular fractures present unique problems due to the bony anatomy and varied functions associated with the intact mandible. Mandibular fractures can be the most difficult to manage of all facial fractures and require a thorough understanding of mandibular anatomy, dental occlusion, and various stabilization techniques. Additionally, bacterial contamination of mandibular fractures is the rule rather than the exception, and initial attention must be directed to this problem. While recent advances in stabilization with rigid intraoral skeletal and external skeletal fixation have been welcome additions to the surgeon's armamentarium, traditional methods remain the technique of choice for most mandibular fractures. Certainly there is no substitute for attention to the details of occlusion, proper application of arch bars, appropriate internal fixation, and excellent wound care. Experience has shown that with careful adherence to these principles, successful treatment outcome can be expected. The objectives of mandibular fracture treatment remain reestablishment of normal facial esthetics, proper mandibular form, and good oral function. With accurate diagnosis, diligent care and application of the principles outlined in this chapter, the surgeon can predictably achieve these objectives in the therapy of mandibular fractures.

SUGGESTED READING

Bertz JE: Maxillofacial Injuries Clin Symp 33:4, 1981

Dingman RO, Natvig P: Surgery of Facial Fractures. W.B. Saunders, Philadelphia, 1964

Gerlock AJ, Sinn DP, McBride KL: Clinical and Radiographic Interpretation of Facial Fractures. Little, Brown & Co., Boston, 1981

Huelke DF, Burdi AR, Eyman CE: Association between mandibular fractures and site of trauma, dentition and age. J Oral Surg 20:478, 1962

Leake D, et al: Definitive treatment of mandibular fractures in young children. Oral Surg 36:164, 1973

Mathog RH: Maxillofacial Trauma, 1st Ed. Williams & Wilkins, Baltimore, 1984

Neal DC, et al: Morbidity associated with teeth in the line of mandibular fractures. J Oral Surg 36:859, 1978

Osbon DB: Facial trauma. p. 214–241. In Irby WB (ed): Current Advances in Oral Surgery. C.V. Mosby, St. Louis, 1974

Rowe NL: Fractures of the jaws in children. J Oral Surg 27:497, 1969

Rowe NL, Killey HC: Fractures of the Facial Skeleton. 2nd Ed. Williams & Wilkins, Baltimore, 1970

Schneider SS, Stern M: Teeth in the line of mandibular fractures. J Oral Surg 29:107, 1971

Walker RV: Effect of traumatic mandibular condyle fracture dislocations on growth in the Macaca Rehsus monkey. Am J Surg 100:850, 1960

Zallen RD, Curry JT: A study of antibiotic usage in compound mandibular fractures. J Oral Surg 33:431, 1975

Rigid Internal and External Fixation of Mandibular Fractures 10

Peter A. Hilger

Although many techniques have been devised for treatment of mandibular fractures, any method selected must include anatomic reduction and adequate immobilization if an osseous union with proper occlusion is to be achieved. Simple fractures of the dentate mandible are most frequently managed with some form of intermaxillary fixation. If satisfactory reduction and immobilization are not obtained with this method alone, open reduction and internal fixation (usually in the form of interosseous wiring) are required. Occasionally, the simpler fixation techniques will not provide adequate immobilization. This may be due to the type of fracture, as seen in injuries that produce multiple small fragments which preclude open reduction and interosseous wiring. Alternate forms of fixation may also be indicated because of the patient's condition prior to the fracture.[1] This is exemplified by fractures of the atrophic edentulous mandible in patients without dentures.

Rigid internal and external fixation provide better immobilization than interosseous wiring. Rigid external fixation methods were introduced for orthopedic injuries as early as 1898.[2] Application of this principle to maxillofacial injuries was developed during World War II. In 1949, Hall Morris refined this technique and added acrylic as part of the appliance thus eliminating much of the cumbersome external metallic device.[3] Few modifications of the technique have occurred since that time. The internal fixation technique has been recently developed, and an application of this technique for maxillofacial surgery was reported by Spiessl in 1979.[4]

Several different internal and external fixation systems are commercially available. Examples of internal fixation systems include the Mouly bone plate technique, the Swiss A-O plating system, and the Champy monocortical miniplate system.[5] External fixators include those of Rogers Anderson and Hall Morris. Rigid fixation is not needed for most mandibular fractures, and the techniques require expensive, complex surgical equipment, as well as advanced surgical skills.

INDICATIONS

A common feature of both rigid internal and external fixation is elimination of the need for interdental fixation. The most common indication for rigid fixation is a fracture of the edentulous mandible. This is especially true when the patient has had no dentures prior to injury or when the dentures are lost at the scene of the accident. Many elderly patients tolerate interdental fixation with dentures very poorly and are much easier to manage and maintain in positive nitrogen balance with rigid fixation. Due to preexisting dental disease or trauma, some patients have an inadequate number of teeth to establish interdental fixation and normal occlusion. Fractures in these patients can also be managed with rigid fixation. Occasionally, patients who have sustained a head injury grind their teeth for variable lengths of time following injury. When these patients have sustained a mandibular fracture, it may be difficult to maintain interdental fixation. Constant jaw motion can pull dental appliances off the teeth, repeatedly break fixation bands, and cause dental and gingival injury. Rigid fixation can reduce these problems by eliminating the need for interdental fixation.

Careful consideration should be given to the use of interdental fixation in patients with a seizure disorder because of the potential of airway obstruction and aspiration. Again, rigid fixation may be an appropriate method of treatment for mandible fractures in this group. Intermaxillary fixation is uncomfortable and severely restricts the patient's diet. Some less compliant patients, therefore,

refuse to maintain interdental fixation. This can lead to a malunion, nonunion, and/or osteomyelitis. Rigid fixation is also a useful option for management of these patients.

Severe maxillofacial injuries can cause a loss of mandibular bone. These injuries are usually associated with extensive skin and mucosal lacerations. Bone grafting at the time these injuries are initially repaired is avoided because of an increased risk of infection. An external fixation device will maintain proper anatomic alignment while the mucosa and soft tissues heal (Fig. 10-1). The defect is grafted at a later time, when the wounds have stabilized and healed.

If an injury has produced a badly comminuted fracture rather than loss of bone, it is preferable not to attempt open reduction and internal fixation of the fragments. Extensive periosteal stripping may devitalize the bone. Rigid external fixation will maintain reduction and fixation without opening the fracture site.

Some patients develop delayed union or nonunion because of inadequate immobilization. In these instances, rigid internal or external fixation can provide suitable immobilization to allow bony union.

In the patient with osteomyletis of the mandible, debridement of the involved bone may result in a segmental mandibular defect. The external fixation

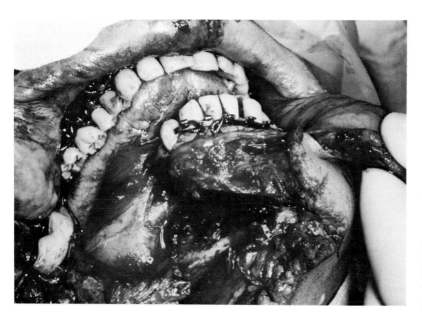

Fig. 10-1. This patient sustained loss of the right mandibular body and oral mucosa in a motor vehicle accident. A Morris biphase apparatus can be used to maintain proper anatomic relationship of the remaining fragments while the soft tissues heal. Bone grafting is performed as a delayed procedure.

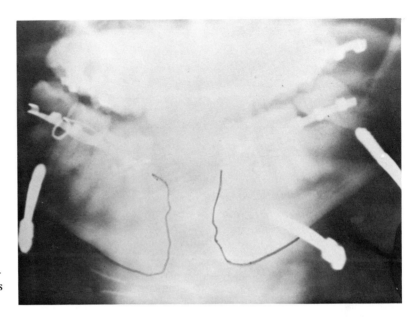

Fig. 10-2. Symphyseal defect following osteomyelitis, with screws in place for rigid external fixation.

device can be used to maintain proper anatomic relationships until the mandible is reconstructed (Fig. 10-2). Both the internal and external rigid fixation devices are useful for repair of the mandible following osteotomy for resection of an oral or pharyngeal tumor. These methods provide excellent immobilization yet allow jaw mobility that facilitates nutrition, wound care, and airway maintenance.

troughs intersecting at an obtuse angle (Fig. 10-4). Each half of the plate contains screw holes with the inclined planes sloping medially. The screw heads are hemispheres. When tightened, the head first engages the sloping portion of the screw hole and glides toward the fracture site. This action causes the fracture to be immobilized and compressed. Researchers have studied bone healing in fractures under compression and have termed the healing process *primary bone healing*. This differs from the usual healing process because of a lack of callus

RIGID INTERNAL FIXATION

Principles of Action

The most popular rigid internal fixation system is the dynamic compression plate developed in Switzerland (manufactured by Synthes Corp.). The plate used for mandible fractures is a smaller version of the plates used for orthopedic surgery. They are commercially available in various lengths with different numbers and patterns of holes (Fig. 10-3). In cross section each screw hole resembles two

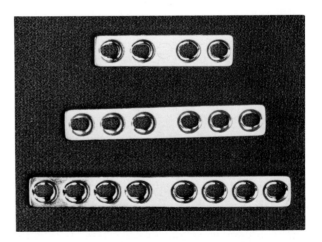

Fig. 10-3. Dynamic compression plates (DCP) are available in several sizes. Three examples are shown.

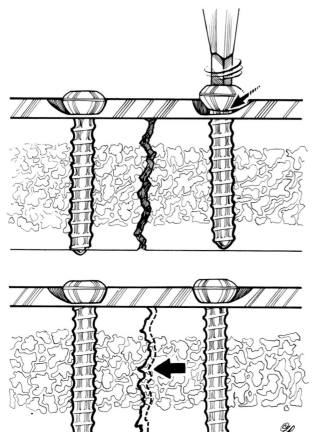

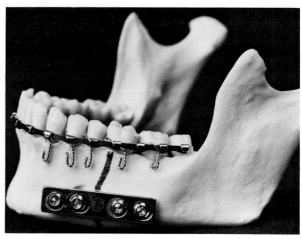

Fig. 10-5. In the dentate mandible, an arch bar combined with the compression plate provides more uniform compression along the line of fracture.

Fig. 10-4. The sloping screw holes of the DCP cause compression of the fracture when the screws are tightened.

formation. In the fracture under compression, simultaneous bone resorption and axial osteogenesis occur.

The greatest amount of axial compression can be produced if the plate is applied to the midportion of the facial cortex. Unfortunately, such placement can cause screws to traverse the alveolar canal leading to neurologic or vascular injury. Application near the alveolar surface of the mandible is also inappropriate because screw placement may cause dental injury. Therefore, the plate must be applied near the inferior mandibular margin. This produces eccentric compression and distraction of the fracture near the alveolar surface. Modifications of the technique have been devised to overcome this problem. If the fracture occurs through the dentate portion of the mandible, an arch bar or tension

band can be applied to the teeth before the plate is placed. This provides more even distribution of compression (Fig. 10-5). If the fracture occurs in an edentulous area, a two-hole plate can be applied above the alveolar canal; this in combination with the inferiorly positioned plate provides more axial compression (Fig. 10-6). The edentulous mandible poses special problems. In most cases, significant mandibular atrophy has occurred, and the mandible has insufficient height to permit the placement of two plates. Therefore, a second type of plate has

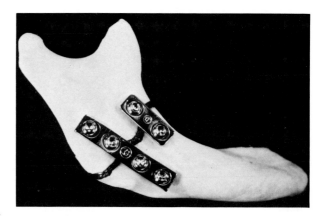

Fig. 10-6. Axial compression can be produced in the edentulous portion of the mandible with the use of a two-hole plate near the superior margin of the mandible and a multihole DCP placed below the alveolar canal.

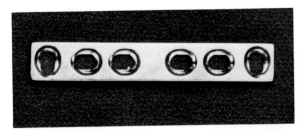

Fig. 10-7. Eccentric dynamic compression plate (EDCP). Screws placed in the most lateral holes cause rotation of the bone fragments around medially placed compression screws. The combination of forces provides adequate axial compression with one plate.

been developed. In this plate the two most lateral screw holes have the trough oriented perpendicular to the axis of the plate (Fig. 10-7). This plate has been labeled the eccentric dynamic compression plate (EDCP). The remaining holes in this plate are oriented in the axis of the plate. Screws placed in the lateral holes of an EDCP cause slight rotation of the mandibular fragments and compression of the alveolar surface. Tightening of the remaining screws causes compression of the fracture near the inferior margin of the mandible. This combination of forces provides adequate compression and immobilization.

Fractures of the condylar portion of the mandible can cause special problems. Most fractures in this region can be managed with soft diet or interdental fixation. However, occasionally an injury produces significant fracture dislocation of the mandibular condyle. This can lead to loss of mandibular vertical height and an open-bite deformity. This is particularly true with bilateral condylar fractures. Several authors have advocated open reduction and internal fixation with interosseous wiring for this type of injury. If the condylar head has been displaced from the glenoid fossa, the pull of the lateral pterygoid muscle tends to retain the condylar head in a medially displaced position. Interosseous wiring of the fracture may fail to maintain proper reduction, and the wire may form a hinge with the condylar head displaced medially. Recently a West German group has devised a method of rigid internal fixation which helps maintain proper reduction.[6] This technique utilizes a lag screw that traverses the vertical ramus (Fig. 10-8). The distal end has cortical threads which firmly

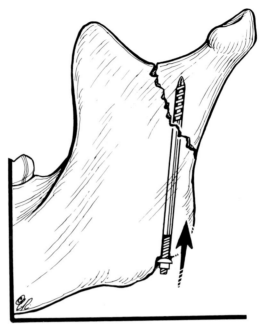

Fig. 10-8. Lag screw fixation. Cortical threads in the tip of the screw engage the condylar fragment. Tightening the nut at the end of the screw compresses the ramus and condylar fragments.

hold the condylar fragment. The portion of the screw traversing the vertical ramus has finer screw threads which do not engage the bone. After the lag screw has been placed into the condylar fragment, a nut tightened beneath the vertical ramus causes the vertical ramus to move superiorly with compression of the fracture site. The designers of this technique feel that it provides more reliable reduction and superior fixation.

Technique

Several manufacturers produce instrumentation for rigid internal fixation. The technique described utilizes the dynamic compression plating system manufactured by the Synthes Corporation. The specialized instruments required for compression plating are reduction-compression forceps, drill guides, twist tap, depth gauge, screwdriver, and bone-holding forceps (Fig. 10-9). Variable length titanium screws are also available (Fig. 10-10). The plates are also constructed of titanium to avoid

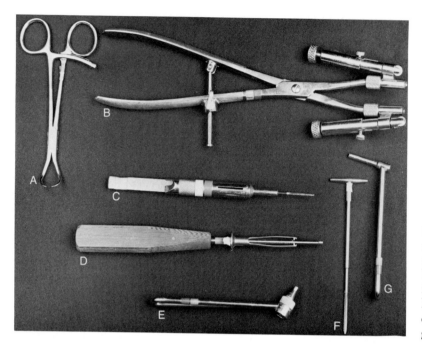

Fig. 10-9. Instruments required for mandibular plating (Synthes Corp.) (**A**) Reduction forceps for small bones. (**B**) Reduction-compression forceps. (**C**) Depth gauge. (**D**) Hexhead screwdriver. (**E**) Eccentric drill guide. (**F**) Twist tap. (**G**) Drill guide.

electrolytic osteolysis. A standard dynamic compression plate (DCP) appliance has all of the holes oriented so that tightening the screws creates axial compression. The eccentric dynamic compression plates are constructed so that screws tightened in the lateral holes create a force perpendicular to the plate. This force, in concert with the screws in the other holes creates uniform axial compression.

Fractures between the ascending ramus and the mandibular symphysis can be treated with this form of fixation. When the surgeon elects to use the plating system, the location of the fracture and status of the dentition dictate the details of the surgical technique, the goal of which is the reestablishment of normal occlusion. At the beginning of the procedure, those patients who have adequate

dentition are placed in intermaxillary fixation with arch bars and wire ligatures. Rigid internal fixation can then be established through an intraoral or extraoral approach, depending upon the location of the fracture and preference of the surgeon. An intraoral exposure can be considered for those fractures anterior to the mental foramen. If the fracture is located posterior to this location, adequate intraoral exposure may be difficult. After the fracture has been identified, the soft tissues are elevated sufficiently to allow placement of the plate near the inferior margin of the mandible. A four- or six-hole DCP or EDCP will provide sufficient fixation for most fractures. If the injury has produced several fracture lines and bony fragments, a larger plate may be required. Screw holes are drilled into the inferior margin of the mandible approximately 1 cm on each side of the fracture line. These holes are created with a hand drill or variable speed power drill and are directed toward the alveolar surface of the mandible. The holes are tapped, and 10-mm screws are used to secure the bone reduction forceps to the mandible. With the aid of the reduction forceps, the fragments can be manipulated and proper reduction established (Fig. 10-11). A compression plate is selected and molded with a bending pliers to fit the contour of

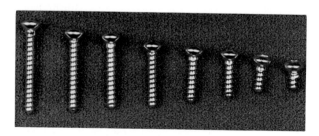

Fig. 10-10. Hex-head screws of varying lengths.

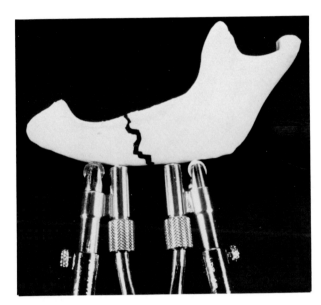

Fig. 10-11. The reduction-compression forceps are secured to the margin of the mandible, and the fragments are reduced and compressed.

the mandible (Fig. 10-12). The plate should be slightly more concave than necessary to provide evenly distributed compression on both the lingual and facial cortices. The compression plate is then placed near the inferior margin of the mandible and held in position with a plate-holding clamp. With the aid of an eccentric drill guide placed in the plate holes, a drill can be used to penetrate both mandibular cortices. The holes must be placed so that as the screw is tightened the compressive forces are properly directed. For those holes oriented in the axis of the plate, the drill holes must be placed in the lateral aspect of the screw holes. For those holes oriented perpendicularly to the axis of the place, the hole must be placed in the inferior aspect of the plate hole. After the mandibular holes are created, they are tapped and a measuring device is used to determine the thickness of the mandible (Fig. 10-13). Appropriate length screws are selected so that the threads will engage both facial and lingual cortices of the mandible. Screws are inserted but not tightened. After all screws are placed, they are tightened on alternate sides of the fracture line (Fig. 10-14). The reduction forceps and screws holding it in place can then be removed. If the surgeon has elected to use a transoral approach, it may be difficult to place the most posterior screws through limited oral exposure. When this occurs, the holes can be drilled and the screws placed through a percutaneous stab incision. Long drill guides are available to protect soft tissues. After placement of the plate, a suction drainage system may be beneficial. If interdental fixation was initially established, the patient is taken out of interdental fixation at the conclusion of the procedure. Appliances on the maxillary dentition can also be removed. If a mandibular arch bar has been placed, and the fracture is located in the tooth-bearing portion of the mandible, it is left in place to act as a tension band to aid axial compression. Some surgeons even elect to place a layer of acrylic over

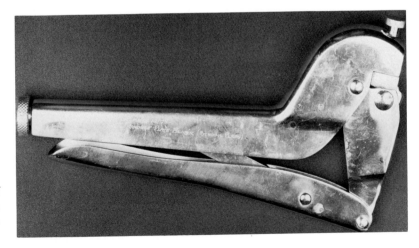

Fig. 10-12. One of several types of plate benders used to mold the plate to the contour of the mandible.

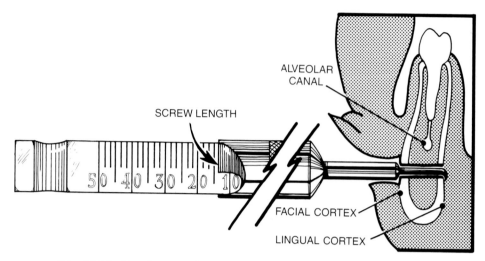

Fig. 10-13. Depth gauge for measuring the thickness of the mandible.

the mandibular arch bar to prevent stretching of the metal.

Surgical intervention with this technique, like all others, should occur as early as possible following injury. When the injury has produced extensive soft tissue loss, or if the patient has marked dental or gingival disease, repair with rigid internal fixation is delayed until the patient's condition is improved. An alternate technique such as rigid external fixation may also be selected.

Advantages and Disadvantages

Rigid internal fixation using compression plates has been found to produce primary bone healing compared to healing by callus formation associated with other methods of mandibular repair. In primary bone healing, bone is absorbed along the fracture site, and osteocytes immediately bridge the defect. This technique provides several advantages over interdental fixation. The patient is allowed to resume a normal diet on the first postoperative day, thereby shortening the patient's catabolic phase. Because fewer oral appliances are used, there is a significant improvement in ease of oral hygiene and a reduction in the incidence of postoperative gingival and dental disease. Many patients who sustain maxillofacial trauma have nasal obstruction due to nasal injuries or nasal packing. Rigid fixation provides the patient with an adequate oral airway and may eliminate need for tracheotomy.

Application of the compression plate in rigid internal fixation requires a specific set of expensive instruments. It may be difficult to justify the cost of

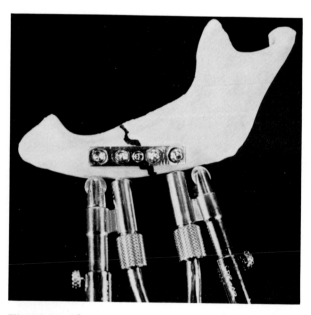

Fig. 10-14. The compression plate is applied to the facial cortex of the mandible. The screws engage both the lingual and facial cortical plates. After they are tightened, the reduction-compression forceps are removed.

this equipment in a hospital where there are a limited number of mandibular fractures. In addition, the surgical technique is much more complicated than more traditional methods of internal fixation, and some reports in the literature have indicated an increased complication rate with its use.[7] Placement of the compression plate requires a larger skin incision and more soft tissue stripping than that required for placement of interosseous wires. Consequently there is a larger scar. The compression plate is applied to the facial cortex of the mandible. In a thin person this may be cosmetically significant. Use of the plate for an edentulous mandibular fracture can create difficulties with the fit of a denture.

It is recommended that the plate be removed approximately 1 year after it is placed. This requires a second surgical procedure with its associated risks and morbidity. Those patients who have had dentures remodeled to avoid impingement on the plate may find their dentures again need remodeling following plate removal. Some authors have found that accurate restoration of normal occlusion can be difficult with the compression plate technique, and therefore they suggest that it has limited use in the dentate jaw.[8] Finally, presence of a metallic device can cause jaw pain in cold weather.

RIGID EXTERNAL FIXATION

Principles of Action

As previously noted, external fixation devices have been utilized for a longer time than rigid internal fixation devices. Numerous systems are available, but the system used most frequently is the Hall Morris biphase apparatus.[9] This method utilizes percutaneous cortical screws to secure the device to bone. Screws should be placed so that the threads engage both cortices. Whenever possible two pins should be placed on each side of the fracture line to provide adequate immobilization. In addition, screws should be placed at least 1 cm apart. Following pin placement, an adjustable bar and linkage apparatus is affixed to each pin. The fracture is then reduced manually, and the bar and linkage system is tightened to maintain reduction. This completes the first phase of application. In the second step a cold cure acrylic bar is applied to the pins. The acrylic bar can be molded in a tray and allowed to harden to a semisolid consistency before being placed on the pins. After the acrylic has hardened, the metal bar and linkage system can be removed, and fixation will be maintained with the percutaneous screws and acrylic bar (Fig. 10-15).

Technique

The instrumentation required for external fixation is much simpler than that required for compression plating (Fig. 10-16). Although general anesthesia is preferred, application can be performed under local anesthesia. The first portion of the technique involves placement of percutaneous screws. At least two screws should be placed on each side of the fracture line, 1 to 2 cm away from the fracture, whenever possible (Fig. 10-17). If injury has produced multiple fragments, it may be possible to place pins only in larger fragments. Pins should be directed so they avoid injuring dental structures and the neurovascular bundle in the mandibular canal. Once location of a pin site has been selected, a stab wound is made through the skin to the mandibular periosteum. A pediatric nasal speculum can be placed in the incision to protect the soft tissues when holes are drilled in the bone (Fig. 10-18). A hand drill with a 5/64″-diameter twist drill is used to perforate both mandibular cortices. Vitalium biphase pins have a shaft diameter of 5/64″ and are available with cortical thread lengths of 1/4″, 1/2″, and 3/8″. The surgeon should select a screw that has cortical threads long enough to penetrate the facial cortex of the mandible and engage the lingual cortex. For example, in the symphyseal region a 3/8″ length thread may be necessary, while at the mandibular angle a 1/4″ thread would be appropriate (Fig. 10-19). Holes are drilled with a hand drill to avoid generating heat at the pin site, which can

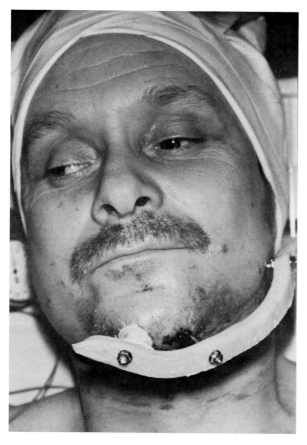

Fig. 10-15. Morris biphase device used for mandibular fixation.

cause osteonecrosis and later loosening of the pins. Remaining pins should be placed so that they are at least 1 cm apart (Fig. 10-20).

Once the pins have been secured, the adjustable bar and linkage system is applied. Before tightening the system, fragments are manually reduced. Tightening the bar and linkage system maintains reduction (Fig. 10-21). Reduction is evaluated by visual inspection or intraoperative radiographs. Occasionally, this form of fixation can be supplemented with open reduction and interosseous wire fixation. An extraoral approach is preferred when interosseous wire fixation is chosen. After the fracture is reduced, an acrylic splint is molded and placed on the pins. An adjustable acrylic mold is available with the instrument set. The mold should be greased with a light layer of Vaseline before the acrylic is formed to prevent later adherence of the splint to the mold. Cold cure acrylic can be obtained from many dental supply houses, or orthopedic bone cement can be used. A mixture that hardens in approximately 10 minutes allows adequate working time (Fig. 10-22). Powder and liquid components of the system are mixed together until a paste consistency is achieved. This mixture is placed in the mold, allowed to become semisolid, and then applied to the fixation pins. A small amount of bone wax applied to the pins can facilitate later removal of the splint. The acrylic cures

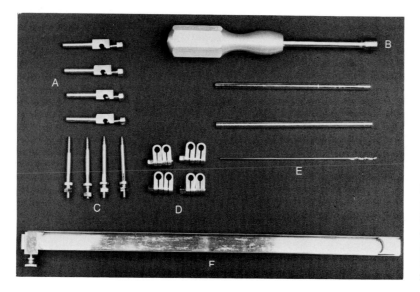

Fig. 10-16. External fixation instrumentation (Richards Manufacturing Co.) **(A)** Percutaneous pins with cortical threads of varying length. **(B–D)** Bar and linkage apparatus. **(E)** Wrench. **(F)** Adjustable acrylic mold.

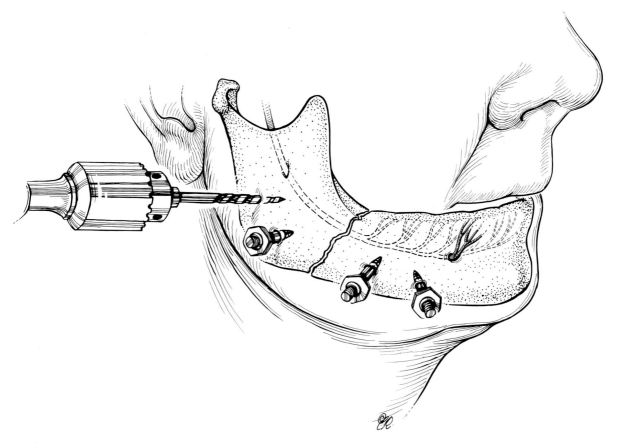

Fig. 10-17. Placement of pins. Two pins are placed on each side of the fracture and at least 1 cm from the fracture site.

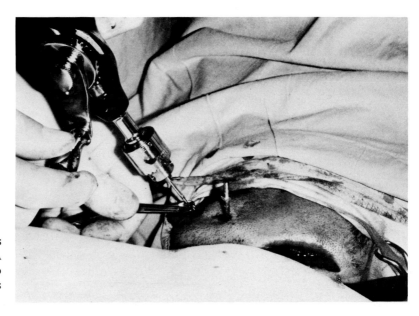

Fig. 10-18. A 5/64″ twist drill is used to place holes for the pins. A pediatric nasal speculum is used to protect the soft tissues during this portion of the procedure.

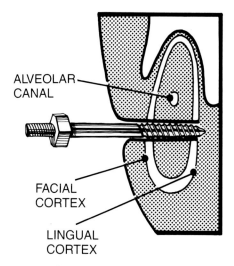

ALVEOLAR CANAL

FACIAL CORTEX

LINGUAL CORTEX

Fig. 10-19. A threaded pin is tightened so that its threads engage both cortical plates of the mandible.

with an exothermic reaction, necessitating the application of ice to the acrylic and pins for several minutes to avoid thermal injury to the skin or bone. Nuts are placed on the lateral ends of the pins to hold the splint in place, before the acrylic has solidly set.

An alternate acrylic splint utilizes a polyvinyl chloride endotracheal tube. If one elects to use this method, a #7 or #8 endotracheal tube is selected, and perforations are made in the tube at the pin sites. The endotracheal tube can then be placed on the pins and gently secured with nuts, but not tightened so as to obstruct the lumen of the tube. The acrylic is mixed and placed in a urethral catheter syringe that is used to inject the acrylic into the endotracheal tube (Fig. 10-23). After the acrylic has hardened, the bar and linkage system is removed (Fig. 10-24).

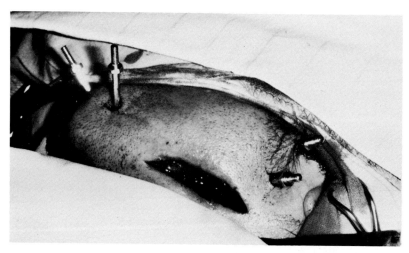

Fig. 10-20. The pins should be placed at least 1 cm apart.

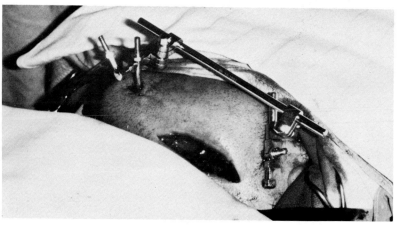

A

Fig. 10-21. (A) The metal bar and linkage system is applied to the pins. After the bony fragments are reduced, tightening of the links maintains reduction. This completes the first phase of the procedure. (*Figure continues.*)

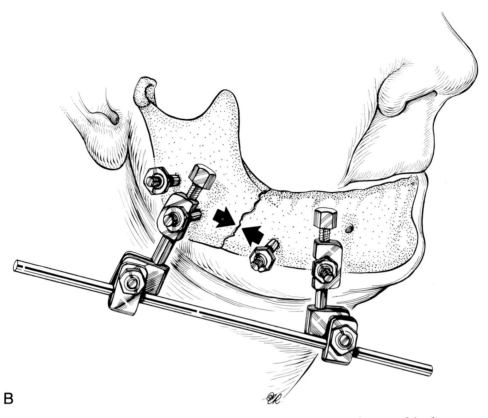

B

Fig. 10-21 (*continued*). (**B**) The metal bar and linkage system maintains reduction of the fragments until an acrylic bar has been applied.

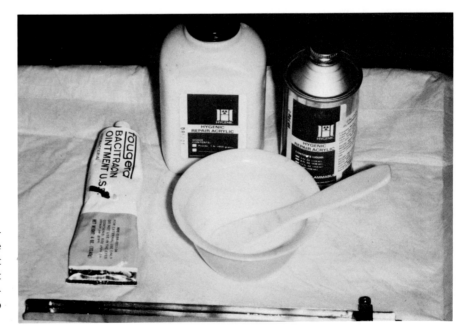

Fig. 10-22. Cold cure acrylic, Vaseline, mold, and mixing bowl are used to prepare an acrylic bar that will be placed on the pins. A light layer of Vaseline in the mold prevents the acrylic from adhering to the mold.

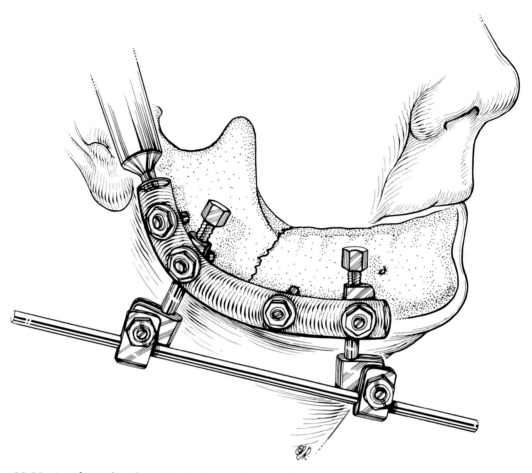

Fig. 10-23. A polyvinyl endotracheal tube can be modified to fit over the pins. Liquid acrylic can be injected into the tube via a urethral catheter syringe.

This technique may be used for difficult cases where osseous union may be delayed beyond the usual 4 to 6 weeks. Before the external fixation device is removed, the acrylic splint is split with a Gigli saw or oscilating saw, and stability of the fracture is assessed. Radiographic evaluation can also be performed at this time. If the fracture has not healed, the acrylic splint can be repaired to again produce rigid fixation. After healing, the splint and pins can usually be removed in the clinic without anesthesia.

This system is useful for fixation of some malar fractures, a limited number of frontal sinus and nasoethmoid fractures, as well as mandibular fractures (Fig. 10-25). As previously noted, rigid external fixation is useful for maintaining the proper anatomic relationship of residual mandibular fragments when bone loss has occurred. In these situations bone grafting is usually performed on a delayed basis. The external fixation device can be removed at the time of bone grafting.

Rigid external fixation devices provide many of the same advantages of rigid internal fixation. Moreover, external fixation devices can be rapidly applied, and in the trauma patient, this can shorten overall anesthesia time.

The external fixation techniques also have their limitations. Because this method utilizes percutaneous pins, facial scars are unavoidable. These scars rarely require revision but can be troublesome. The external fixation device is cumbersome and cosmetically unappealing. Special instrumen-

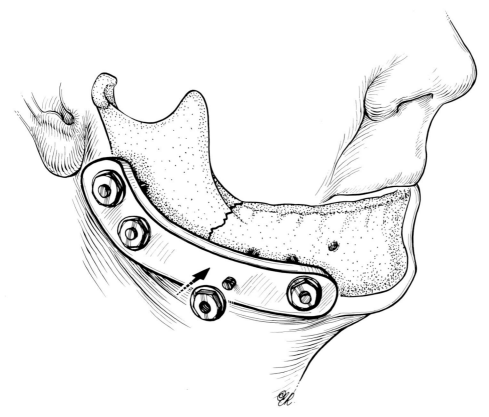

Fig. 10-24. The acrylic bar is secured to the pins with hex-head nuts. After the acrylic has cured, the bar and linkage system is removed.

tation is required for this technique, although it is less expensive and less complicated than that required for rigid internal fixation. Osteitis may develop at the pin sites. This occurs rarely, and when it does occur, osteitis is usually due to a patient's failure to properly care for the wound.

COMPLICATIONS OF BOTH TECHNIQUES

As with any surgical technique, postoperative complications can occur with both rigid internal and external fixation methods. Fractures that occur in the tooth-bearing portion of the mandible are contaminated because the oral mucosa at the fracture site is lacerated. This contamination in combination with the introduction of foreign materials makes use of prophylactic antibiotics necessary. Despite this precaution, postoperative infections do occur. Incidence of soft tissue infections or osteomyelitis is not significantly increased with these methods over traditional techniques.

If the surgeon elects to apply a compression plate through an extraoral approach, a larger incision is required than that required for interosseous wiring. This produces a larger facial scar. Intraoral exposure of the plate is another potential postoperative complication, particularly if the plating technique is utilized for an atrophic edentulous mandibular fracture. Some authors have suggested that if intraoral exposure occurs, the plate need not be removed if it is still rigidly fixed to the mandi-

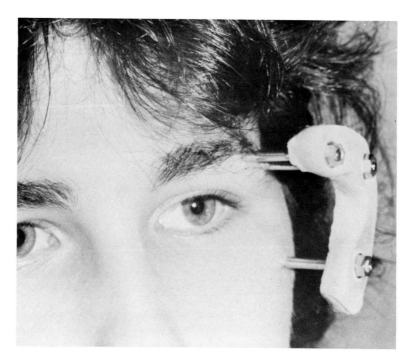

Fig. 10-25. The biphase external fixation system is also useful for other facial fractures. A comminuted malar fracture is immobilized in this photograph.

ble.[4] In this situation, they advise administering local wound care until the mucosa heals.

Dental structures as well as the neurovascular bundle within the mandibular canal can be injured if the plate is not properly positioned near the inferior margin of the mandible. Hypesthesia of the chin can also occur if the surgeon has used an intraoral approach that has produced traction on the mental nerve or if a screw has penetrated the mandibular canal. Paresis of the margin mandibular nerve can occur if an internal fixation device is placed through an extraoral approach and dissection has injured the nerve.

When the external fixation technique is utilized, local hygiene to the pin site consisting of daily hydrogen peroxide and antibiotic ointment application is advised. If proper wound care is not maintained, localized osteitis can occur at the pin sites. This will lead to pin mobility and loss of rigid fixation. Pin placement in the ascending ramus can traverse the parotid gland and result in a postoperative parotid fistula. This can be successfully managed with local wound care. Some scarring does occur at the pin sites. Although small, these scars can be noticable because of the location on the cheek. Scar camouflage may be indicated after osseous union.

If proper reduction is not achieved before either method of rigid fixation is established, a malunion results. Therefore, it is essential that proper occlusal relationships be established prior to fixation.

Mandibular nonunion rarely occurs with these techniques; however, it is more likely to occur if fixation is inadequate or not maintained for an appropriate length of time. The type of injury can also influence the frequency of this complication. Extensively comminuted fractures, and other injuries associated with devascularized bone fragments, are at greater risk of developing of this complication. These techniques are not advised for mandibular fractures in children because unerupted teeth can be injured by the pins or screws.

SUMMARY

Rigid internal and external fixation techniques are useful adjuncts for unusual mandibular fractures. The basic principles of fracture reduction and immobilization apply for these methods as well as the traditional techniques. Before utilizing rigid internal or external fixation, it is important that the surgeon be familiar with the basic principles of action, the complex surgical equipment required, and the details of the surgical technique.

REFERENCES

1. Meyerhoff W, Maisel R: Fractures of the facial skeleton. American Academy of Otolaryngology, Washington, D.C., 1980
2. Anderson R: An ambulatory method of treating fractures of the shaft of the femur. Surg Gynecol Obstet 62:865, 1936
3. Morris JH: Biphase connector, external skeletal splint for reduction and fixation of mandibular fractures. Oral Surg 2:1382, 1949
4. Spiessl B (ed): New Concepts in Maxillofacial Bone Surgery. Springer-Verlag, Berlin, Heidelberg, New York, 1976
5. Hilger P, Duckert L, Boies L: The dynamic compression plate for mandibular fixation. p. 222. In Bernstein L (ed): Rehabilitative Surgery. Vol. 2, 1981
6. Petzel J: Instrumentarium and Technique for Screw-Pin-Osteosynthesis of Condylar Fractures. J Maxillofac Surg 10:8, 1982
7. Wilson K, Christiansen T, Quick C: External fixation in maxillofacial surgery. Otolaryngol Clin North Am 9:523, 1976
8. Strelzow V, Friedman W: Dynamic compression plating in the treatment of mandibular fractures. Arch Otolaryngol 108:583, 1982
9. Becker R: Stable compression plate fixation of mandibular fractures. Br J Oral Surg 12:13, 1974

Evaluation and Treatment of Post-Traumatic Malunion/Malocclusion

11

Paul Hak Joo Kwon
Daniel E. Waite

The care of injuries to the maxillofacial region is a common surgical responsibility for the maxillofacial surgeon. Interference with the facial skeleton and related soft tissues occurs easily in both form and function following injury to this area. Malunion of the jaws may cause marked asymmetry and deformity to the face, altered jaw function, malocclusion, painful teeth and muscles, and pain in the temporomandibular joint. Knowledge of normal facial skeleton and dental occlusion is very important when one evaluates facial and dental harmony, phonetic action, and masticatory function. The axiom that one must know what is normal to observe what is abnormal is so true. The maxilla and mandible are frequently affected by trauma from motor vehicle accidents, domestic injuries, athletics, and ablative surgical procedures. Trauma is the greatest single cause of acquired malocclusion.[1] Injuries may be limited to teeth and/or the alveolar segment, or may involve the mandible, maxilla, and temporomandibular joint. Post-traumatic malocclusion may indicate maxillary and/or mandibular fracture with malposition of fragments. With the possible exception of the greenstick fracture, all jaw fractures may contribute to malocclusion.

The term *malunion* is used to describe a healed fracture, but one in which there is poor or unacceptable alignment (Fig. 11-1). *Nonunion* refers to a complication in management of a fracture wherein a true osseous union does not take place and segments are mobile (Fig. 11-2). *Malocclusion* refers to abnormal tooth-to-tooth position in the jaw that sustained fracture, or in relationship to the opposing jaw (Fig. 11-3). *Tooth malposition* refers to a tooth out of its normal position in the dental arch (Fig. 11-4).

The degree of malocclusion can be minor to extensive. There is probably no fracture so perfectly reduced as to not cause some minor discrepancy in occlusion. The proprioceptive perception of tooth contact is such that any deviation in tooth position is noticed by the patient. The usual complaint is of hypersensitivity from premature contact. The initial injury may interfere with nerve innervation so that patient response may not indicate early pain and discomfort to alert the surgeon to existing malocclusion. In such instances, the more latent complications described below may occur.

A serious complication from malunion is malocclusion. Teeth in malocclusion and malposition may alter functional patterns of jaw movement and

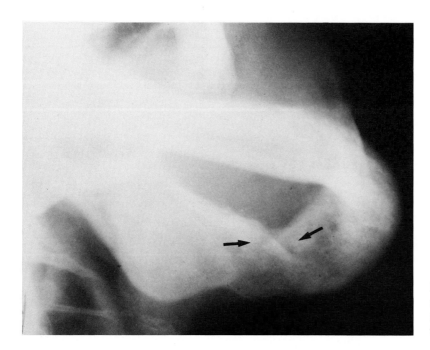

Fig. 11-1. A malunion of the mandible. Note the constriction in the size of the body of the mandible at the point of the union (arrows).

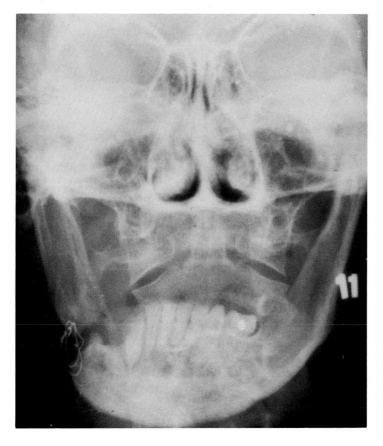

Fig. 11-2. A nonunion of a fracture on the right side. Reduction was achieved with intraosseous wires and no interjaw immobilization. The nonunion is evident in the resorption between the fracture lines.

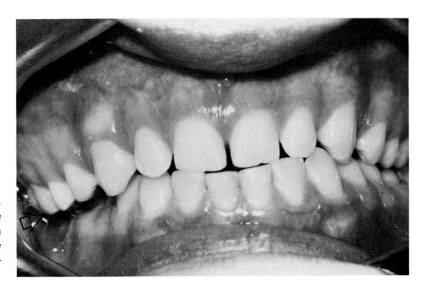

Fig. 11-3. A case of malocclusion. Note the slight anterior open bite and, particularly, the crossbite on the right side (arrow), where the maxillary teeth are in buccal position to the mandibular teeth.

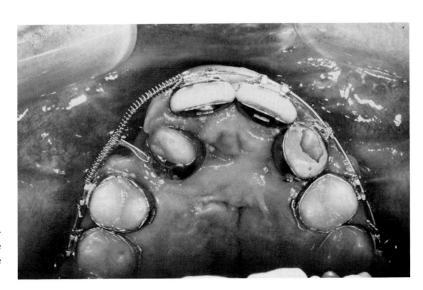

Fig. 11-4. An example of malposition of teeth where the right canine has erupted palatally out of the line of occlusion.

final jaw position. This, in turn, may cause pain in the muscles of mastication. The teeth may also become painful or mobile and result in early tooth loss.

Grossly malunited jaw fractures can cause noticeable asymmetry from acquired malocclusion contributing to deformity of the face. Complicated temporomandibular joint dysfunction, arthritis, and headaches are also common patient complaints.

INCIDENCE

Surgical reduction of fractures of the maxilla and mandible is generally successful, and need for a secondary procedure is unusual. The incidence of post-traumatic malocclusion has been poorly documented in the literature. Steidler et al.[2] reported that occlusal disharmony was present as a residual problem in 19.6 percent of 240 patients with fractures of the maxilla. Mathog and Boies[3] reported a 2.4 percent incidence of nonunion in 577 mandibular fractures seen over a 5-year period. Fifty percent of patients with nonunion were edentulous. In a study conducted by members of the Chalmers J. Lyons Club,[4] 9.2 percent of 120 patients with condylar fractures had posterior displacement and malunion. In addition to these findings, Bruce and Stracham[5] reported a 20 percent incidence of nonunion in 146 patients who had fractures of the edentulous mandible.

ETIOLOGY

Post-traumatic malunion occurs more often in the mandible than in the maxilla. This is partly because the quality of bone in the mandible contributes more to delayed healing than that of the maxilla. The mandible, being a bone in motion, makes fixation more difficult, which contributes both to nonunion and malunion. The mandible is a horseshoe-shaped bone that furnishes key support to the teeth and chewing apparatus and articulates with the skull at its proximal ends.[6,7] This uniquely curved bone, which houses the dental structures and performs the symmetrical and synchronous function of mastication, makes fixation and immobilization for good healing extremely difficult. During the healing period of a jaw fracture, necessary vital functions of swallowing and speaking make stabilization difficult. Malunion is usually caused by improper reduction or ineffective fixation, which may result from failure to recognize or treat these fractures when concentrating on more severe or life-threatening injuries. Malunion may also result when surgical treatment is inadequate or delayed, or when timely treatment is not sought by the patient. A fracture may be adequately reduced and immobilized during the course of the procedure only to have failure occur with a post-recovery anesthetic complication such as extended nausea and retching. This additional strain to the intermaxillary fixation may cause loosening of wires and result in a less than perfect reduction. A secondary accident during the healing period or simple lack of cooperation on the part of the patient may also be contributing factors of malunion.

Imperfect Reduction

It is of primary importance to reduce the bony segments to as near normal position as possible. This is accomplished with both closed and open reduction procedures. If the surgeon cannot be sure of satisfactory closed reduction by palpation of bone for continuity and tooth position, followed by verification by radiographs, then an open approach should be considered. Debridement to remove foreign bodies, blood clots, free small bone segments or interposed soft tissue may be necessary to accomplish reduction. Displacement of bony fragments by muscle pull is a common contributing problem that may lead to poor results.[8] A slight upriding of the posterior segment in an unfavorable jaw fracture near the angle may result in a malunion with malocclusion. Careful attention is necessary to overcome muscle displacement of the segments (Fig. 11-5). Generally, this can be accomplished by restoring adequate occlusion if there are teeth in each of the fractured segments. If this does not adequately reduce the segments, then inferior border wiring, plating, or external fixation may be necessary to immobilize the fracture.

Post-traumatic malunion of the jaws may also result from failure to restore accurate occlusion or jaw relationship due to inadequate dentition or lack of knowledge of the patient's individualized occlusion. When careful attention is given to a patient's personalized bite by observing tooth facets, tooth attrition, anterior midlines, and interdigitation of cusps, restoration of the patient's original jaw position is possible (Fig. 11-6). When teeth are missing, centric relation (i.e., condyles in their most retruded position) is much more difficult to establish. A less than perfect reduction or over-reduction can occur when severe compression forces are applied to the fractured segments. This more frequently occurs when extraoral appliances are

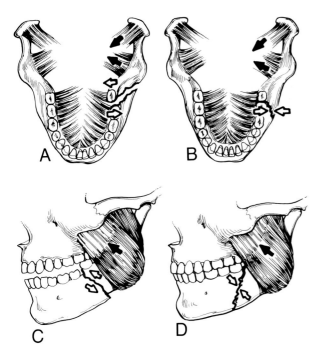

Fig. 11-5. (**A**) A left angle, unfavorable fracture that is displaced by pterygoid musculature. (**B**) A fracture between the second and third molars at the left angle of the mandible. In such cases the muscle pull tends to reduce the fracture and hold it in good position. (**C**) A fracture near the left angle of the mandible in which the masseter muscle pulls the posterior segment superiorly. This is an unfavorable fracture. (**D**) A fracture running from the the posterior part of the alveolus forward in an anterior fashion, thus making the fracture favorable because the masseter muscle tends to reduce the fracture as the muscle is activated.

used. Loss of bony tissue in the line of fracture makes reduction much more difficult and contributes to malposition.

Stabilization

Stabilization of jaw fractures for an adequate period of time is necessary for a normal union to occur. Many methods of fixation are available (see Chapter 9), of which dental arch bar and wire ligation are common. In addition, bone plates or external fixation pins may be indicated in selected cases (see Chapter 10). Bone screws, carefully placed, with good patient cooperation, will often permit

early return to minimal jaw function (Fig. 11-7) and avoid intermaxillary fixation. Splints of varying types, such as the lingual acrylic splint (Fig. 11-8) to minimize collapse of the mandibular arch or palatal splints for the maxilla, can contribute to good fracture stabilization.

Jaw immobilization contributes to poor oral hygiene and requires careful attention by both pa-

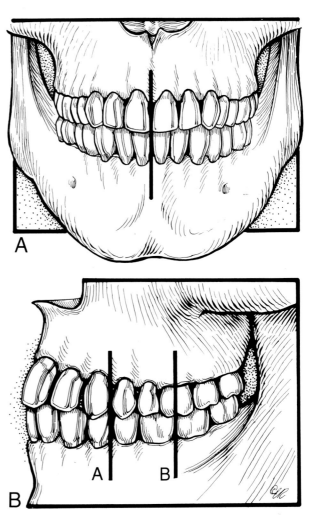

Fig. 11-6. (**A**) An imaginary line drawn between the central incisors of the maxilla, which coincides with the central incisor midline of the mandible, indicates symmetry of the jaws and the anterior teeth in normal position. (**B**) Normal relationship of the maxillary canine to the lower canine and the maxillary first molar to the lower molar is demonstrated. This positioning of the key teeth is referred to as a normal class I canine (*A*) and a class I molar (*B*) occlusal relationship (see Chapter 9).

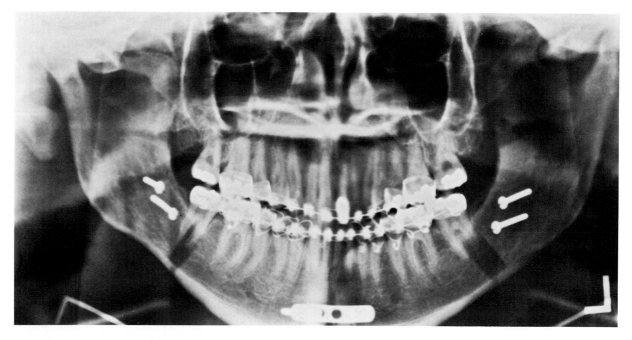

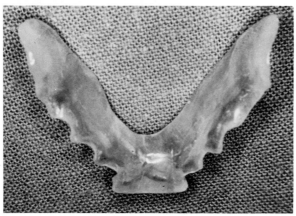

Fig. 11-7. Bone screws in the bilateral segments of the mandible provide a rigid fixation. Note the bone plate in the anterior region that permits the jaw to be mobilized and allows limited jaw function approximately 1 week after the fixation has been applied.

Fig. 11-8. An acrylic lingual splint in mandibular fractures can help prevent collapse of the arch.

tient and clinician throughout the fixation period. The addition of splints, arch bars, and wires make oral hygiene a problem of considerable magnitude, and improved oral hygiene habits are necessary to avoid periodontal disease with resultant loosening or loss of teeth.

Additional Fractures

When only one fracture is present in either jaw, results are usually good. However, multiple jaw fractures are more common. Adequate reduction of a fracture in the body or ramus of the mandible, for example, becomes more complicated when a condylar fracture is present on the opposite side. Condylar fractures frequently contribute to open bite or jaw deviation; however, good post-injury management minimizes these problems. Appropriate reduction and management of condylar fractures and early return to function of the jaws usually serve to reestablish condylar function and prevent ankylosis. In instances of multiple fractures, the surgeon should anticipate post-surgery treatment to restore the patient's occlusion for improved function. Condylar surgery may be required to relieve pain or to correct post-traumatic

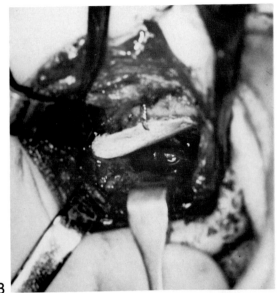

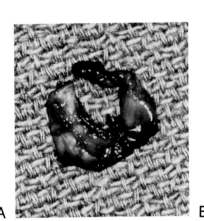

A   B

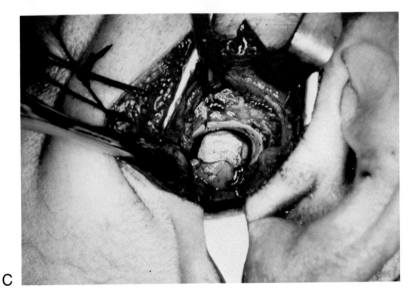

C

Fig. 11-9. (A) The articular disc removed from a patient suffering with degenerative joint disease. Note the center portion of the disc has been eroded completely. (B) A glenoid fossa implant of the Proplast Teflon type is seen lining the glenoid fossa, in position to replace the removed disc from the temporomandibular joint. (C) TMJ surgery showing a glenoid fossa implant and condylar head Proplast implant. The disc has been removed. (Case contributed by Dr. L. Wolford.)

arthritis, degenerative joint disease, internal derangement of the disc (Fig. 11-9).

Infection

Infection is an important consideration in the treatment of jaw fractures and can cause malunion or nonunion. Many times, as a result of the injury, there is contamination which contributes to the infectious process. Endogenous bacteria in the oral cavity are a significant factor when resistance is low and oral hygiene becomes difficult during the post-injury period. The quality of the patient's dentition and general oral hygiene may contribute to infection, or there may be existing infection at the time of injury.

Postoperative management of fractures includes consideration of prophylactic antibiotic coverage, meticulous oral hygiene during the post-injury period and throughout the time of fixation, and nutritional support. If infection does develop during the course of post-surgical management of fractures, it may contribute to malunion. If infection becomes more chronic, it may ultimately give rise to osteomyelitis and nonunion. Predisposing factors to infection at the fracture site are devitalized, infected, or abscessed teeth in the fracture area; hematoma in the fracture area; delayed immobilization with open wound; foreign body contamination in the wound; and poor oral hygiene. Bone healing may be affected by endocrine disorders such as hyperparathyroidism and post-menopausal osteoporosis, developmental disorders such as osteoporosis, and systemic disorders such as reticuloendothelial disease, Paget's disease, osteomalacia, and anemia. Local disorders such as fibrous dysplasia, tumors, and cysts may also affect fracture healing.[7]

Diabetes mellitus exerts a deleterious effect on fracture healing.[10] Powers et al.,[9] utilizing an alloxan diabetes model, demonstrated that fracture healing in growing rats was significantly decreased in the presence of poorly controlled diabetes and deficient diet (as determined by breaking strength measurements of healing femoral shaft fractures).

Bone Atrophy

Bone atrophy usually occurs in the edentulous jaw and becomes so advanced as to be the cause of a fracture (Fig. 11-10). Fracture of the atrophic edentulous mandible is difficult to treat and results in a high incidence (20 percent) of nonunion.[5]

Poor Nutrition

Poor nutritional condition can occur because of lack of normal food intake during intermaxillary fixation. Vitamin C deficiency depresses the formation of bone and collagen, and vitamin D deficiency causes failure of mineralization of new bone.[11] All these factors can contribute to malunion or nonunion of a fractured jaw.

Teeth in Fracture Line

Teeth in the line of fracture may also be a contributing factor to malunion. A tooth may interfere with adequate reduction of the fracture. If the

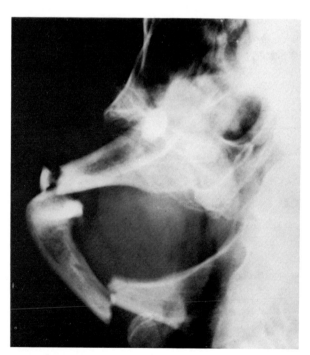

Fig. 11-10. Edentulous fracture. Displacement is due to muscle pull. Complication for fixation-nerve interruption is an indication for use of an extraoral appliance.

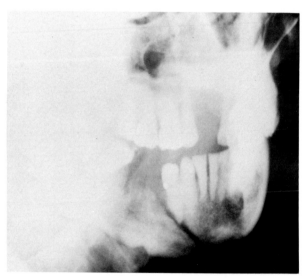

Fig. 11-11. A tooth in the line of a favorable fracture. Note the root end that is exposed in the fracture line.

tooth is a third molar, it may be well to sacrifice it. Other teeth significant to function and continuity of the arch should be evaluated carefully before they are removed. If survival of the tooth is questionable, careful postoperative observation should be instituted to monitor for pulp necrosis. If this occurs with subsequent gangrenous breakdown and root-end contamination, there could be infection of the fracture site. Such infection will contribute to delayed healing and possible nonunion. Treatment of the infection may require endodontic therapy or removal of the tooth. In addition, debridement and extended fixation time may be necessary to recover from the infection (Fig. 11-11).

PATHOPHYSIOLOGY

Pain from Mobility

Neurological complaints are common in the presence of malunion. A neuralgia may exist from impingement of the inferior alveolar nerve if the fractured bone ends do not permit normal repair and healing to take place. When the nerve is severed or severely contused, anesthesia or paresthesia may occur. These injuries may also contribute to the formation of a painful neuroma. If at the time of surgery, a severed nerve is observed, surgical repair should be performed. In most instances, if the bony segments are joined correctly, nerve repair and regeneration will take place. If pain or anesthesia extends beyond a 2-month post-fracture repair period, exploration, decompression, or surgical repair should be considered. Multiple muscular contractile forces operate upon the mandible, with essentially four vectors of pull (see Chapter 6). Depending on the direction of the fracture, these resultant forces may act to make a fracture either favorable or unfavorable in terms of stable bony opposition. Knowledge of this muscular pull is important in determining whether a fracture may be adequately immobilized using only interdental wiring and intermaxillary fixation, as opposed to direct interosseous wiring at the fracture site or other more rigid means of stabilization.

Malunion may present in a number of ways. A vertical malunion, such as those due to condylar fractures or fractures of the mandibular rami, may cause an open bite (Fig. 11-12). Malunion of fractures of the body and angle of the mandible may be responsible for a shortened mandibular arch on the involved side with crossbite malocclusion and retrognathia.[12] These malocclusions can be very

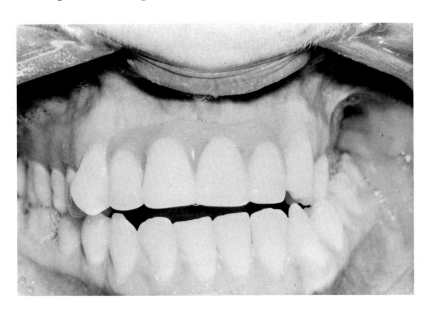

Fig. 11-12. Bilateral condylar fractures in this patient permitted slight overclosure in the posterior region that resulted in an anterior open bite, as evidenced by where the teeth do not touch.

complicated from the standpoint of treatment. Several disciplines may become involved to accomplish final repair and restoration (see section on treatment).

Temporomandibular Joint Syndrome

Another unique consideration of the pathophysiology of jaw fracture is the temporomandibular joint (TMJ). The mandibular articulation is guided by the occlusion of teeth and is important to mastication, mandibular movement, speech, and mandibular growth.[13] The temporomandibular joint is highly specialized and differs from all other bony articulations by the presence of avascular fibrous tissue covering the articulating surfaces and an interposed disc dividing the joint into an upper and lower compartment, which function synchronistically as two joints. It is unique in that both joints act together as one functional unit; no other joint in the body is so dependent on the function of its counterpart.[13] The joint structures can be injured directly from trauma or subsequently from malocclusion

due to malunion of the jaw fracture.

In many mandibular fractures, post-traumatic TMJ pain and discomfort occur. This is usually related to direct transmission of the blow from the symphysis region of the mandible to the temporomandibular joint. The injury may be relatively mild in nature and may not be demonstrable radiographically. Injury to the disc resulting in a tear of soft tissue, microfracture, or bleeding of the joint may set the stage for later internal derangement. Such injury may recover with rest and physical therapy or may lead to traumatic arthritis and degenerative joint disease, requiring joint surgery (Fig. 11-13).

DIAGNOSIS OF MALUNION AND MALOCCLUSION

History

The patient is the best source of information for diagnosing a fracture that has been inadequately reduced. Patients may describe a premature contact of teeth near the fracture site, difficulty in chewing, or simply sore teeth. Patients may describe complaints relating to the temporomandibular joint by stating that in closing the jaw, they have to shift or slide the jaw to be comfortable or to get good closure. They may describe muscle soreness and even headache after chewing. Careful examination of the occlusion and the dentition and palpation of the teeth in the region of the fracture to determine mobility may indicate the malocclusion. A knowledge of the pre-injury occlusal relation is important, particularly when a class I, II, or III occlusion is present.

The surgeon should look carefully at the midlines of the anterior mandibular and maxillary teeth. In the normal occlusion, midlines should coincide, and the patient should be questioned about the teeth's present appearance compared to that of before the injury. To carefully evaluate for premature tooth contacts and a normal occlusal relationship,

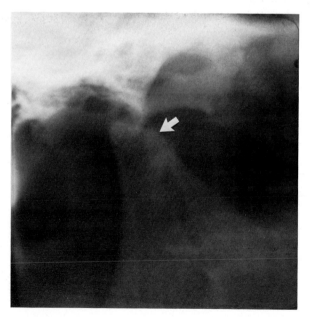

Fig. 11-13. Radiograph of the right temporomandibular joint showing degenerative joint disease. Note the flat and posterior sloping of the eroded condyle (arrow).

the clinician should grasp the symphysis region of the jaw and encourage the patient to relax the muscles while the clinician gently closes the lower jaw against the upper. A gentle tapping of the teeth together by the clinician may demonstrate the premature contacts and determine whether true centric occlusion is possible. This maneuver, when done correctly, places the mandibular condyles in their most retruded position. This pattern of closure is dictated by the musculature, and any interference from the dental units could well indicate malocclusion. The patient should be asked how he or she feels the teeth fit together as compared to before the injury. The intraoral examination should further examine the specific teeth in the region of the fracture and the overlying soft tissue. Percussion of the teeth may elicit apical sensitivity, and palpation of soft tissues in the region of the fracture may indicate tenderness or irregularity of underlying bone, suggestive of malunion. Pulp testing, either electrically or by temperature, may be helpful in determining vitality of the teeth. The use of articulating paper indicates traumatic occlusion and/or loss of tooth contact. Ultimately, study models and jaw relationship records may be necessary as well as a review of the articulated models on an articulator in order to diagnose dental deformity. The patient should be asked to clench the jaw and describe any feeling of movement or other abnormal sensations, as in heavy articulation. In a relaxed manner, the patient should be asked to open and close the jaw, and careful observation should be made for any deviation in movement (Fig. 11-14). Lateral excursions should then be made and measurements recorded. A normal opening, without discomfort, should be in the range of 40 to 45 mm between the incisors, and there should be at least 3 to 5 mm of free excursive movement, as measured from the midlines. By placing a finger in each external auditory canal and asking the patient to go through the same movements, pain and crepitus may be detected, implicating injury of the temporomandibular joint. Finally, if there is any suspicion of nonunion, the surgeon should grasp both segments of the jaw, anterior and posterior to the line of fracture, and carefully observe the teeth proximal to the fracture. Under reasonable examining stress, there should be no spacing, gap, or movement observable between the tooth surfaces.

Radiographic Evaluation

The panographic radiograph is an excellent film to display the mandible. This is a scanning film and will provide a good view of the condyles, rami, and horizontal bodies of the mandible. The symphysis region is much more difficult to view on the panogram, and occlusal films and symphysis views may be necessary. To carefully evaluate the specific area where the line of fracture has occurred and particularly the apices of teeth, the periapical dental film should be used. When questions arise relating to the potential of temporomandibular joint injury, the tomogram is best utilized to demonstrate the bony articulation in depth. The arthrogram (Fig. 11-15A) or magnetic resonance imaging (MRI) (Fig. 11-15B&C) may be necessary to more accurately observe the articular disc and related soft tissues. In instances where facial deformity may be in question, as a result of malocclusion and/or malunion, the lateral cephalogram and the PA head film are necessary.

When all radiographs have been taken and the examination and history including articulated models completed, careful planning for treatment can be contemplated.

TREATMENT

Prevention

The best way to prevent malunion is adequate primary reduction and fixation. Rigid fixation and careful reproduction of the patient's original occlusion, prior to injury, are significant factors in prevention of malunion or malocclusion. There will be situations where missing teeth will complicate reduction, and acceptance of a less than ideal occlusion may be necessary to assure good bony union. In addition, loss of bony substance in the region of fracture may require bone grafting and/or use of bone plates to maintain appropriate bony

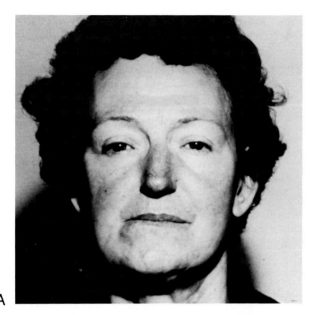

A

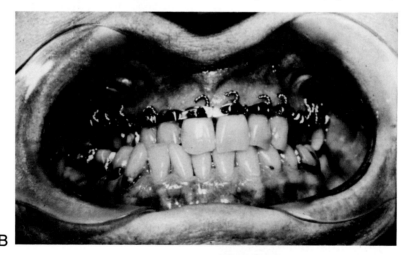

B

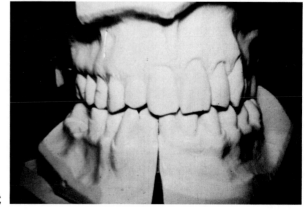

C

Fig. 11-14. (A) Asymmetry of the face. The mandible moved to the right side as a result of a jaw fracture on the right side. **(B)** Note the intraoral mandibular asymmetry and the right side crossbite where the mandibular occlusion is outside the maxillary occlusion. The maxillary arch bar is in position and ready for surgical management. **(C)** Model surgery demonstrating a midline surgical osteotomy and a ramus osteotomy that permit the mandibular occlusion to be more carefully fitted to the maxillary occlusion. (*Figure continues.*)

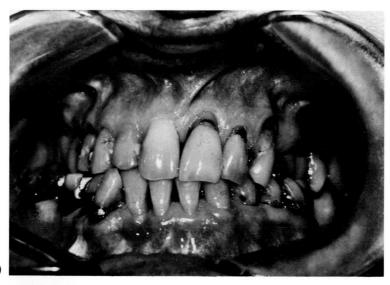

Fig. 11-14 (*continued*). (D) View 1 year after surgery showing the midline symmetry of the maxillary and mandibular teeth and the corrected posterior crossbite. **(E)** View 1 year after surgery. Facial features are balanced and the asymmetry corrected.

D

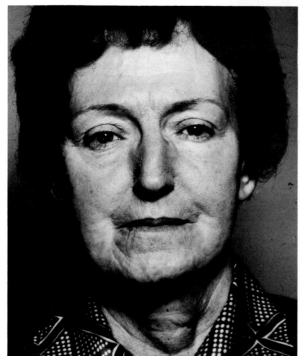

E

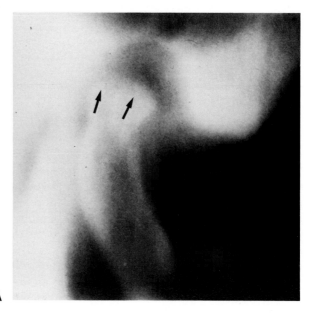

Fig. 11-15. (A) A tomogram of a temporomandibular joint. The patient has degenerative joint disease and several bone spurs on the superior surface (arrows). These bone spurs cause crepitus and considerable pain. At the time of surgery, there was a perforation of the disc, as seen in Figure 11-9A. (*Figure continues.*)

A

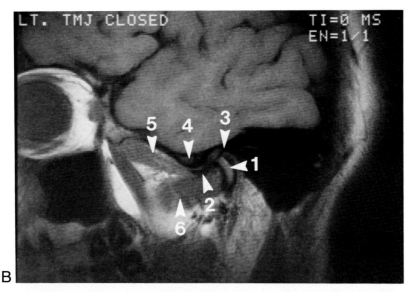

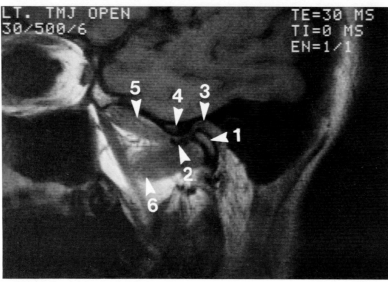

Fig. 11-15 (*continued*). (B & C) Open and closed nuclear magnetic resonance imaging in a patient with TMJ injury. (1) Displaced condyle. (2) Mandibular condyle. (3) Glenoid fossa. (4) Eminence. (5) Superior lateral pterygoid muscle. (6) Inferior lateral pterygoid muscle. (Case contributed by Dr. Don Chiles.)

continuity or tooth alignment. A completely edentulous patient, particularly an older person with mandibular atrophy, may require extraoral fixation, a prosthesis, or splint with circumferential wiring to effect an acceptable reduction. In young patients, a mixed dentition further complicates fixation methods. This is due to the presence of multiple tooth buds and deciduous and permanent teeth in various stages of development. Occasionally, overlay acrylic splints can be placed on the arch with quick-cure acrylic lining, which forms an immediate impression within the splint, to lock in the mixed dentition. This is further stabilized by circumferential wiring in either arch to maintain the dental occlusion. Nevertheless, in such instances the bite will be slightly opened and a malocclusion may occur. Fortunately because it is a mixed dentition, the loss of deciduous teeth and the eruption of the successors may salvage an otherwise compromised occlusion disharmony. These are but a few examples of the complicating problems that present to the clinician and may prevent ideal results. The reader is encouraged to carefully review Chapter 9.

Specific Treatment Modalities

Tooth Malposition

Tooth malposition can occur either as one or more teeth out of position, contributing to a malocclusion, or as an individual cusp in premature contact. Inspection of the occlusion and careful questioning of the patient as well as observation of the patient articulating in a relaxed position probably will indicate the teeth in question. Further delineation of this problem can be accomplished with the use of articulating paper. After carefully noting the teeth and/or cusps in question, equilibration may be sufficient treatment. Equilibration entails selective grinding with a high-speed rotary stone burr under a continuous flow of coolant liquid until the disharmony is corrected. Such correction should only be done within the enamel. Any grinding of teeth that would necessitate involvement of the dentin is probably an indication of a more major dental correction. In special situations where a tooth is sufficiently malposed to require extensive reduction of the tooth's surface or where it is contributing to traumatic occlusion, a more complete restoration of the tooth should be considered. This may involve cast gold inlays and/or crowns. A tooth acutely tender from traumatic occlusion usually involves hypersensitivity. Necrosis and death of the pulp may follow, which require endodontic treatment to save the tooth (Fig. 11-16).

Tooth extractions may have to be considered in some cases. When this occurs, immediate attention should be given to maintaining the interdental space in order to provide for bridge construction. Should this not be done, it will only be a matter of time before the teeth proximal to the fracture will tip into the space, complicating the occlusion and jaw function on the side of fracture.

Occasionally, premature tooth contact may be due to myofascial pain and muscle spasm. If clinical examination verifies this, attention should be given to reducing myofascial pain through physical therapy methods and muscle relaxants before tooth surfaces are ground away or other tooth structures removed. Temporomandibular joint injury, which may have occurred at the time of the original fracture, may need to be considered in relation to premature tooth contact. Degenerative joint disease, internal derangement, or simple hemorrhage into the joint may cause slight jaw deviation and/or altered function after the intermaxillary fixation is removed. In such instances, temptation to correct the teeth may be in error. Physical therapy to the joints and related musculature, treatment splints, or ultimate surgery of the joints may have to be considered.

Surgical Reoperation

Early Problems. When recognition of malposition or malocclusion is determined early, immediate restoration should be considered. This may be accomplished by adjusting fixation to overcome the malposition. If muscles are the problem, as in the instances of unfavorable fractures, then additional fixation, such as inferior border wiring, plating, or external fixation, may be necessary (Fig. 11-17). If a collapse of either arch occurs, it may be necessary to use palatal splints in the maxilla or a lingual splint

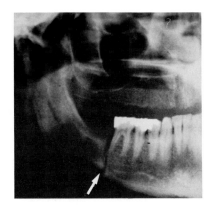 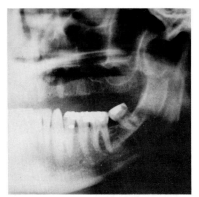

Fig. 11-16. An unfavorable fracture. Note the straight-line fracture behind the first molar. Because the root tip is so close to the fracture line, the blood supply is compromised, and the possibility exists for developing a tooth abscess, which would require root canal treatment of the tooth, an alternative preferable to the tooth's removal.

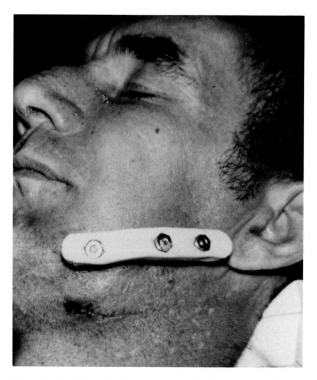

Fig. 11-17. Mandibular fracture that has been reduced and immobilized by the external biphase pin fixation unit.

in the mandible. Lingual splints in the mandible are particularly helpful to avoid tipping of the fractured segments, displacement, and malposition. In early discrepancies, usually a tightening of wires or readjustment of the occlusion will be sufficient to overcome such problems.

Delayed Problems. To correct a long-standing malunion and/or malocclusion, many factors need to be considered.

The patient's interest in extensive dental correction and cooperation may be a factor. Whenever possible, restoration of the occlusion, if it adequately corrects the problem, is a good choice. This may be costly and involve placing many or all of the teeth in crowns, bridges, porcelain jackets, etc.

The extraction of teeth, which would then be replaced with partial or full prosthesis, is a possibility. If extensive periodontal disease exists and there remains little bone support around the teeth, or if the patient is poorly motivated, there may be no choice but surgical removal of the dentition. Except in such situations, removal of the teeth should not be a first choice of treatment.

It may be possible to correct a deformity by a reoperation. Sectioning through the region of the fracture or at some other point in the osseous region may permit a better realignment of the jaw. For example, in the case of anterior mandibular collapse a step osteotomy with or without a bone graft may be indicated (Fig. 11-18). After the appropriate osteotomy and placement of the jaws in the new position, rigid fixation must be monitored throughout the healing period.

When malocclusion and/or malposition of the jaws is extensive, such as in posterior or anterior open bite or deviation of the jaws, very complex surgical correction may be indicated. Such correction encompasses the principles of orthognathic surgery. The use of diagnostic casts and surgical models, bite registration, face bow transfer, and cephalometric radiographs with prediction tracings are all important and fundamental to careful planning for the correction of complex jaw deformity (Fig. 11-19).

In mandibular asymmetry resulting from mandibular fracture, correction will most likely have to be within the mandible. This can be accomplished by sagittal split osteotomies of the ramus or vertical osteotomies together with repositioning of the jaw in correct symmetrical position. If as a result of injuries a condylar intracapsular type fracture has occurred, TMJ surgery may be necessary. This may include reconstruction of the entire temporomandibular joint. Such correction could well encompass removal of the disc and reconstruction of the joint to include a Proplast insert into the glenoid fossa and implant to the condylar head.

The problem of anterior open bite, whether due to problems relating to a mandibular fracture or a fracture of the maxilla, is often best corrected in the maxilla. The tendency for relapse when closing the open bite through ramus procedures is high. Maxillary repositioning through LeFort I osteotomy has proven to give excellent results for the treatment of open bite[14] (Fig. 11-20).

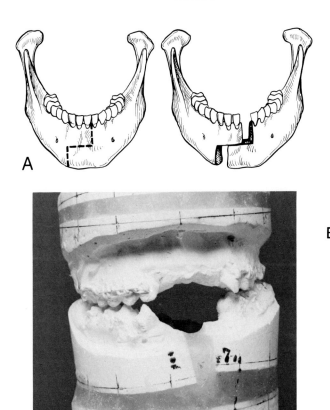

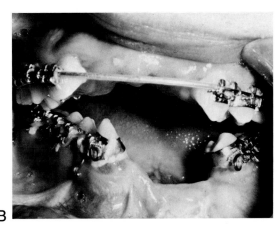

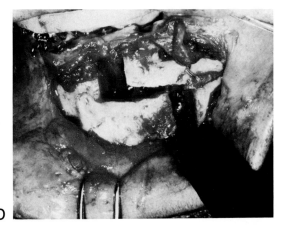

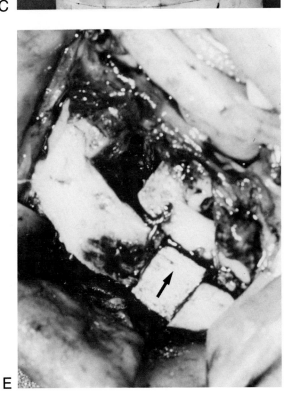

Fig. 11-18. (**A**) A representation of a step-osteotomy procedure. This surgical procedure is utilized when there has been collapse of the arch. The surgical approach is to widen the arch through the surgical design. (**B**) A patient with a post-traumatic malunion in the region of the mandibular symphysis. The malunion causes a narrowing of the mandibular arch with resultant arch and resultant malocclusion. (**C**) The model surgery in preparation for management of this type of fracture. The bone section is in the midline of the mandible, which permits an expansion of the lower jaw until the occlusion is in acceptable relationship to the maxillary occlusion. (**D**) The surgical procedure on the same patient. Note the step osteotomy permitting the widening of the jaw in this region. (**E**) The step osteotomy is completed, with a bone graft in position near the inferior border to hold the separated segments in their new positions (arrow).

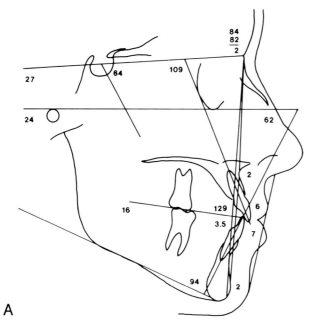

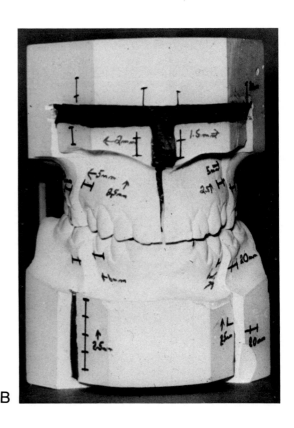

Fig. 11-19. **(A)** Cephalometric tracing showing a standard analysis for normal facial, skeletal, and dental relationships. These profiles and figures are helpful when compared with an abnormal analysis and can also aid in determining areas where correction is indicated. **(B)** An example of standard model surgery, which is used prior to surgical procedures to indicate areas where osteotomies can be used to correct occlusal disharmonies.

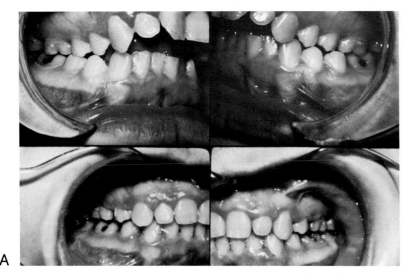

Fig. 11-20. **(A)** The upper photographs demonstrate the anterior open bite and malocclusion that were corrected by a LeFort I maxillary osteotomy; the lower photographs demonstrate the post-surgical occlusion that resulted from this surgical technique. The maxilla is surgically disarticulated into two, three, or four pieces, which permits the maxilla to be reassembled into an acceptable position in relationship to the lower jaw. (*Figure continues.*)

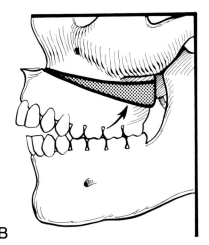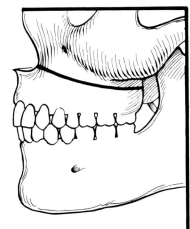

Fig. 11-20 (*continued*). (**B**) Schematic drawings of a LeFort I maxillary osteotomy demonstrating the down-fracture technique.

Special Considerations in Children

Jaw fractures in children fortunately heal very rapidly and often without complication. Because the alveolus of the jaws is filled with teeth in various stages of development and eruption, the loss of teeth as a result of fracture and/or their malposition may occur. Following injury, careful observation through the eruptive stages of the teeth is important to ensure normal healing and development.

Injuries to the jaws often create condylar problems that may be demonstrated in growth disturbances (Fig. 11-21).

Whenever a condylar fracture occurs, the family and patient should be aware of the possibility of interference in growth patterns of the jaws.[15] The condyle is the center of growth that contributes to the downward and forward growth of the mandible. This growth occurs at the periosteal surface of the condyle by apposition to the superior and posterior surfaces of the condylar head.[16] Because of lack of growth on the side of trauma, asymmetry and inadequate oral opening or ankylosis may develop. If condylar neck fractures occur, specific fracture treatment will be significant[17] (see Chapter 9). Orthodontic consultation is an integral part of most treatment plans, particularly in pediatric injuries. Functional appliances may be indicated, as soon as fixation and healing are complete, to provide further stimulation and development (Fig. 11-22).

Kwapis and others[18] summarized their experience regarding a malunited condylar fracture that was treated with a subcondylar osteotomy in a young patient. In this case, despite severity of injury to the condyle and surgical intervention, the mandible has continued to grow normally. If ankylosis develops, early surgery may be indicated to prevent progressive facial deformity. The goal of

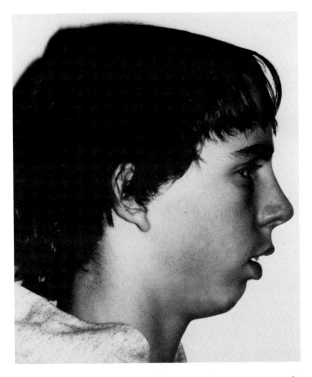

Fig. 11-21. A retrognathic facial profile showing inadequate growth of the mandible subsequent to a childhood condylar injury. The dental occlusion in such a patient is referred to as a class II malocclusion.

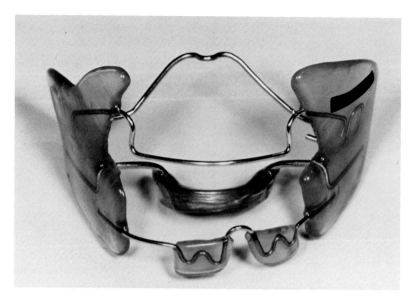

Fig. 11-22. A functional pediatric dental appliance is used to stimulate growth and provide guidance for jaw position.

surgery at an early age is twofold: to resolve the ankylosis and allow normal growth in the future, and to overcome the growth deficit that has already occurred.[19] Careful follow-up care in pediatric fractures is especially important for detection of further problems of malocclusion as teeth erupt and continued growth takes place.

SUMMARY

Malunion and malocclusion will occur as complications to fracture management. Restoration to normal function should be the primary goal when evaluating a post-fracture complication. After careful review of the patient's records, interview, history, and examination, the clinician is able to determine the course of further treatment, if indicated. Treatment methods may be minimal and involve only the dentition or may be complex affecting the bite, jaws, muscles, and the temporomandibular joint.

REFERENCES

1. Harrigan WF: Occlusion and surgery. Dent Clin North Am 25(3):446, 1981
2. Steidler NE, Cook RM, Read PC: Residual complications in patients with major middle third facial fractures. Int J Oral Surg 9:259, 1980
3. Mathog R, and Boies L: Non-union of mandible. Laryngology. 86:908, 1976
4. Members of the Chalmers J. Lyons Club: Fractures including the mandibular condyle: a post-treatment survey of 120 cases. Int J Oral Surg 5:45, 1947
5. Bruce RA, Stracham DS: Fractures of the edentulous mandible: The Chalmers J. Lyons Academy study. Int J Oral Surg 34:973, 1976
6. Walker R, Bertz J: Facial & Extra-Cranial Head Injuries. Care of the Trauma Patient. McGraw-Hill, New York, 1966
7. Kruger G: Textbook of Oral and Maxillofacial Surgery, 6th Ed. C.V. Mosby, St. Louis, 1984
8. Thomas, Kurt H: Traumatic Surgery of the Jaws. C.V. Mosby, St. Louis, 1942
9. Powers HH, Hirscham JC, Shaften GW: Retardation of fracture healing in experimental diabetes. J Surg Res 8:424, 1968
10. Singer AR, Udupa KN: Some investigations on the

effect of insulin in healing of fractures. Indian J Med Res 54:1071, 1966

11. Sevitt S: Bone Repair and Fracture Healing in Man: Etiology and Pathogenesis of Non-Union of Fractures. Churchill Livingstone, Edinburgh, 1981
12. Conley H: Complications of Head and Neck Surgery. W.B. Saunders, Philadelphia, 1979
13. Guralnick WC: Textbook of Oral Surgery. Little, Brown & Co, Boston, 1968
14. Kwon HJ, Bevis RR, Waite DE: Apertognathia (open bite) and its surgical management. Int J Oral Surg 13(4):278, 1974
15. Waite DE: Pediatric fractures of jaw and facial bones. Pediatrics 51:551, 1973
16. Enlon DH: The Human Face. Harper & Row, New York, 1968
17. MacLennan WD, Simpson W: Treatment of fractured mandibular condylar process in children. Br J Plast Surg 18:423, 1965
18. Kwapis BW, Dyer MH, Knox JE: Surgical correction of malunited condylar fracture in a child. J Oral Surg 31:465, 1973
19. Profitt WR, Vig KWL, Turvey TA: Early fracture of the mandibular condyles: Frequently and unspected cause of growth disturbances. Am J Orthod 78:1, 1980

Craniofacial and Panfacial Fractures

12

Richard A. Pollock
Joseph S. Gruss

The number of patients who survive the initial insult of complex trauma has increased, in great part owing to the efficiency of helicopter and ground transport systems.[1] As a result, surgeons are now often called upon to treat patients with combined injuries of the cranium and face. In cases where the skull, midface, and mandible are affected, fractures involve the entire osseus infrastructure of the head and neck. These injuries, panfacial in the true sense of the word, are a challenge to even the most energetic and well-trained reconstructive surgeon.

CLINICAL EXAMINATION

Instability and deformation are the hallmarks of craniofacial fractures. Mobility of the fracture site is a major clue to the presence of craniofacial injury. Dislocated bone fragments are detectable even in the presence of ecchymosis and soft-tissue contusion.[2,3]

Pattern of Injury

The frontal, ethmoid, and sphenoid bones form a major structural complex at the junction of the midface and cranial base (Fig. 12-1). Involvement of this complex and adjacent buttresses of the facial skeleton establishes the pattern of craniofacial injury.[4-8]

Sturla[7] has conveniently classified complex fractures into two groups: patients with central fractures and those with predominantly lateral fractures.

Central Craniofacial Fractures

Force directed over the frontonasal region creates a central fracture.[7,8] Fracture lines involve the frontonasomaxillary (medial) and perhaps the frontoethmoidal-vomerian (central) buttresses, then extend to enter the frontal sinus and ethmoidal complex. Fracture lines involve nasal, vomer, maxillary, ethmoid, and frontal bones (Fig. 12-2). The infraorbital rim and medial wall of the orbit are often severely comminuted. The frontal sinus is involved to a varying degree, and intracranial exten-

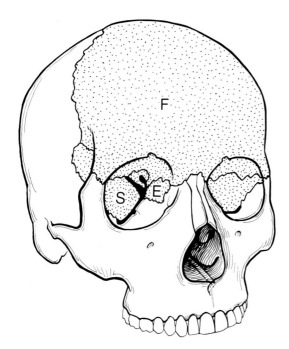

Fig. 12-1. The frontal, ethmoid, and sphenoid bones are highlighted. The involvement of these structures establishes the pattern of craniofacial injury. F, Frontal; S, Sphenoid; E, Ethmoid.

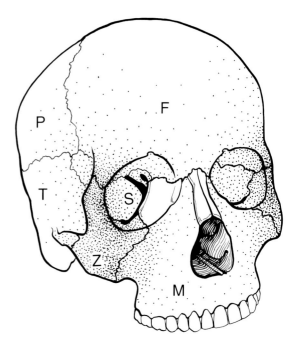

Fig. 12-3. Lateral craniofacial fractures involve the maxillary, zygomatic, and frontal bones as well as the sphenoid, parietal, and temporal bones. P, Parietal; F, Frontal; T, Temporal; S, Sphenoid; Z, Zygomatic; M, Maxillary.

sion is often present, manifested by fractures of the posterior table.

Lateral Craniofacial Fractures

When force is applied to the frontozygomatic area, fractures are initiated in the lateral aspect of the face and cranium.[7,8] Fracture lines involve the frontozygomaticomaxillary (lateral) buttress and extend across the greater wing of the sphenoid. Fractures of this type commonly involve maxillary, zygomatic, frontal, and sphenoid bones. In some instances, the fracture extends to involve the parietal bone. The lateral aspect of the frontal sinus and orbit are often severely comminuted and on occasion outwardly displaced, which causes orbital dystopia (Fig. 12-3).

Combined Central and Lateral Fractures

With marked force, fractures involving both the central and lateral skull and face may be produced.[7,8] In such cases profound dislocation and

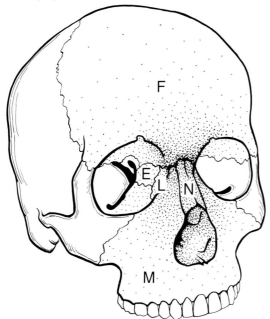

Fig. 12-2. Central craniofacial injuries involve the nasal, vomer, maxillary, lacrimal, ethmoid, and frontal bones. F, Frontal; E, Ethmoid; L, Lacrimal; N, Nasal; M, Maxillary.

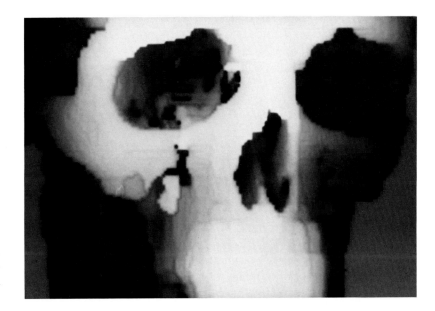

Fig. 12-4. This three-dimensional radiograph was reproduced from high-resolution CT scans of a patient with maxillary, zygomatic, and orbital fractures.

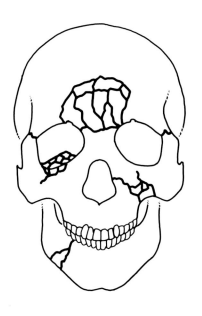

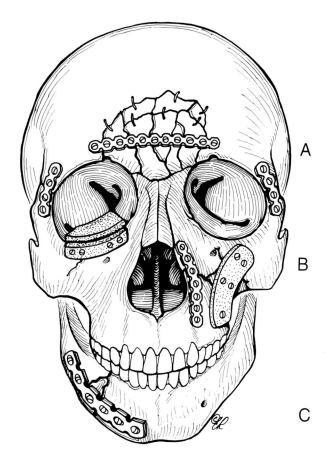

Fig. 12-5. Cranial bone has not been lost. The repair sequence moves downward. First, the cranial vault is repaired (**A**). Then, the reconstituted facial complex is reattached to the cranium (**B&C**).

instability are present. The plastic surgeon and neurosurgeon are well advised to suspect fracture extension into the anterior or middle fossa. Only rarely do combined fractures involve the posterior fossa.

into three-dimensional images (Fig. 12-4). Three-dimensional radiographs have more lifelike characteristics and free the examination from the restriction of biaxial interpretation. Reconstruction can be planned preoperatively with greater detail and accuracy.

RADIOGRAPHIC STUDY

High-resolution computerized tomography (CT), available since the early 1980s, offers greater detail than conventional CT scan techniques. By choosing "wide-window" focus, the computer is programmed to enhance bone detail. Craniofacial fractures, which would otherwise be occult, can thus be identified prior to surgery.

Three-dimensional tomography has recently been made available. It converts the multidirectional 1 mm-views of high-resolution CT scans

PRINCIPLES OF SURGICAL MANAGEMENT

Most patients with craniofacial or panfacial injuries undergo treatment within 24 to 48 hours, even in the presence of coma. When possible, maxillofacial and craniofacial repairs are accomplished at the time of neurosurgical exploration, and aided by use of steroids, barbiturates, hyperventilation, and intracranial pressure monitors.

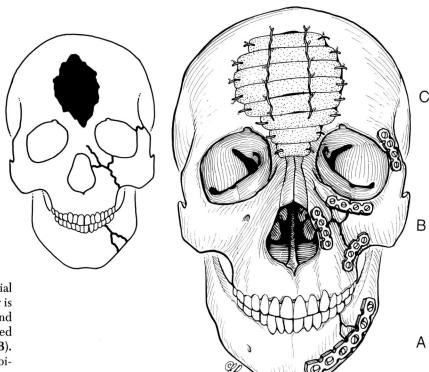

Fig. 12-6. There is loss of cranial bone, and the sequence of repair is reversed. First, the mandible and maxilla are repaired and reattached to stable residual cranium (**A & B**). Bone grafts are then used to stabilize the cranial vault (**C**).

Sequence of Repair

Force is seldom singularly and solely applied to the midline; usually one side of the craniofacial skeleton is more involved than the other. The surgeon should repair the less damaged hemifacial structures first. More severely injured areas of comminution or bone loss on the opposite side are then reconstructed.

The following sequence is recommended once wide exposure and periosteal elevation are achieved:

If there is no loss of cranial bone, fractures of the cranial vault must be stabilized. Work then progresses downward to reconstruct the midface and mandible (Fig. 12-5).

If cranial bone is missing or if massive cranial comminuation is present, repair of the cranial vault should be placed last in the sequence (Fig. 12-6). First, the mandible is repaired, then the maxilla. Next, the midface is reattached to the remaining stable segments of the cranial vault. The amount of missing frontoethmoid and sphenoid bone can then be assessed. Bone grafts are then used to reconstruct the cranial vault.[9]

In the combined presence of craniofacial fractures and bilateral condylar neck fractures of the mandible, the order is reversed. The surgeon first repairs the midface to determine appropriate midfacial height. The mandible is then repaired.

Rigid internal fixation with bone-graft support makes use of external fixation devices relatively unnecessary. In patients with bilateral condylar neck fractures associated with severe midfacial injury, external fixation devices may be used when

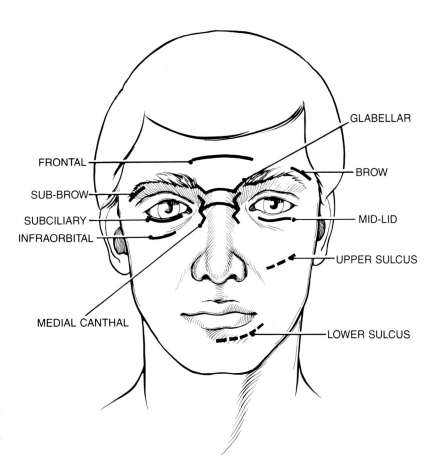

Fig. 12-7. On occasion, craniofacial fractures may be localized and approached through singular or local incisions. These incisions, however, should not be used because they eliminate the flexibility of further exposure and do not offer the possibility of harvesting cranial bone grafts.

intermaxillary fixation cannot be accomplished and when open reduction of condylar neck fractures is not performed.

Surgical Incisions and Exposure

Isolated craniofacial fractures (e.g., those restricted to the frontal bone or fronto-orbital area) may on occasion be successfully approached through local incisions.[2] (Fig. 12-7).

Complex fractures are more often exposed through incisions that permit wide periosteal elevation and exposure of a broad expanse of bone[10] (Fig. 12-8). The mandible in the area of the symphysis is approached through an intraoral incision. Fractures of the mandibular body, angle, or ramus are best approached through external incisions. When necessary, the masseter is released from its insertion, using a periosteal elevator and beginning posteriorly.

The maxilla is very readily exposed through a gingivobuccal incision.[11] Access is gained to each medial and lateral buttress for repair, stabilization, or replacement. The infraorbital nerve and rim are readily visualized through the gingivobuccal incision, but exposure is too indirect to permit repair of fractures of the orbit.

Since ethmoid, sphenoid, and frontal bones make major contributions to the orbital bone structure, craniofacial fractures often involve the orbit. Exposure and repair of these fractures are critical. The subciliary incision is the incision most frequently used; however, translid, transconjunctival, and canthotomy incisions are alternatives.[2,3,12,13]

The orbital roof, frontozygomatic structures, frontal bone, and nasoethmoid complex are best reached through a transcranial (bicoronal) incision. The incision extends from pinna to pinna. The

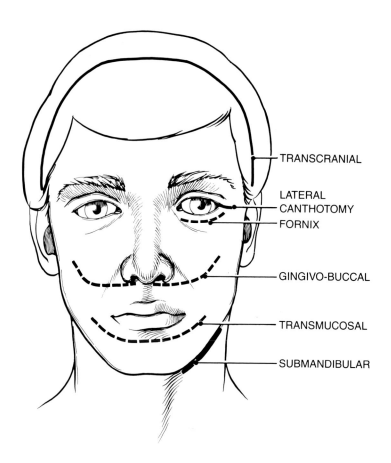

TRANSCRANIAL

LATERAL
CANTHOTOMY

FORNIX

GINGIVO-BUCCAL

TRANSMUCOSAL

SUBMANDIBULAR

Fig. 12-8. Craniofacial fractures are usually exposed through multiple incisions and broad periosteal elevation. These larger incisions offer improved visibility and control. Metal plates, rib grafts, and screws are more readily applied to the fractured segments.

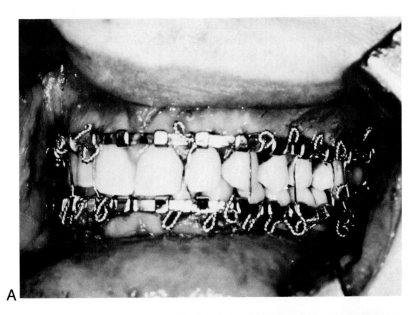

Fig. 12-9. Intermaxillary fixation may be accomplished using (**A**) arch bars and wire ligatures or (**B & C**) Ernst ligatures.

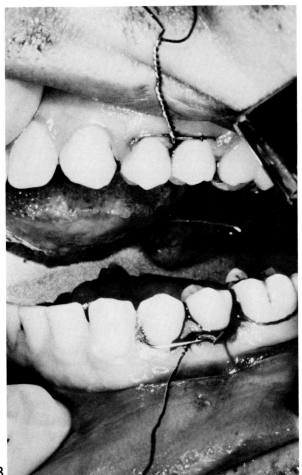

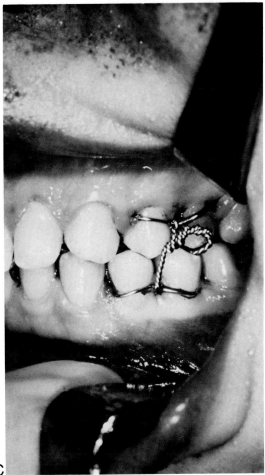

plane of dissection is subperiosteal so as to preserve the blood supply to the pericranium and protect the supraorbital vessels and nerves.[13]

The operative plan is finally formulated after the periosteum is widely elevated and the fractures fully exposed.

Debridement

Pulverized bone and small bone sequestra, including those of the midface or posterior table of the frontal sinus, are discarded; bone otherwise is preserved. Foreign bodies and mucosal shreads, which after 48 hours are potential nidi of infection, are meticulously removed. Copious irrigation is required.

Like Dingman,[14] Dickinson,[15] and Schultz,[16] we favor the preservation of the frontal sinus cavity and do not obliterate the nasofrontal duct.[8]

Intermaxillary Fixation

In most patients, an attempt is made to place the jaws in occlusive fixation. The dental occlusive pattern serves as a template for reconstruction and provides a modest element of stabilization.

Erich arch bars and connecting interarch ligatures (Fig. 12-9A) may be used to accomplish intermaxillary fixation. When intermaxillary fixation is to be temporary, we prefer to use Ernst ligatures (Fig. 12-9B,C).

Intermaxillary fixation is often removed at the end of the procedure. In other cases, rubber-band or wire fixation is maintained for 6 to 7 days, until trismus, muscle spasm, and discomfort abate.

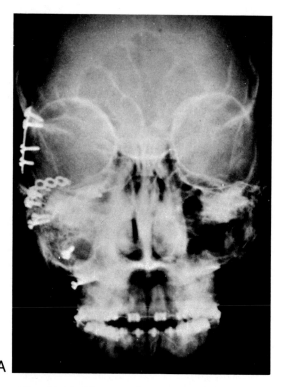

A

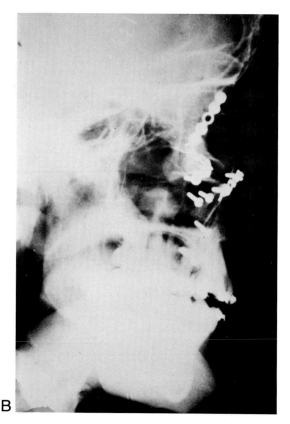

B

Fig. 12-10. Plates and screws provide rigid stabilization of bone fragments. This additional stability is critically important in patients with inherently unstable, combined injuries of the cranium and face.

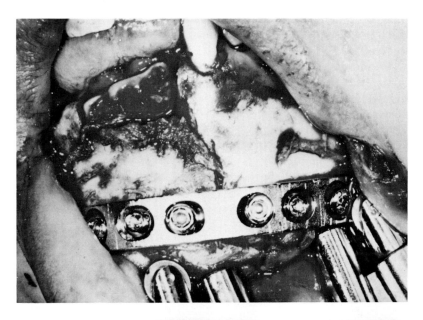

Fig. 12-11. Unfavorable fractures of the mandible are rigidly stabilized using plates that apply compression at both the mandibular margin and the alveolar margin. Reduction forceps are present in the lower portion of the photograph.

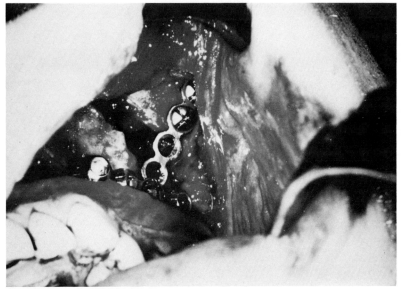

Fig. 12-12. The lateral (frontozygomaticomaxillary) buttress in this patient has been stabilized with a vertical plate and screws. A transverse plate has been used to anchor the lateral maxilla to the medial buttress. A section of pulverized, comminuted bone has been debrided prior to the application of a stabilization plate.

Wire, Plates, Screws

Comminuted fragments of bone are wired together[2,17] or stabilized using plates and screws.[18,19] Direct interosseus wiring, as a singular means of reducing bone fragments, can cause telescoping and offers less rigid stabilization of complex fractures than that provided by plate application.

Circumzygomatic, circumfrontozygomatic, circumorbital wires, and other methods of craniofacial suspension have been described. Suspension wires are used to suspend the maxilla or jaw complex (maxilla and mandible) to a stable portion of the skull, zygoma, or orbit.[3] These techniques when unaccompanied by reconstruction and realignment of the midfacial buttresses tend to cause midfacial collapse and posterior displacement of the maxilla. The post-surgical patient is prone to suffer from midfacial compression and lack of anterior projection.

Plates are contoured to match the bone anatomy.

Drill holes are made, then tapped, and screws are used to apply the plate to the reduced fragments of bone (Fig. 12-10).

Mandibular plates are usually thicker than those used elsewhere on the facial skeleton, and the screws are larger in diameter. Special reduction forceps and compression plates are utilized to approximate fractured segments, both at the inferior mandibular margin and at the alveolar crest. (Fig. 12-11) (see Chapter 10).

Medial and lateral buttresses of the midface, frontozygomatic suture, infraorbital rim, and other areas of the upper skeleton may be rigidly stabilized using metal plates less than 1 mm in thickness. These plates are more malleable and can be readily adjusted prior to application (Fig. 12-12).

Bone Grafting

Missing bone is replaced by selected grafts. Potential donor areas include the iliac crest, ribs, and skull. Split cranium is probably the graft of choice for skull and perhaps all upper facial injuries, particularly if the traumatic defect has a small surface area. In extensive defects, rib has the distinct advantage of offering a large volume of graft with minimal morbidity to the patient (Fig. 12-13).

Split rib also has the advantage of malleability. Rib may be contoured to match medial or lateral buttresses of the midface, infraorbital rim, or walls of the orbit (Fig. 12-14). The split rib graft is molded to stabilize bone compromised by comminution, such as the midfacial buttresses of the

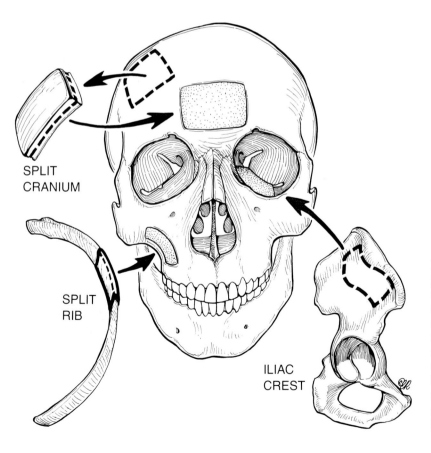

SPLIT
CRANIUM

SPLIT
RIB

ILIAC
CREST

Fig. 12-13. Missing bone is replaced by grafts selected from one of three sites: the cranium, the iliac crest, and the thorax. Split cranium appears to have a lower resorption rate, but the volume of skull grafts may not be sufficient in patients with large bone deficits. Split rib or iliac crest is chosen, perhaps in combination with cranial grafts, to replace missing bone in large defects.

Fig. 12-14. (A) A defect in the infraorbital margin is replaced by a carefully measured and contoured split rib graft. (B) The rib graft is wired into place, and further bone grafts replace the orbital floor and medial wall. These bone grafts can alternatively be fixed in place using lag screws.

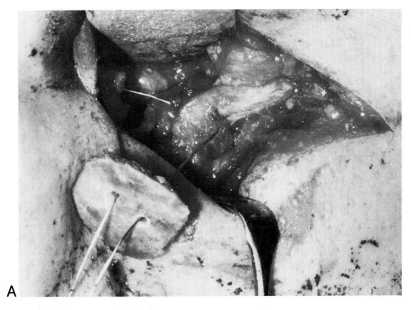

A

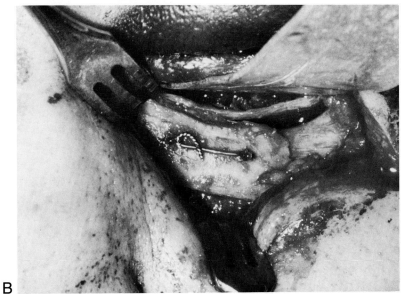

B

Fig. 12-15. Nasoethmoid fractures and subsequent collapse have caused a saddle nose deformity. (A) A cantilevered graft is fashioned from split cranium. *(Figure continues.)*

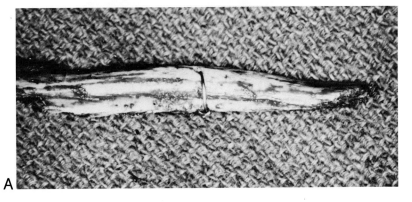

A

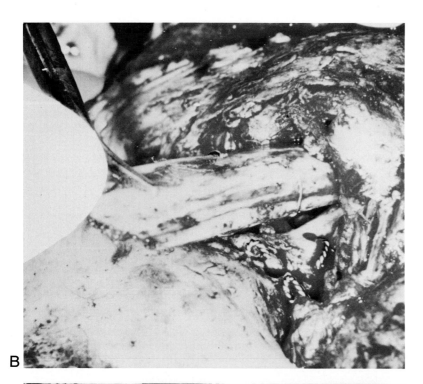

B

Fig. 12-15 *(Continued)*. **(B)** It is inserted as an onlay graft to be secured by screws.

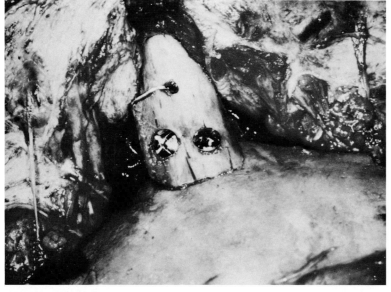

Fig. 12-16. In this patient, a cantilevered graft has been constructed from split ribs. It is secured to the base of the frontal bone using screws.

maxilla. Grafts are "lagged" to underlying bone using screws.

Bone grafts are often necessary to maintain nasal contour and projection, particularly in the presence of saddle-nose deformities and nasoethmoid collapse. The graft is anchored to the base of the frontal sinus using screws (Figs. 12-15, 12-16).

The following case studies exemplify three types of complex fractures: cranio-orbital-frontal fractures (forehead with split cranial grafts) (Figs. 12-17 to 12-20); cranio-midfacial fractures (forehead with split rib) (Figs. 12-21 to 12-24); and panfacial fractures (cranium-midface-mandible) (Figs. 12-25 to 12-28).

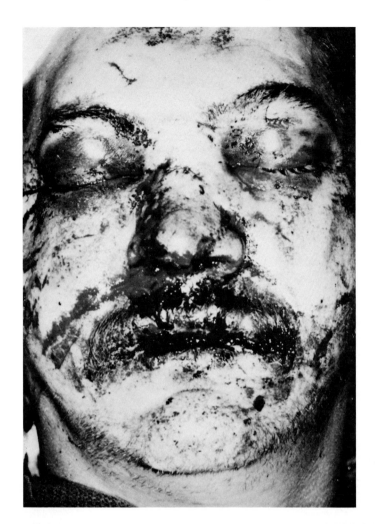

Fig. 12-17. This patient suffered fractures of the maxilla, palate, orbit, and frontal sinus in a high-speed vehicular accident.

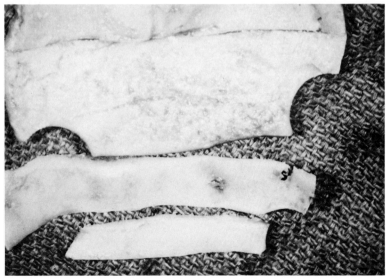

Fig. 12-18. The cranium (frontal bone) is removed to provide neurosurgical exposure. The inner and outer tables are split. The inner table will be used to stabilize bones of the midface.

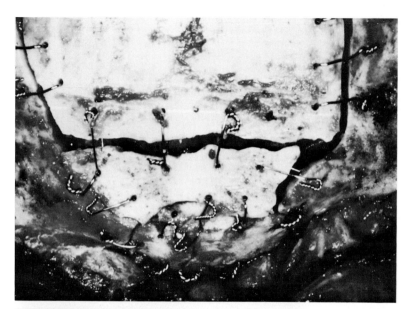

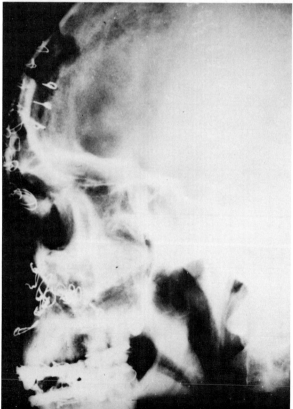

Fig. 12-19. First the outer table of the frontal bone is placed in position and secured with wires. The lower, imploded glabellar segment is reduced and stabilized. Then, the maxillary fractures are reduced and stabilized, with the jaws in intermaxillary fixation. The reconstituted maxilla is then secured to the repaired cranial vault.

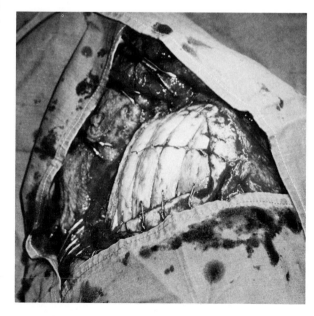

Fig. 12-20. This lateral radiograph depicts the realignment of the frontal convexity and the stabilization of the midfacial buttresses using wires. Intermaxillary fixation was abandoned on the fifth postoperative day.

Fig. 12-21. Complex panfacial injury with loss of large area of left frontal orbital bone. A primary split rib cranioplasty using chain-link wiring reconstructs the large cranio-orbital defect.

Fig. 12-22. Contour restoration can be obtained by bending and utilizing the natural spring of split rib grafts.

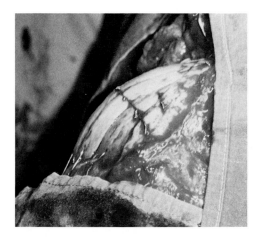

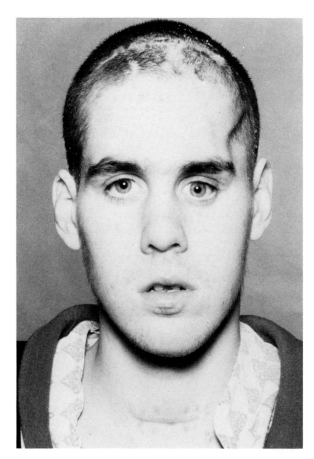

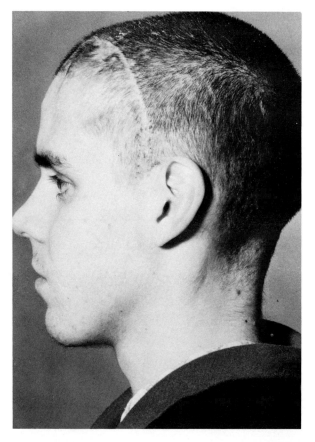

Fig. 12-23. Early postoperative appearance showing good restoration of fronto-orbital contour and anatomy. Note the inadequate correction of the left orbital dystopia. The severity of oculo-orbital displacement or dystopia in association with cranio-orbital injury may frequently be underestimated.

Fig. 12-24. Lateral view showing contour restoration of the cranio-orbital region.

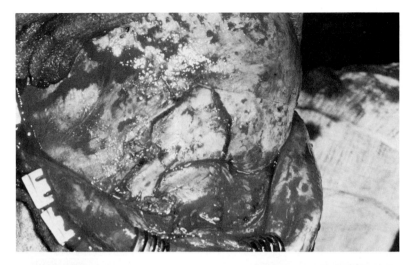

Fig. 12-25. Massive panfacial injury following boating accident. The coronal flap retracted downwards reveals multiple comminuted fractures of the cranio-orbital and frontal sinus region.

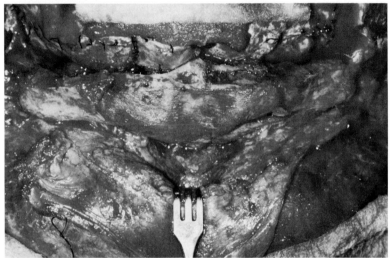

Fig. 12-26. Following neurosurgical exploration and dura repair, multiple fractures along the entire cranio-orbital frontal sinus and glabellar region are seen.

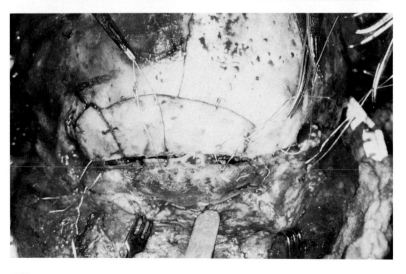

Fig. 12-27. All fractures are carefully reduced following exenteration of frontal sinuses, and repair is completed.

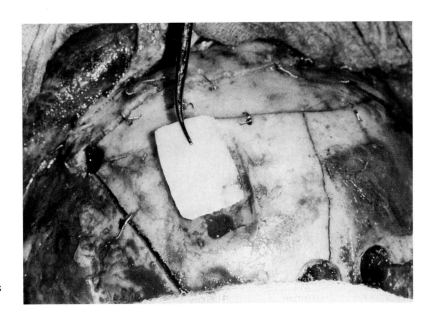

Fig. 12-28. A split cranial graft is harvested for orbital floor repair.

TECHNICAL PITFALLS IN RECONSTRUCTION

Management of frontal sinus fractures remains controversial. Like some other investigators[13-15] we have chosen not to obliterate (with fat) the frontal sinus or the nasofrontal ducts in acute trauma cases. The anterior and posterior tables are preserved. The sinus cavity is maintained, with the expectation that the nasofrontal duct will continue to function.[8]

In cases of severe injury of the anterior and posterior tables of the frontal sinus, an attempt is made to further segregate dura from the frontal bone. In these circumstances, we have been favorably impressed by the ease with which a "pericranial curtain" may be interposed as an extra barrier between cranial contents and facial skeleton[8] (Fig. 12-29).

Pericranium may also be successfully utilized to isolate the nares and sinuses from cantilevered grafts, which are used to reconstruct the nasal dorsum.[19,20]

All bone grafts undergo remodeling and to some degree are resorbed. Loss of bone volume probably occurs less following transplantation of skull than with use of rib or iliac crest. The degree to which an excess of bone is inserted to compensate for resorption becomes a matter of clinical judgement.

When rib grafts are used along the supraorbital ridge, there is a tendency to underestimate the amount of rib required to reestablish a normal contour. To obtain appropriate postoperative projection, the surgeon uses a full rib or an extra layer of split rib.

Deficits in the orbital floor and lateral or medial orbital walls must be filled with bone grafts. Care is taken to insert sufficient volume to reconstruct the normal upward slope of the orbital floor as the apex is approached. The surgeon must compensate for anticipated bone resorption but at the same time not overfill the orbit and place the optic nerve at risk (Figs. 12-30, 12-31).

Orbital roof fractures need not be repaired unless the posterior sinus wall is missing or not intact. When grafts *are* needed to repair the orbital roof, a limited volume of bone is inserted. An excessive volume of graft material tends to push the orbit down (Fig. 12-32).

On rare occasions the orbit can be displaced inferiorly en bloc by the traumatic event. This dislocation may be missed during cursory examination.

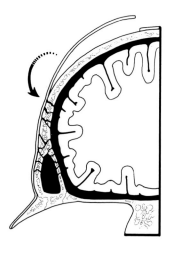

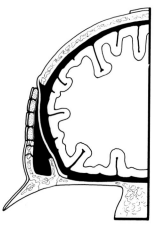

Fig. 12-29. A "pericranial curtain" may be interposed to further isolate the cranial contents from the facial skeleton, after repair of the dura.

Fig. 12-30. Bone grafts are used to reconstruct the (**A**) orbital floor and (**B**) medial orbit wall. The normal, upward slope of the orbital floor is reconstructed.

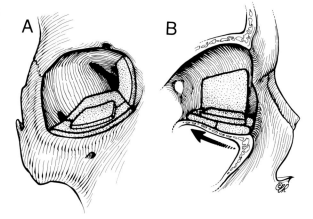

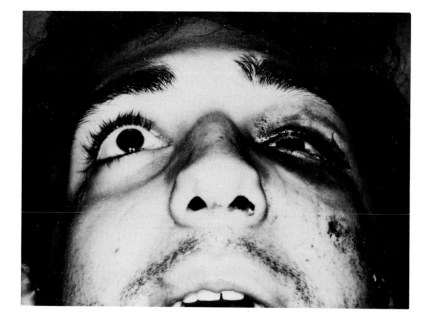

Fig. 12-31. The insertion of an insufficient volume of graft, graft resorption, and progressive fat atrophy may combine to create enophthalmos.

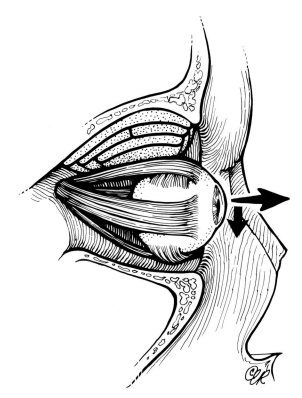

Fig. 12-32. The insertion of excessive bone grafts in the superior orbit may push the orbital contents downward and outward.

REFERENCES

1. Fischer RP, Flynn TC, Miller TW, Duke KH: Urban helicopter response to the scene of injury. J Trauma 24:946, 1984
2. Gruss JS: Fronto-naso-orbital trauma. Clin Plast Surg 9:577, 1982
3. Pollock RA, Dingman RO: Management and reconstruction of athletic injuries of the face, anterior neck, and upper respiratory tract. p. 592. In Schneider R, Kennedy JC, Plant ML (eds): Sports Injuries: mechanisms, prevention and treatment. Williams & Wilkins, Baltimore, 1985
4. LeFort R: Experimental study of fractures of the upper jaw. I and II. Rev Chir 23:208, 1901 (Plast Reconstr Surg 50:497,600, 1972)
5. Huelke DF, Harger JH: Maxillofacial injuries: Their nature and mechanisms of reduction. J Oral Surg 27:451, 1969
6. Merville L: Multiple dislocations of the facial skeleton. J Maxillofac Surg 2:187, 1974
7. Sturla F, Absi D, Buquet J: Anatomical and mechanical considerations of craniofacial fractures: an experimental study. Plast Reconstr Surg 66:815, 1980
8. Gruss JS, Pollock RA: Combined injuries of the cranium and upper face. (Submitted for publication.)
9. Gruss JS, Mackinnon SE, Kassel EE, Cooper PW: The role of primary bone grafting in complex craniomaxillofacial trauma. Plast Reconstr Surg 75:17, 1985
10. McCord CD Jr, Moses JL: Exposure of the inferior orbit with fornix incision and lateral canthotomy. Ophthalmic Surg 10:59, 1979
11. Casson PR, Bonanno PC, Converse JM: The midface degloving procedure. Plast Reconstr Surg 53:102, 1974
12. Tessier P: The conjunctival approach to the orbital floor and maxilla in congenital malformation and trauma. J Maxillofac Surg 1:3, 1973
13. Pollock RA, Borges AF, Munro IR: Craniofacial incisions and exposures. (Submitted for publication.)
14. Dingman RO: Supraorbital and glabellar fractures. Plast Reconstr Surg 45:227, 1970
15. Dickinson J: Frontal sinus fractures. Laryngoscope 83:1291, 1973
16. Schultz RC: Supraorbital and glabellar fractures. Plast Reconstr Surg 45:27, 1970
17. Munro IR: Craniofacial surgical techniques for asthetic results in congenital and acute traumatic deformities. Clin Plast Surg 8:303, 1981
18. Schmoker RR: The eccentric dynamic compression plate: an experimental study as to its contribution to fixation of the lower jaw. Swiss Association for the Study of Internal Fixation, Bern, 1975
19. Gruss JS, McKinnon SE: Complex maxillary fractures: Role of buttress reconstruction and immediate bone grafts. (Submitted for publication.)
20. Argenta LC, Friedman RJ, Dingman RO, Duus EC: The versatility of pericranial flaps. Plast Reconstr Surg 76:695, 1985

Injuries to Specialized Structures 13

Haim Y. Kaplan
Daniel C. Baker

EAR TRAUMA

Anatomy

The external ear consists of the pinna, the external auditory meatus, and the tympanic membrane. The pinna or auricle has a thin convoluted skeleton of elastic cartilage to which the skin envelope is tightly adherent. The external ear is located approximately one ear's length posterior to the lateral orbital wall. The long axis parallels the dorsal axis of the nose, which is about 20° off the vertical axis. The vertical dimension of the ear equals the vertical dimension of the nose. The convolutions of the skin follow those of the cartilage. The anterior-lateral skin is much more adherent to the cartilage than the posterior-medial skin. The external ear is prone to trauma because of its narrow attachment to the head at the hard temporal bone and its position away from the skull.

The ear can be described as a cup-like concha surmounted by encircling scapha and further rimmed by the helix (Fig. 13-1). The main buttress of the ear is the Y-shaped antihelix.[1] The caudal extension of the antihelix is the antitragus. The car-tilage curves down to form the concha and comes up again as the tragus, which serves to protect the opening of the external auditory meatus. The ear lobule is basically a skin flap that contains fibro-fatty tissue and projects from the tip of the anti-tragus. The external auditory canal extends from the concha to the tympanic membrane. The lateral wall of the canal is composed of cartilage, while the medial wall of the canal is bone. The cartilage of the canal is a continuation of the tragal cartilage, and is connected to the helix through a narrow bridge called the isthmus.[2] This special anatomic design leaves a gap in the cartilaginous structure of the auricle. The gap, called the trago-helicine incisure, is a weak area where avulsions usually occur (Fig. 13-1).

The cartilage of the meatus does not form a tube but rather it forms the posterior-inferior wall of the meatus. The anterior-superior wall of the meatus is a recess in the temporal bone. The cartilage extends halfway along the meatal canal to form a lazy S-shaped tunnel in the temporal bone.

The tympanic membrane (ear drum) has a downward and inward slope, making the posterior wall of the canal 6 mm shorter than the anterior wall, which is about 25 mm in length or depth.

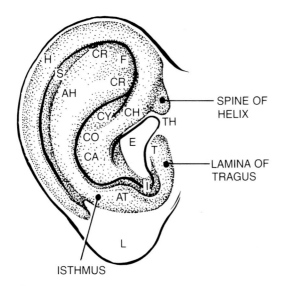

Fig. 13-1. The anatomy of the external ear and cartilage skeleton. F, Triangular fossa; H, Helix; AH, Antihelix; T, Tragus; AT, Antitragus; S, Scapha; L, Lobule; E, External auditory meatus; CY, Cymba of concha; CA, Cavum of concha; CO, Concha; CR, Crura of antihelix; I, Intertragic notch; CH, Crus of helix; TH, Trago-helicine incisure.

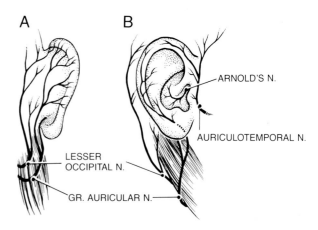

Fig. 13-2. (A & B) The sensory innervation of the external ear.

Innervation

The sensory innervation of the external ear is from several nerves. The lower two-thirds of the auricle is supplied by the great auricular nerve[2,3] (Fig. 13-2), which emerges from the posterior aspect of the sternocleidomastoid muscle and runs superficial to the external jugular vein beneath the platysma toward the auricle. At the lower part of the auricle, the nerve divides to form the anterior and posterior branches, which supply their respective surfaces of the auricle. The auriculotemporal nerve supplies the anterior-superior aspect of the auricle and the superior aspect of the auditory canal. The posterior-superior skin is supplied by the lesser occipital nerve. The concha and the posterior aspect of the auditory canal are supplied by the nerve of Arnold, which originates from the superior jugular ganglion and contains fibers of the fifth, ninth, and tenth cranial nerves. The nerve enters the meatus between the cartilaginous and the bony portions of the canal.

Blood Supply

The vascular supply to the auricle is abundant, enabling the auricle to survive on small bridges of skin.[3] The main blood supply to the auricle derives from the posterior auricular and the superficial temporal arteries. The posterior auricular artery originates either from the external carotid or occipital artery and travels along the posterior belly of the digastric muscle where it branches to the parotid glands mastoid air cells, and the posterior aspect of the auricle. The anterior aspect of the auricle is supplied by a branch of the superficial temporal artery.

The venous drainage of the lower two-thirds of the ear is to the external jugular vein. The superior third of the ear drains to the posterior facial vein.

General Considerations

The auricle is a complicated structure that makes reconstruction difficult. The ear drum and the external auditory meatus should be evaluated in every case of ear trauma. Under local anesthesia, the auricle is irrigated with a saline-betadine or Zephiran solution. If necessary, a very conservative debridement is performed. Even small fragments of tissue that appear to be partially compromised should be repaired if they are structurally important. Antibiotic treatment should be used in comminuted, fragmented, or contaminated ears.

Classifications of Trauma

Simple Laceration

Laceration of the auricle is by far the most common type of trauma. If involved, the rim should be sutured first to assure the accurate reconstruction of the auricle. If the rim is not involved, the posterior skin is sutured first using absorbable suture material (chromic 4-0 or 5-0). In small lacerations, there is no need to suture the cartilage framework; however, it is sometimes necessary to suture the cartilage to provide skeletal support for the ear. The preferable suture for keeping the edges of lacer-

ated cartilage in apposition is absorbable 5-0 material in simple or figure-of-eight sutures. The anterior skin is sutured with 5-0 nylon. The sutures are usually removed after 7 days.

Segmental Loss

Occasionally a segment of full-thickness external ear can be missing or hanging by a narrow soft-tissue bridge. The segment should then be treated as a composite graft in which the segment is returned and secured to its proper anatomic position. It is critical to provide the segment with adequate dermal contact for revascularization, which sometimes necessitates beveling the incision or resecting a piece of cartilage to ensure adequate dermal contact. It must be determined whether the segment of the auricle is too large (no larger than 2 to 3 cm) to be replanted as a composite graft (Fig. 13-3) and, in

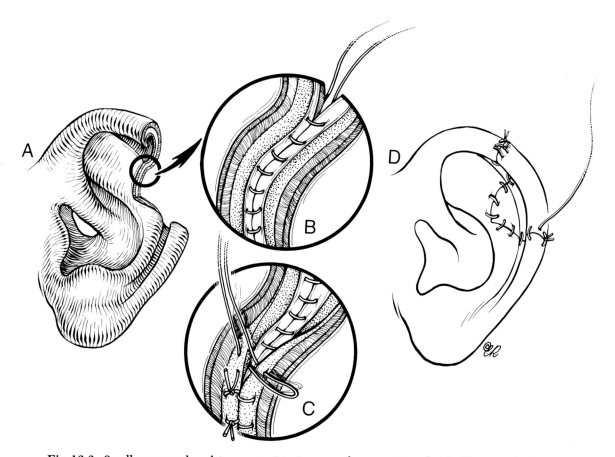

Fig. 13-3. Small segmental avulsions up to 2 to 3 cm may be repositioned and will revascularize as composite grafts. **(A)** Schematic drawing of a small segmental avulsion and the **(B–D)** meticulous, layered closure of postauricular skin, cartilage, and lateral ear skin.

the event the graft is unsuccessful, whether there is a way to use the cartilage to reconstruct the auricle.

In deciding whether to replant a segment of the auricle, the surgeon should consider his or her own experience with segmental ear replantation, the age of the patient (the chances of successful composite graft decreases with age), and the status of the recipient bed. Other factors to consider are medical or surgical problems that might delay proper healing and the use of heparin, ice packing, and antibiotics.

Postoperative treatment should include bed rest, use of a supportive bandage, application of ice to cool the replanted part (thereby decreasing its metabolic rate), heparin anticoagulant treatment, and antibiotics to cover gram-positive bacteria.

When replantation of the auricle is not possible, an attempt should be made to preserve the cartilage framework (Fig. 13-4). The skin is removed by dissection or dermabrasion, and the cartilage is buried under a posterior retroauricular skin flap. If the concha is not involved with the laceration, the tunnel technique as described by Converse can be used.[4] If the severed part is in good condition, and the posterior auricular skin is undamaged, one option is to use the "pocket principle." This involves dermabrading the auricular skin, reattaching the amputated segment, and covering it under a retroauricular skin flap. The segment receives increased blood supply through the dermabraded area in the critical first few days after replantation. Ten to twelve days after replantation, the auricle is delivered out of the pocket to allow the dermabraded skin to reepithelialize.

Abraded Avulsion

Avulsion of the auricle is characterized by loss of skin and minimal involvement of cartilage. In cases where the perichondrium still covers the cartilage, a skin graft can be applied to cover the defect. A good donor site is the retroauricular skin of the contralateral ear. When perichondrium is missing, the best treatment is coverage with a retroauricular skin flap.

Occasionally the cartilage will be tatooed with grease or asphalt and have total or partial loss of skin and cartilage. The external ear should be carefully irrigated (sometimes a soft brush will help),

and debridement should be conservative. The ear can be treated with wet dressings until spontaneous epithilialization occurs. The ear should be reassessed a few months later for possible reconstruction.[5]

In avulsion injuries, the laceration goes through the external auditory canal. The skin of the canal should be sutured with fine absorbable sutures of 4-0 or 5-0 chromic, and a stent should be kept in the canal for 5 to 7 days.

Otohematoma

An otohematoma is a subperichondrial hematoma of the ear. Since the cartilage is totally dependent on the perichondrium for its survival, a collection of blood separating the cartilage from the perichondrium might result in necrosis of the cartilage. Blunt trauma to the ear in boxers and wrestlers can result in otohematoma. Recurrent hematoma results in fibrosis between the cartilage and the perichondrium that obliterates fine detail in the underlying framework and leads to a "cauliflower" ear. Treatment of the hematoma entails evacuation of the hematoma either by aspiration or by surgical incision. Following evacuation of the hematoma, a well-molded pressure dressing must be applied. The patient must be followed closely for any reaccumulation of blood.

Total Amputation

Total amputation of the external ear occasionally presents with scalp avulsions. The only way to revascularize the ear is by using microsurgical techniques, namely microvascular anastomosis of the superficial temporal or posterior auricular arteries. These arteries are of small caliber (0.4 to 1.0 mm). The primary problem of revascularization is venous drainage, which is very difficult to locate and secure.[6]

In 1980 Pennington et al. successfully replanted an avulsed ear (Fig. 13-5). The four points they emphasize are:

1. Using a bench technique to explore the avulsed ear, injured vessels are tagged and debrided.
2. Extensive use is made of interposition vein grafts to eliminate tension at the anastomotic suture line.

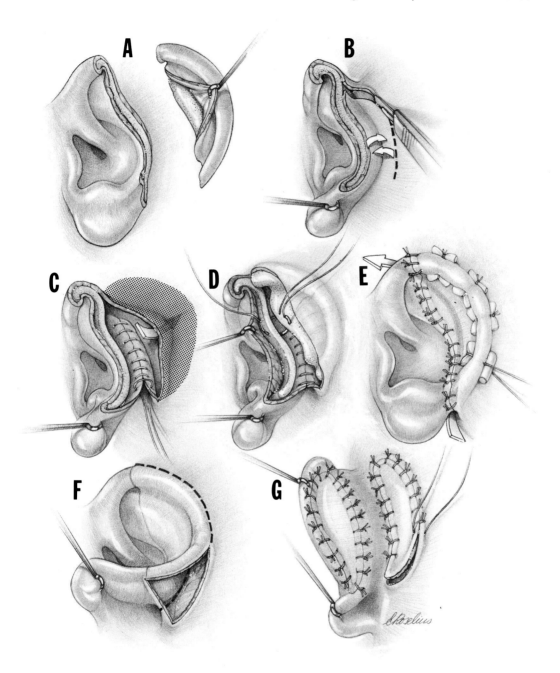

Fig. 13-4. Schematic drawing of a large segmental loss and the use of the cartilage framework to reconstruct the pinna. (**A**) Skin is removed from the large segmental avulsion. (**B & C**) The retroauricular flap is prepared. (**D**) The cartilage is coapted. (**E**) The skin is sutured, taking care to eliminate any "dead space." (**F & G**) Two weeks later, the retroauricular flap is separated, the helix elevated, and the postauricular defect repaired by skin graft. (Redrawn from Converse JM: Reconstruction of the auricle. Plast Reconstr Surg 22:150, 1958. © 1958 The Williams & Wilkins Co., Baltimore.)

SUPERF. TEMPORAL A. & V.

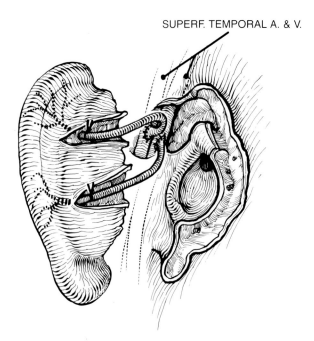

Fig. 13-5. External ear replantation entailing vein grafts to the superficial temporal artery.

3. The anastomosis is performed between the single suitable artery of the amputated ear and the vein graft on the bench.
4. By completing the arterial anastomosis first, small veins to be used for venous drainage (0.4 mm) can be more readily identified.[7]

As in replantation of other body parts, a two-team approach is indicated, when possible. The anastomosis of the artery should be performed first to aid in the identification of the tiny thin-walled veins. Extensive use of interpositional vein grafts in both the arterial and venous anastomoses will aid in obtaining tension-free anastomoses.

FACIAL NERVE TRAUMA

The facial nerve (cranial nerve VII) conveys motor innervation to the facial muscles, excretory function to the salivary and lacrimal glands, and taste to the anterior two-thirds of the tongue.[8] The most unfortunate sequela of facial nerve injury is facial muscle paralysis. Loss of orbicularis oculi muscle function may cause exposure keratitis and blindness. Paralysis of the orbicularis oris results in drooling, disturbances in speech and eating, and a hypotonic cheek. Paralysis of the muscles of facial expression, with its concomitant grotesque disfigurement of the face, causes significant emotional distress.

Anatomy

The facial nerve leaves the cerebellopontine angle with the eighth cranial nerve. Both leave the posterior cerebral fossa to enter the internal auditory meatus (Fig. 13-6). The fallopian canal is 33 mm long and courses through the petrous portion of the temporal bone to end at the stylomastoid foramen. Along its course, the nerve gives off three branches:

1. Greater petrosal complex. This nerve complex comprises greater superficial, external, and smaller petrosal nerves, which come off the geniculate ganglion. The complex regulates secretomotor function of the lacrimal gland and conveys taste to the soft palate.
2. Motor nerve to stapedius. This nerve provides a damping effect on vibration reaching the middle ear.
3. Chorda tympani. This nerve arises 5 mm proximal to the stylomastoid foramen and courses superiorly back through the middle ear. It exits the ear through the petrotympanic fissure and supplies secretomotor fibers to the sublingual and submaxillary glands, and taste to the anterior two-thirds of the tongue.

The first branches of the facial nerve as it leaves the fallopian canal at the stylomastoid foramen are the motor nerves to the six rudimentary muscles of the auricle, and the motor nerve to the posterior belly of the digastric muscle.[9] Along the fallopian canal, the nerve is well protected from trauma by the bony pyramid of the petrous bone. Fractures of the petrous bone involve the facial nerve and cause paralysis in 20 to 40 percent of cases.

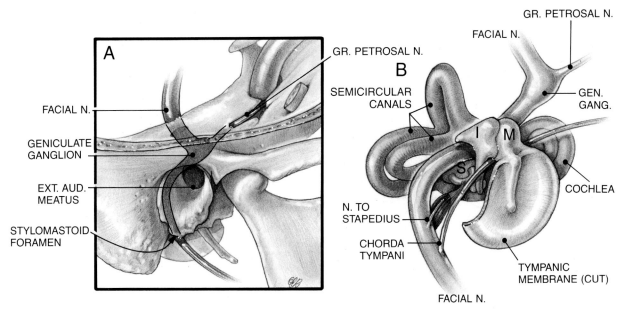

Fig. 13-6. (**A**) The course of the facial nerve in the temporal bone. (**B**) The anatomic relationship between the facial nerve and the middle and inner ear. I, Incus; M, Malleus; S, Stapes.

Exiting the stylomastoid foramen, the facial nerve runs in an upward concave course. It passes in front of the posterior belly of the digastric muscle and lateral to the stylomastoid process, external carotid artery, and posterior facial veins. Reaching the mandibular ramus, the nerve turns upward and forward within the substance of the parotid gland and divides to form its terminal branches. The average length of the trunk is 13 mm.[10] The trunk of the nerve passes 2.5 to 3.5 cm above the mandibular angle and bifurcates into two main divisions: the temporofacial and cervicofacial trunks.[11] The temporofacial trunk is usually twice as thick as the cervicofacial division. The two main subdivisions of the facial nerve further divide to form five terminal branches: temporal, zygomatic, buccal, marginal mandibular, and cervical. Davis et al.[11] describe six main types of ramification of the facial nerve based on the anastomoses between branches (Fig. 13-7).

Type I (13 percent). No anastomosis between branches.

Type II (20 percent). Anastomosis within branches of the temporofacial division only.

Type III (28 percent). A single anastomosis between temporofacial and cervicofacial divisions,

with the anastomotic branch usually passing in front of the parotid duct.

Type IV (24 percent). A combination of types II and III (i.e., anastomosis within the temporofacial division and between the temporofacial and cervicofacial divisions).

Type V (9 percent). Two anastomoses between temporofacial and cervicofacial divisions.

Type VI (6 percent). Extensive interconnection between the various branches.

The branch with the most interconnections is the buccal branch. The temporal and marginal mandibular branches have the least collateral contributions, which makes these branches more prone to irreversible trauma. Anterior to the parotid gland, nerve branches lie under the superficial masseteric fascia or the superficial musculo-aponeuritic system (SMAS). At this site, the nerve is most susceptible to trauma. Medial to a vertical line drawn from the lateral angle of the eye, spontaneous neurotization will occur, particularly with the zygomatic and the buccal branches. However, a long laceration that transects several neighboring rami may result in permanent palsy. The mandibular and cervical branches lie deep to the platysma muscle. The

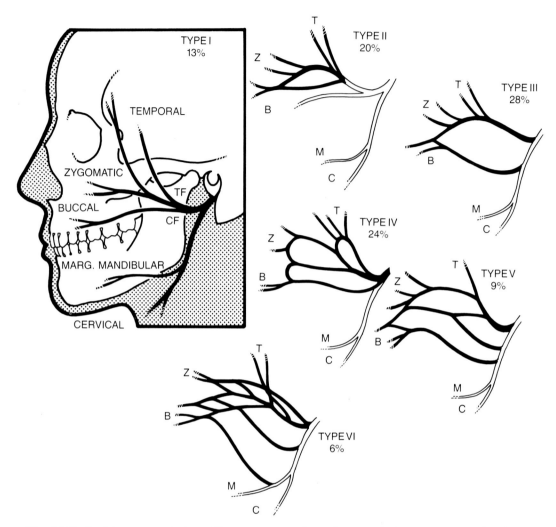

Fig. 13-7. Facial nerve variations. The anastomotic branches are dark. TF, Temporofacial; CF, Cervicofacial.

mandibular branch passes along the body of the mandible. Based on cadaver dissections, Dingman and Grabb[12] described the maximal downward displacement of the nerve as being 1 cm below the mandibular body. However, Baker and Conley[13] clinically observed during parotidectomy that the average downward position was 2 cm. In cases where skin and muscle were atrophic and lax, the mandibular branch was inferiorally positioned as much as 4 cm.

Other branches susceptible to trauma are the temporal and zygomatic divisions. As these branches leave the parotid gland, they course over the zygomatic arch under the thin superficial fas-

cia, penetrate the temporalis fascia, and innervate the frontalis muscle. Transection of the temporal branch will cause palsy in 85 percent of cases. Transection of the zygomatic division is less likely to have a detected clinical effect due to its multiple interconnections with other facial nerve branches.

Classifications of Facial Nerve Injuries

Facial nerve injuries have been classified[14] by etiology into four major types: birth injury, laceration, surgical trauma, and temporal bone fracture.

Birth Injury

Facial nerve paralysis in the newborn may be due to congenital anomaly or traumatic delivery. Because the mastoid bony prominence of the newborn is not fully developed, a forceps delivery may cause injury to the facial nerve if it is squeezed between the forceps and the vertebral column. In most cases the injury will be a neuropraxia with complete recovery expected within 2 to 4 weeks.

Clinical diagnosis of facial paralysis in babies is made only when the baby cries, as asymmetry may not be seen in a newborn at rest because of the high tonus of the soft tissues. If repeated conductive tests fail to show improvement, exploration of the nerve is advisable.

Laceration

Facial laceration with laceration of the underlying nerve is the most frequent cause of peripheral segmental nerve paralysis. The etiology is usually a windshield laceration in a motor vehicle accident, or a knife wound. It is important to document the functional integrity of each of the five major nerve branches before injection of local anesthesia. In severe head injury or multiple trauma, it is often difficult to establish correct diagnosis. The face is bruised, edematous, and painful to move. The patient may be comatose, or agitated and uncooperative. In multiple trauma victims, facial laceration and facial paralysis receive low priority. An effort should be made to repair the nerve within the first 48 to 72 hours. During the first few days post-injury, the distal nerve endings retain their ability to transmit an electrical impulse to the facial muscles. Using a nerve stimulator, the surgeon can identify these endings. When definitive repair is not possible, the distal nerve endings should be tagged with a suture at the time of primary exploration. This aids in identification and retrieval of the transected end at a later date.

Surgical Trauma

The facial nerve may be included in an en bloc resection for malignant tumors of the parotid gland. In such cases, facial paralysis is a predicted outcome. Immediate nerve grafting provides the best results. A division of the nerve or its branches may be interrupted inadvertently in a superficial parotidectomy, or while performing a biopsy. If nerve interruption is detected, repair is mandatory. If a gap exists, an interposition nerve graft is the treatment of choice. Grafts can be harvested from either the greater auricular nerve or the sural nerve (Figs. 13-8, 13-9). If paralysis is detected in the early postoperative period, the etiology may be inadvertent sectioning of a branch, or neuropraxia due to intraoperative traction, electrocoagulation, or pressure. Nerve conduction tests are helpful in determining the nature of injury. The various electrodiagnostic tests are discussed below.

During mastoidectomy and ear canal surgery,

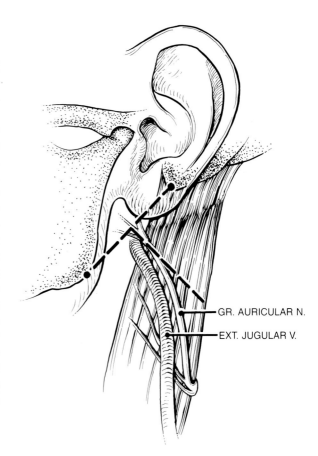

GR. AURICULAR N.

EXT. JUGULAR V.

Fig. 13-8. The position of the greater auricular nerve is identified as Erb's point. This is found by drawing a line from the mastoid tip to the angle of the mandible. A perpendicular line bisecting this first line is drawn on the neck. Erb's point is approximately 6 cm below the intersecting lines.

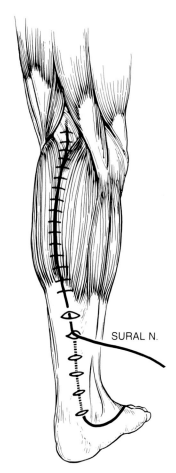

SURAL N.

Fig. 13-9. Harvesting of the sural nerve as a free graft.

the nerve is vulnerable from the level of the geniculate ganglion to the stylomastoid foramen. The incidence of facial nerve palsy from ear surgery is 0.6 to 3.7 percent.[15] The fallopian canal forms a prominent rounded eminence between the niche of the oval window and the bony horizontal semicircular canal. The tympanic wall is thin or in some cases, dehiscent. The nerve is then covered by a thin lining of mucoperiosteum, which can easily be injured during a stapes operation. In mastoidectomy, the most susceptible segment of the nerve is the last 13 mm in the fallopian canal.[16]

The incidence of partial facial paralysis following rhytidectomy is about 0.7 percent.[13] Castanares lists the possible etiology of facial nerve injury in face lift.[17] If nerve injury is detected at surgery, a fascicular nerve repair is indicated. When palsy is

documented postoperatively, conduction studies will suggest the nature of the nerve injury. However, since 80 percent of patients experience spontaneous recovery within 6 months, watchful monitoring accompanied by reassurance of the patient is the treatment of choice.[13] If facial paralysis persists for more than 6 months with no evidence of improvement, exploration of the nerve and repair is the treatment of choice.

Temporal Bone Fracture

May[18] found that in 16 percent of 218 patients with facial paralysis, where paralysis was due to trauma, the majority had temporal bone fractures. Facial paralysis occurs in 40 percent of the transverse and 20 percent of the longitudinal fractures of the petrous pyramid. Longitudinal fractures are more common than transverse fractures.[19] A good prognosis for recovery can be expected with incomplete traumatic palsy and with total palsy that has a delayed onset. In both situations, the nerve is contused with concurrent secondary edema (neuropraxia).[20] Fisch recommends surgery only if the motor fibers have reached 90 percent degeneration, as demonstrated by electroneurography within a week following onset of palsy.[21] It is essential to visualize the fracture line radiographically or by computed tomography, as facial paralysis following head injury may be due to different etiologies such as midbrain damage, or avulsion of the nerve from the cerebellopontine angle. These are conditions in which reparative surgery has very little to offer.

ELECTRODIAGNOSTIC TESTS

Clinical tests that assess the integrity of various functions of the facial nerve branches may help to establish the level of injury (Fig. 13-10). These tests are designed to objectively document facial paralysis, differentiate the type of nerve injury, and prognosticate recovery. Since the facial nerve

LEVEL OF PATHOLOGY

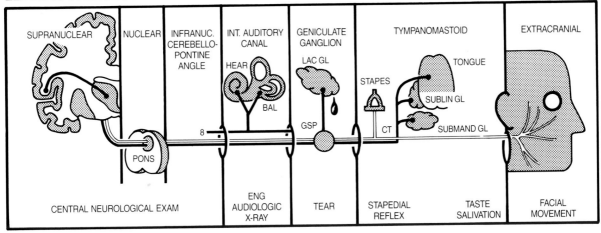

Fig. 13-10. Schematic drawing illustrating the lesion testing site in the diagnosis of a facial nerve injury. HEAR, Hearing; BAL, Balance; LAC GL, Lacrimal gland; GSP, Greater superficial petrosal; CT, Chorda tympani; SUBLIN GL, Sublingual gland; SUBMAND GL, Submandibular gland.

retains its conductivity for approximately 72 hours following nerve transection, most tests will indicate nerve injury only following that lag period. It is essential to perform the first electrodiagnostic test as soon as possible to serve as a base line.

Conduction Test

The facial nerve is maximally stimulated at the angle of the jaw when a recording electrode is placed in the frontalis or orbicularis muscles. Latency of the distal muscle potential is measured from onset of stimulus, first on the normal side and then on the abnormal side. Latency greater than 3.8 msec is considered abnormal. If normal response is obtained only with a current twice the normal threshold, nerve conduction is said to be absent. The length of latency period suggests the nature of nerve injury—neurapraxia, axonotmesis, or neurotmesis.

Strength-Duration Curves

Strength-duration curves are graphic measurements of nerve and muscle excitability. Two vari-

ables are measured: the amount of current required to cause a minimal perceptible contraction, and the threshold of contraction at progressively shorter durations. In normal muscle, fine intramuscular nerves will respond. In denervated muscle, response will be that of a direct muscle stimulation. During reinnervation, a broken curve is obtained that shows elements of both muscle and nerve stimulation. The curve roughly demonstrates a quantitative determination of the degree of reinnervation.

Chronaxie

Chronaxie is the duration of a stimulus (twice the minimal stimulus acting over an infinite period of time) that evokes a mechanical muscle twitch (rheobase). Normal chronaxie is less than 1 msec. Any pathologic process that impairs conductivity of lower motor neurons will produce an abnormal chronaxie. It takes a longer stimulus to get a direct reaction from muscle fibers. This is a gross test, and there has to be substantial nerve damage before the nerve shows abnormality.

Electromyography

Electromyography is a technique of recording muscle potentials without external stimulation. It can determine nerve muscle pathways and intrinsic muscle pathology. Using needle electrodes in the facial muscles, the electrical interference is recorded. Normal muscle at rest does not have electrical potentials. Fibrillation in a muscle at rest indicates denervation. Following partial voluntary muscle contraction, motor unit potentials of 500 to 800 mV in amplitude and 4 to 8 msec in duration, are generated. On maximal contraction all motor neurons fire simultaneously, but asynchronously, in a pattern known as the interference pattern. Two weeks following complete nerve transection, fibrillation is seen in muscles at rest, although no change is observed in voluntary contraction. In partial nerve laceration, fibrillation is seen in muscles at rest. On slight voluntary contraction, multiple polyphasic potentials appear, with some giant forms, as evidence of reinnervation. On maximal voluntary contraction, the number and size of potentials remain about the same. In myopathy, the characteristic finding is low voltage and an inability to recruit additional motor units on voluntary contraction.

Electroneurography

Electroneurography[22] is a means of measuring and recording compound action potentials of a given muscle. This test can be performed only if the facial nerve on the other side of the face is uninjured. The test is useful in quantitating degree of nerve dysfunction.[20]

In acute facial nerve trauma, nerve conduction testing and electroneurography are the tests most helpful in determining degree of denervation in the first week after trauma. Intensity-duration curves at 15 days following trauma give better information as to the degree of denervation. To assess the degree of reinnervation, the most sensitive test is electromyography. Reinnervation patterns are detected in electromyography weeks before facial movement can be seen.

TREATMENT

The goal of treatment in all cases is restoration of anatomy. Whenever possible, the lacerated nerve should be sutured, primarily without tension, or grafted using a greater auricular nerve or sural nerve graft. Surgical repair should be performed as soon as possible after injury. Not only is macroscopic anatomy more easily identified soon after injury, but microscopic orientation is more evident. Contraindications to immediate nerve repair are high velocity wounds, extensive tissue destruction, contaminated wounds, and life-endangering multiple trauma. If it is necessary to delay primary repair, the ideal time for reexploration is 3 to 4 weeks post-injury. This provides enough time for proper debridement and control of infection and schedules repair at a point when there is little fibrosis and minimal neuroma formation.[23,24] Although nerve repair should be performed as soon as possible, facial nerve restoration can be accomplished as late as 2 to 3 years after facial nerve transection.[25,26]

COMPLICATIONS

Results of nerve repair are usually good. One of the complications of repair is synkinesis, the unintentional muscular movement of one portion of the face when another part of the face moves voluntarily.[27] Most commonly, there is an upward movement of the oral commissure and upper lip during blinking or winking of the eye, or closure of the eye during talking and smiling. In an attempt to reduce the incidence of synkinesis, intraneural topographic anatomy has been studied. Sunderland describes fascicles as being diffusely distributed,[28] whereas May[29] and Miehlke[15] believe that discrete fascicles may be present proximal to the stylomas-

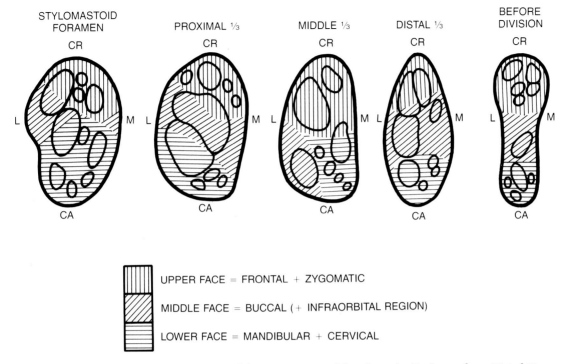

STYLOMASTOID FORAMEN — PROXIMAL ⅓ — MIDDLE ⅓ — DISTAL ⅓ — BEFORE DIVISION

UPPER FACE = FRONTAL + ZYGOMATIC

MIDDLE FACE = BUCCAL (+ INFRAORBITAL REGION)

LOWER FACE = MANDIBULAR + CERVICAL

Fig. 13-11. The intraneural anatomy of the extratemporal facial trunk. (Redrawn from Meissl G: Facial nerve suture. p. 209. In Fisch U: Facial Nerve Surgery. Aesculapius, Birmingham, AL, 1977.)

toid foramen. Meissl,[30,31] in his studies of extratemporal facial nerve topography, found that in spite of plexiform arrangement and changing fascicular pattern, there are areas in which certain neuromuscular units predominate (Fig. 13-11).

As Millesi has written, it is critical that nerve repair be performed without tension. Tension results in fibrosis, which blocks nerve regeneration. If an end-to-end anastomosis cannot be achieved without tension, an interposition nerve graft that will relieve tension along the suture line will achieve better results.[32,33] Millesi describes four basic steps in nerve anastomosis:

1. Sufficient resection of the damaged or fibrotic fibers. The circumferential fascicular epineurium is excised in a strip-like fashion, which entails separation of the nerve into fascicular groups.
2. Approximation by a single epineural stitch (Fig. 13-12).
3. Coaptation of nerve ends in which they are brought into optimal contact. In some cases, it is better to compromise on less accurate coaptation rather than increase surgical trauma.
4. Maintenance of coaptation. This is usually achieved with fine 9-0 or 10-0 nylon sutures.

Baker and Conley reported 70 percent good to excellent results using epineural sutures with 4× loop magnification.[34] For patients in whom only some of the distal nerve can be identified, a combined masseter or temporalis muscle transfer with partial nerve repair seems to give good results. Immediately after surgery, the patient gains good tonus, and muscle neurotization is enhanced.

In most traumatic nerve injuries, it is possible to identify nerve ends and to restore nerve continuity with either primary repair or interpositional nerve graft.[35,36] However, in some cases it is impossible to use the ipsilateral nerve. Cross-facial reinnervation is an alternative that has good physiologic rationalization.[37,38] Another procedure for establishing good muscle tone with mass movement is the hypo-

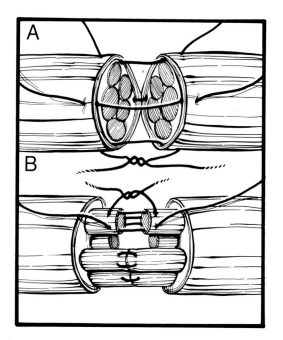

Fig. 13-12. Facial nerve repair. **(A)** Epineural repair. **(B)** Polyfascicular repair, which is used frequently in nerve grafts.

glossal to facial anastomosis (7–12 hook-up)[39,40] or use of the temporalis and masseter muscles to improve movement of the orbicularis oculi and orbicularis oris. Although all patients gain immediate tonus on the affected side, it takes some time to gain voluntary control of the muscles. Static techniques such as dermal suspension, slings tarsorrhaphy, lid loading, and face lift should be performed in combination with facial reanimation muscle transfers.

PAROTID DUCT INJURIES

The parotid duct carries the saliva of the parotid gland to the oral cavity. The duct is 6 to 7 cm in length, and 2 to 4 mm in diameter. It leaves the gland at its anterior-superior border, crosses the face anteriorly, then overlies the masseter muscle.

At the anterior border of the masseter the duct turns sharply toward the oral cavity and passes through the buccal fat pad and penetrates the buccinator muscle. It then runs obliquely under the oral mucosa for about 5 mm to open at the tip of the parotid papilla[41] (Fig. 13-13).

The duct is narrow at the opening of the papilla and creates a valve-like mechanism. The papilla itself is located opposite the upper second molar tooth. In 20 percent of cases[41] the proximal parotid duct is accompanied by an accessory gland, which is usually superior to the duct. The accessory gland drains into the main duct via multiple small ducts.

The distal duct is thin as it exits the gland and becomes thicker as it passes over the masseter muscle. Along its course the duct is accompanied by a branch of the buccal division of the facial nerve and the transverse facial artery. The course of the duct approximates a line drawn from the mid-tragus to the corner of the mouth. The papilla is located just lateral to a vertical line that passes through the lateral canthus.

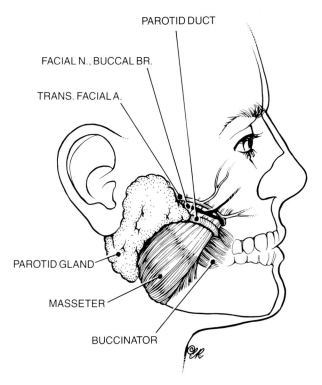

Fig. 13-13. Schematic drawing showing the relationship of the parotid gland, parotid duct, masseter muscle, and facial nerve.

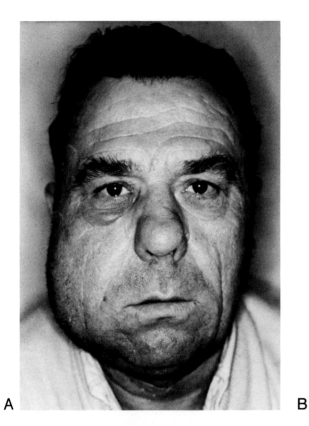

A

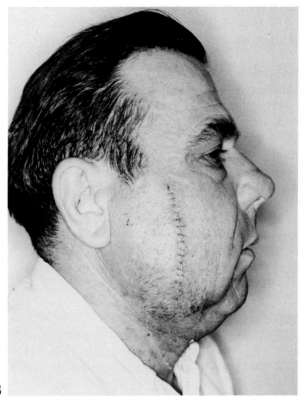

B

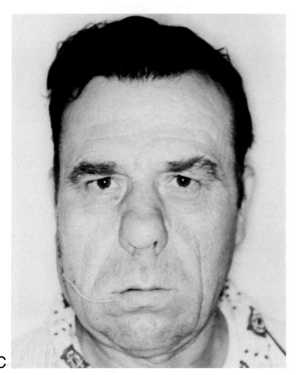

C

Fig. 13-14. Acute laceration of Stenson's duct, which when left unrepaired, caused parotid swelling. (**A**) Frontal view. (**B**) Lateral view. (**C**) View after reexploration, repair, and canulation of Stenson's duct.

Diagnosis

The most common cause of injury is a deep laceration of the face by a broken windshield, knife, or bullet. Laceration and transection of the parotid duct can be easily missed because there are no symptoms or obvious signs of an acute laceration of the parotid duct. A missed diagnosis might lead to parotid swelling, saliva leakage, wound infection, pseudocyst, or fistula formation (Fig. 13-14). Any injury that crosses the course of the parotid duct may lacerate or transect the parotid duct. A high index of suspicion and careful evaluation under optimal conditions will assure correct diagnosis.

Rarely, transection may be the result of blunt trauma. In these cases blood in the parotid duct papilla is suggestive of the diagnosis. Since the buccal branches of the facial nerve follow the course of the duct, paralysis of the buccinator and the levator muscles of the corner of the mouth will indicate possible concomitant injury. Definitive diagnosis is made by cannulating the duct with a lacrimal dilator and a probe. If the duct is transected, the tip of the probe will be seen exiting the wound. With injection of methylene blue through a polyethylene or silicone catheter into the papilla, laceration or transection will be detected by extravasation of dye.[42] The proximal end of the lacerated duct can be located by simply squeezing the

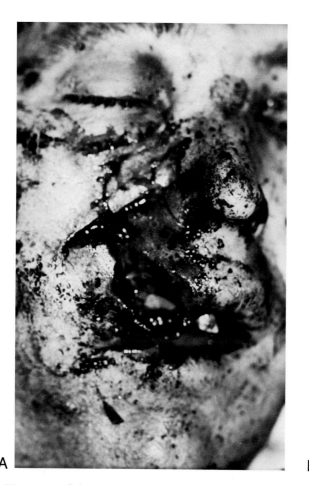
A

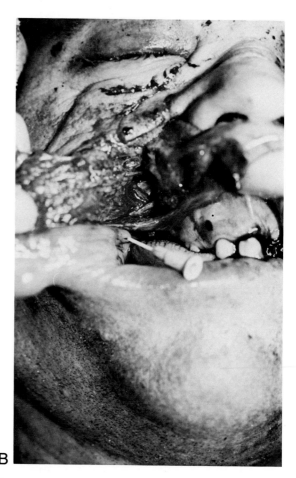
B

Fig. 13-15. (A) Patient with a LeFort III facial fracture and a mandibular fracture with soft tissue injury. A parotid duct injury should be suspected and ruled out. (B) Photograph showing the intubation of the parotid duct with a #20 angiocatheter, which is used to test the integrity of the duct.

parotid gland. Saliva will be seen flowing from the proximal cut end.

Treatment

Proximal Third of the Duct

At this level, the duct is thin walled and sometimes engulfed by accessory parotid tissue. Reanastomosis of the duct is difficult and not always successful. The preferred procedure in a difficult situation is ligation of the proximal and distal segments of the duct. The gland will then undergo reflex atrophy. Irradiation is needed on rare occasions when the gland remains swollen and painful for a prolonged period of time.

Ligation of the duct is also the procedure of choice in cases in where a segment of the duct is missing. An interposition vein graft can be applied, but results for this procedure are poor, while the alternative of duct ligation is usually successful.

Distal Two-Thirds of the Duct Overlying the Masseter Muscle

At this level the duct is well formed and can be easily dissected from the surrounding tissues. A polyethylene or silicone catheter is introduced to the parotid gland through the papilla and into the duct. The anastomosis is performed under magnification while the catheter is in place, using interrupted sutures of 9-0 nylon. The catheter is left in place for drainage and stenting of the anastomosis (Figs. 13-15, 13-16).

The Region of the Duct Distal to the Masseter

A laceration in this area is difficult to repair. It is simpler to suture ligate the distal cut end of the duct and to reinsert the proximal end into the oral cavity. The reinsertion should be performed so that the sphincter mechanism will be reestablished. The duct is passed through the buccinator muscle so that it obliquely enters the oral cavity. Following the suturing of the duct, an adequate-sized catheter is left in the duct proximal to the anastomosis to assure proper drainage of the saliva and to prevent stenosis. Formerly, the draining catheter was

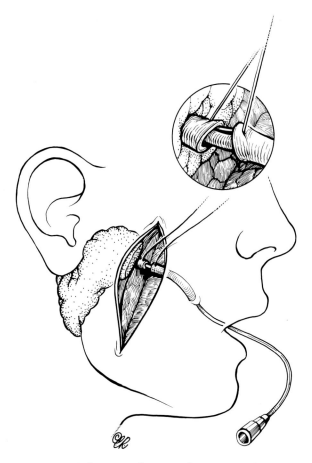

Fig. 13-16. Schematic drawing showing intubation of the duct and the repair closing over a polyethelene catheter.

left in place for 3 to 4 weeks to overcome edema formation and late scarring.[43-46] However, with use of precise microsurgical techniques, a watertight anastomosis with exact apposition of the duct wall can be achieved. Inflammatory reaction and edema formation is less, and thus there is no need for prolonged stenting. Usually under these circumstances, stenting is not necessary after 5 to 7 days.

The muscle layer is carefully approximated using 5-0 chromic catgut, and the skin is sutured as well. A pressure bandage is applied over the parotid area. It is advisable to use prophylactic antibiotics, such as penicillin and cephalothin, that cover anaerobic flora and penicillinase-producing stapholococcus, which are the usual causes of parotitis.

Postoperatively, leakage from the lacerated gland or duct with accumulation of saliva is treated with aspiration and pressure dressings.

REFERENCES

Ear Trauma

1. Tolleth H: Artistic anatomy dimension, and proportions of the external ear. Clin Plast Surg 5(3):337, 1978
2. Hollinshead WH (ed): Anatomy for surgeons. Hoeber-Harper, New York, 1960
3. Allison GR: Anatomy of the external ear. Clin Plast Surg 5(3):419, 1978
4. Converse JM: Reconstruction of the auricle. Plast Reconstr Surg 22:150, 1958
5. Mladick RA, Horton CE, Adamson JE, Cohen BI: The pocket principle, a new technique for reattachment of the severed ear part. Plast Reconstr Surg 48:219, 1971
6. Nahai F, Hayhurst JW, Salibian AH: Microvascular surgery in avulsive trauma to the external ear. Clin Plast Surg 5:423, 1978
7. Pennington DG, Lai MF, Pelly AD: Successful replantation of a completely avulsed ear by microvascular anastomosis. Plast Reconstr Surg 65:820, 1980

Facial Nerve Injury

8. Bell C: On the nerves, giving an account of some experiments on their structure and functions, which leads to a new arrangement of the system. Trans Royal Soc London 3:398, 1821
9. Goss CM (ed): Gray's Anatomy of the Human Body. 29th Ed. Lea & Febiger, Philadelphia, 1973
10. Dargent M, Duroux P: Donnees anatomiques concernant la morphologie et certains rapports du facial intra parotidien. Presse Med 54:523, 1946
11. Davis RA, Anson BJ, Budinger JM, Kurth LE: Surgical anatomy of the facial nerve and parotid gland, based upon a study of 350 cervicofacial halves. Surg Gynecol Obstet 102(4):385, 1956
12. Dingman RO, Grabb WC: Surgical anatomy of the mandibular ramus of the facial nerve, based on the dissection of 100 facial halves. Plast Reconstr Surg 29:266, 1962
13. Baker DC, Conley J: Avoiding facial nerve injury in rhytidectomy. Plast Reconstr Surg 64(6):781, 1979
14. McCabe BF: Symposium on trauma in otolaryngology. I. Injuries to the facial nerve. Laryngoscope 83:1891, 1972
15. Miehlke A: Surgery of the facial nerve. Urban and Schwarzenberg, Munich, 1973
16. Paporella MM, Shumric DA: Otolaryngology. 2nd Ed. W.B. Saunders, Philadelphia, 1980
17. Castanares S: Facial nerve paralysis coincident with or subsequent to, rhytidectomy. Plast Reconstr Surg 54:637, 1976
18. May M: Trauma to the facial nerve, Symposium on trauma to the head and neck. Otolaryngology Clin North Am 16(3):661, 1983
19. Fisch U: Current surgical treatment of intratemporal facial palsy. Clin in Plast Surg 6:377, 1979
20. Glasscock ME, Wiet AJ, Jackson CG, Dickin JRE: Rehabilitation of the face following traumatic injury to the facial nerve. Laryngoscope 89:1389, 1979
21. Fisch U: Surgery for Bells palsy. Arch Otolaringol 107:1, 1981
22. Hughes GB: Electroneurography: Objective prognostic assessment of facial paralysis. Am J Otol 4:73, 1982
23. Millesi H: Nerve suture and grafting to restore the extratemporal facial nerve. Clin Plast Surg 6(3):333, 1979
24. Lee KK, Terzis JK: Management of acute extratemporal facial nerve palsy. In Symposium on Peripheral Nerve Microsurgery. Clin in Plast Surg 11(1):203, 1984
25. Conley J: Long-standing facial paralysis rehabilitation. Laryngoscope 84:2155, 1974
26. Bunnell S: Surgical repair of the facial nerve. Arch Otolaryngol 25:235, 1937
27. Crumley RL: Mechanisms of synkinesis. Presented at the annual meeting of the American Academy of Facial Plastic and Reconstructive Surgery, April 27, 1978
28. Sunderland S: Mass movement after facial nerve injury. p. 285. In Fisch U (ed): Facial Nerve Surgery. Aesculapius Publishing, Birmingham, Alabama, 1977
29. May M: Anatomy of the facial nerve (spatial orientation of fibers in the temporal bone). Laryngoscope 83:1311, 1973
30. Meissl G: Die itraneurale topographie des extrakraniellen nervus facialis. Acta Chir Austr 25(suppl 5), 1979

31. Meissl G: Facial nerve suture, p. 209. In Fisch U (ed): Facial Nerve Surgery. Aesculapius Publishing, Birmingham, Alabama, 1977

32. Millesi H, Meissle G, Berger A: Further experience with interfascicular grafting of the median, ulnar, and radial nerves. Bone Joint Surg (Am) 58:209, 1976

33. Millesi H: Nerve suture and grafting to restore the extratemporal facial nerve. Clin Plast Surg 6:333, 1979

34. Baker DC, Conley J: Facial nerve grafting: A thirty year retrospective review. Clin Plast Surg 6:343, 1979

35. Orgel MG, Terzis JK: Epineural versus perineural repair in ultrastructural and electrophysiological study of nerve regeneration. Plast Reconstr Surg 60:80, 1977

36. Hudson AR, Hunter D, Kline DG, Bratton BR: Histological studies of experimental interfascicular graft repair. J Neurosurg 51:333, 1979

37. Scaramella L: L'anastomosi tra i due nervi facciali. Arch Otolaryngol 82:209, 1971

38. Anderl H: Cross-facial nerve transplantation in facial palsy (principle and further experience). Transcription of the sixth International Congress of Plastic and Reconstructive Surgery. Masson, Paris, 1975

39. Conley J, Baker DC: Hypoglossal facial nerve anastomosis for rehabilitation in facial paralysis. Plast Reconstr Surg 63:66, 1979

40. Conley J: Hypoglossal crossover in one hundred twenty two cases. Trans Am Acad Olaryngol 84:763, 1977

Parotid Duct Injuries

41. Davis RA, Anson BJ, Budinger JM, Kurth RE: Surgical anatomy of the facial nerve and parotid gland, based upon a study of 350 cervico facial halves. Surg Gynecol Obstetr 102:385, 1956

42. Van Sickles JE, Alexander JM: Parotid duct injuries. Oral Surg 52:364, 1981

43. Takeshi K, Kiyoshi T: Surgery of the stensen's duct. Arch Otolaringology 93:189, 1971

44. Newman S, Seabrook D: Menegement of injuriesto Stensen's duct. Ann Surg 124:544, 1946

45. DeVylder J, Carlo J, Stratigos GT: Early recognition and treatment of the traumatically transected parotid duct: report of a case. J Oral Surg 36:43, 1978

46. Hendler BH, Quinn PD, Moon A: Primary repair of Stensen's duct after hemifacial transection: Report of a case. Oral Surg 39:587, 1981

Index

Note: Page numbers followed by t denote tables; those followed by f denote figures.

275